atlas of lymphography

Dr. T. de Roo

atlas of lymphography

Dr. T. de Roo, radiologist

Central Hospital, Alkmaar, The Netherlands

with foreword of

Prof. Dr. A. Rüttimann, radiologist

Stadtspital Triemli, Zürich, Switzerland

H.E. Stenfert Kroese bv, Leiden 1975

Acknowledgements

ISBN-13:978-94-010-1591-2   e-ISBN-13:978-94-010-1589-9
DOI:10.1007/978-94-010-1589-9

Part of the patient material was acquired during my study at the University Hospital, Department of Radiology, Leiden (Head of the Department: Prof. Dr. J.R. von Ronnen).

The logetron prints of the radiograms and colour photographs were made by Mr. C. Th. Ruygrok (Department of Radiology, University Hospital, Leiden).

The reproductions for the chapter HISTORY were obtained through the services of Dr. A. M. Luyendijk-Elshout (National Museum for the History of Natural Sciences, Leiden).

The radiograms in figs. 278, 282, 287, 289, 290, 303 and 381 are from the collections of S.H. van Minden, M.D. (Binnen Hospital, Eindhoven) and J.M. van Nouhuys, M.D. (Red Cross Hospital, The Hague).

English translation by Mrs. G.P. Bieger-Smith.

Graphic Design Flor Silvester gvn / printed by Targa bv
's-Hertogenbosch, The Netherlands.
© 1975 Dr. T. de Roo.
Softcover reprint of the hardcover 1st edition 1975
This book has been published in co-operation with SANDOZ bv., Holland, who distributed a separate edition.

Foreword

Today the diagnosis of malignant diseases and determination of the causes of 5 lymphoedema are inconceivable without lymphography. The radiologist now has a new method of examination at his disposal which offers him broad new diagnostic possibilities; on the other hand however, it also demands of him a thorough knowledge of the topographical anatomy, histology and physiology of the lymphatic system, the effects of contrast fluids and the appearance of complications, as well as an extensive clinical knowledge of every possible disease of the lymphatic system.

The Atlas in question is a survey of this new branch of science.

The author is a pioneer in the field of lymphography. He has contributed to its development: the improvement and detailed refinement of technique and diagnosis was his special hobby. In particular he compared and evaluated selective supplementary roentgenological examination methods in lymphography in large patient series. With singular intensity he worked on the possibilities and limitations of the visualization of tumour metastases. This Atlas is based on ten years of experience. Its special value lies in the possibility of rapid orientation as well as a precise representation of lymphography as radiological method of examination.

Dr. Tom de Roo has thus attained the objectives he had set for this book and, within the field of radiological methods of examination, he has accorded lymphography the position and recognition it deserves.

A. Rüttimann, Zürich 1974

Contents

Introduction

For years there was little interest in the study of the lymphatic system in man.
The answer to the question of why this important organic system had barely
been explored lies in the lack of roentgenological visualization of the lymphatic
system.

Kinmonth's revolutionary discovery in 1952 brought about a considerable
change. He used a subcutaneous injection of blue dye to visualize the lymphatic
vessels; the lymphatics, which normally could not be differentiated from the
surrounding tissue, absorbed the blue tissue fluid and became visible. As a result, a direct injection of contrast fluid was possible.

Initially the diagnostic possibilities remained limited because water-soluble
contrast media were used. In 1961 however significant progress was achieved
when oily contrast fluids were introduced. By using these oily contrast media,
which do not mix with lymph, it became possible to visualize anomalies of the
thoracic duct as well as the lymphatic channels and lymph nodes of the extremities, pelvis, the lumbar and aortic regions, and the axillary, subclavicular and
supraclavicular regions. This sudden development has caused such an overwhelming amount of specialized literature in the past few years that a critical
evaluation is scarcely possible. It has become clear that with practice anyone
can master the technique; but considerable experience is required to evaluate
lymphograms – in particular when the presence or absence of metastatic carcinoma, especially in borderline cases, must be established.

The purpose of this atlas is to review the use of lymphography in practice with
reference to the lymphographic examination of almost 1500 patients. Two
other aspects are also considered: what are the exact indications and what can
the physician, who requests a lymphographic examination, expect? In this con-
text, cervical lymphography and lymphography of the mammae are not discussed since, however interesting they may be, the present techniques are difficult
and the diagnostic results disappointing.

In fact an examination is only worthwhile if the number of faulty diagnoses can
be kept within acceptable limits. For these reasons, selective supplementary
methods of examination, such as tomography, phlebo-cavography, aortography
and arteriography as well as follow-up radiograms, are considered in detail. The
correct use of these supplementary examination methods is a prerequisite if the
number of faulty diagnoses is to remain within acceptable limits.

It is my hope that this atlas will fulfill the need for a survey of the diagnostic
possibilities in lymphography – a survey based on personal experience. In this
type of atlas, it is inevitable that certain aspects receive more attention than
others and when opinions differ as to technique or method, the personally preferred approach is chosen. My aim is however to offer a justifiable appraisal of
present-day lymphography and particularly, to stress its proven diagnostic value
in practice.

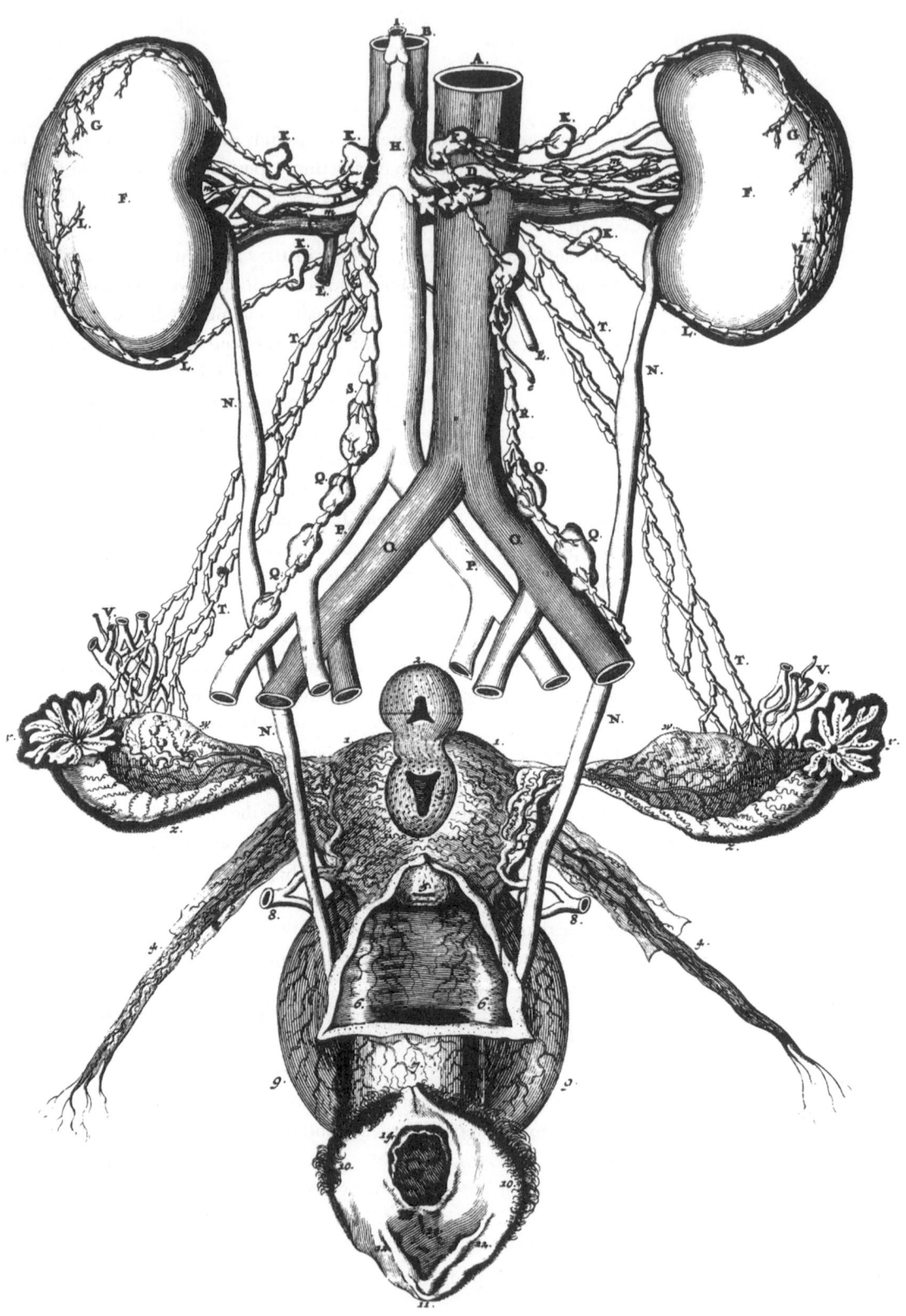

fig. 1 Lymphatic system of the kidneys and female reproductive organs. Illustration from the book "Adenographia Et Uteri Foemenei Anatome Nova" by A. Nuck (1692).

History

The existence of lymphatic channels was already known in ancient times. Aristotle (384-322 B.C.) described vessels containing a colourless fluid. Erasistratus and Herophilus (± 300 B.C.), physicians of the Alexandrian school, used the term ductus lactei for these channels in man as well as animals. It was 2000 years later before further study of these vessels was undertaken.

Fallopio (1523-1562) described the lymphatic channels in the liver; Eustachio (1513-1574) discovered the thoracic duct in the horse and in the mesenterium of the dog, Aselli (1581-1627) found numerous vessels filled with a milky fluid which he called vasa chylifera. Johannes van Horne (1621-1707), appointed Professor of Anatomy in Leiden in 1651, discovered the thoracic duct in man. Independently of Pecquet, who found the cysterna chyli in dogs, van Horne gave a detailed description of the large lymphatic channels in man in his treatis "Novus ductus chyliferus" (1652). Other investigators of that period are Thomas Bartholinus (1630-1702) and Olaus Rudbeck (1616-1680) who reported the results of their work almost simultaneously. Rudbeck's monograph (1653) on the lymphatic system is important because he was the first to mention the valves. He also suggested that constriction of the lymphatics could cause ascites and oedema. In order to distinguish the vessels from the surrounding tissue, they were filled with air, milk or coloured fluid. Joannis de Wale (1604-1644), lecturer in physiology in Leiden, was the first anatomist to study the lymphatic system in relation to Harvey's theory of the circulation of blood. His most important work was "Epistolae duae de motu chyli et sanguinis" (1645).

Antonius Nuck (1650-1692), appointed Professor of Anatomy in Leiden in 1677, was the first to succeed in visualizing practically the entire lymphatic system. His technique, the injection of mercury, made it possible to conserve the lymphatic channels in order to study their course and interrelationship. His book "Adenographia curiosa et uteri foemenei anatome nova" (1692) can still be considered the basis of our knowledge of this material. Jan Swammerdam (1637-1680) and Frederik Ruysch (1638-1731) also made important contributions to the discovery of the lymphovascular system.

Mascagni (1781) and Cruikshank (1789), building on the work of Nuck, dealt with the topography of the lymphatic system in all parts of the body.

After these publications in the 17th and 18th centuries, it was many years before the finer morphological structure of the lymphatic system was also known and a reasonably clear picture began to emerge. It was believed that the lymph node parenchyma contained large hollow spaces with afferent vessels leading in and efferent vessels leading out (Noll, 1850). Many diseases were ascribed to spoiled or stagnant lymph, including also the swelling of lymph nodes. Not until the detailed studies of Kölliker (1852), Billroth (1858, 1861, 1862), Teichman (1861), Frey (1861), Hansen (1871) and His (1860, 1862) was it shown that lymph nodes were part of a special organic system that can be clearly differen-

10

tiated from other lymphoid tissues. In fact, even today His' basic principles relating to the histological architecture of the lymphatic channels and lymph nodes have barely changed. Nuck's technique, the injection of mercury, was difficult and time-consuming; therefore others looked for a simpler method. In 1896, Gerota introduced a new solution: Prussian blue oil paint highly diluted with terpentine and ether. After diverse improvements, this method was generally used in cadavers. On the basis of this technique, Jossifow (1930) wrote a monograph on the total lymphatic system in man: a monograph which is still worth reading. In 1932, Rouvière also published an excellent handbook on the same subject.

The above-mentioned investigations were carried out on cadavers; Dalmady was the first to study the lymphatic vessels in vivo (1911).

To visualize the lymphatic channels and lymph nodes for roentgenological examination, use was made of:

A *"The indirect method"* Numerous authors attempted to visualize lymphatics by injecting contrast fluids into body cavities (peritoneal, pericardial, pleural, subarachnoidal, subdural and nasal) or soft tissues (uterus, joints, bronchi,

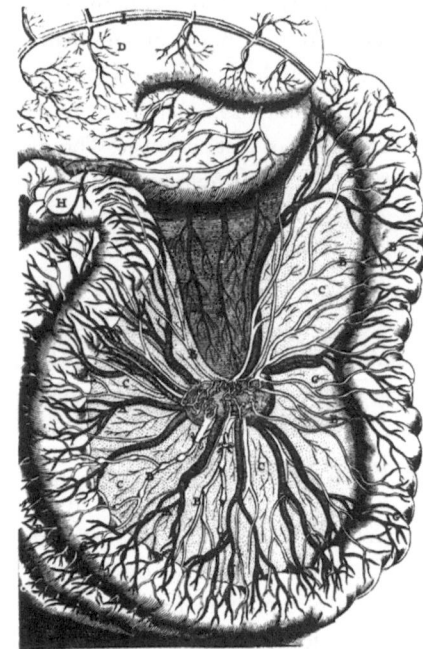

2

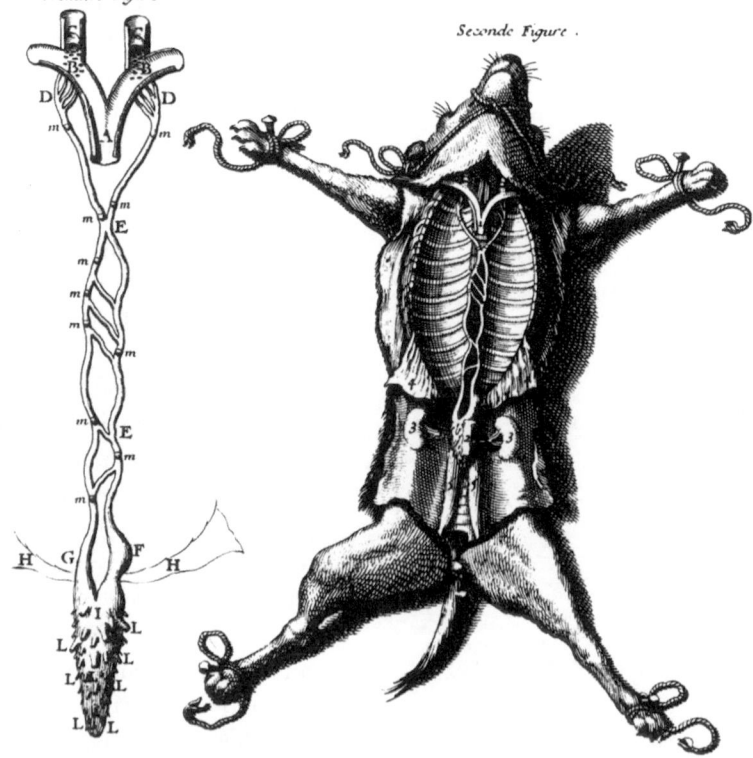

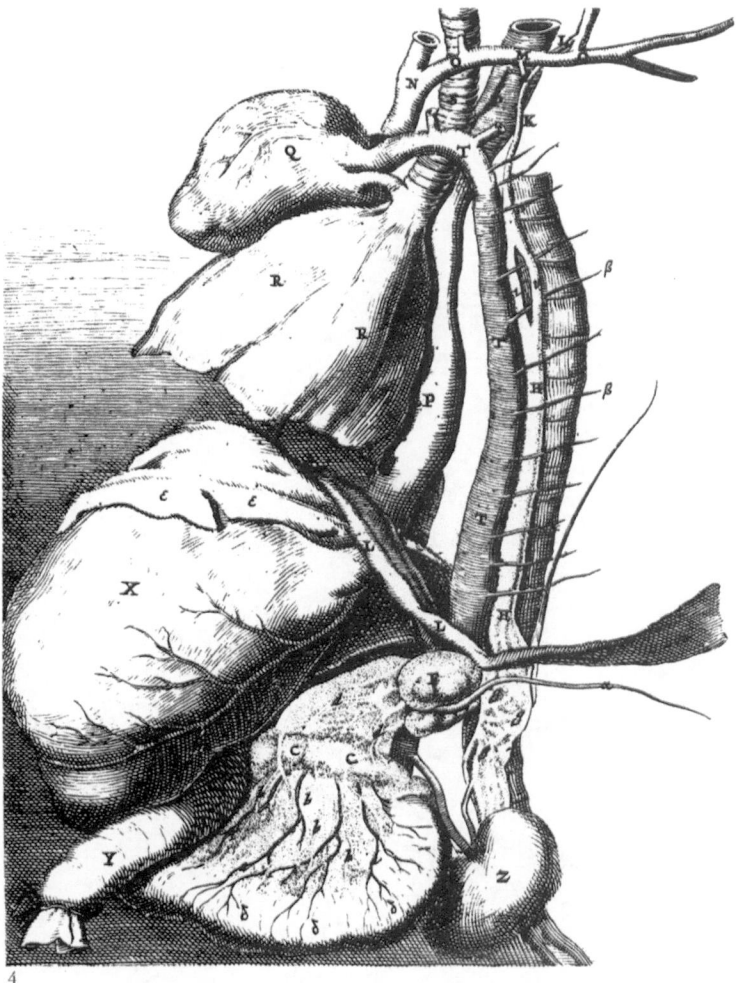

4

fig. 2 Drawing of the mesenterial lymph vessels, taken from the letters by Joannis de Wale "Epistolae Duae De Motu Chyli Et Sanguinis" (1641-1645).

fig. 3 Discovery of the cysterna chyli in dogs. Illustration from the book "Joannis Pecqueti Experimenta Nova Anatomica Parisiis" by J. Pecquet (1651).

fig. 4 Discovery of the thoracic duct (HH) by J. v. Horne. Illustration from his work "Novus Ductus Chyliferus (1652)."

muscles, tendons, tongue, tonsils, testes and epididymis). The contrast media used were colloidal solutions of thorium-dioxide such as thorotrast, oily solutions such as lipiodol and water-soluble solutions such as urografine, biligrafine, joduron and collargol.

Pfahler (1932) was the first to show lymphatic vessels in man roentgenologically; one week after an injection of lipiodol into the maxillary sinus, the lymphatic vessels leading away from this region could be observed. The lymphatics and lymph nodes in the thorax were visualized in 1933 by Saito who injected thorotrast into the peritoneal cavity and in 1934 by Bartolotti and Torelli by means of an injection into lung tissue. Menville and Ané (1933) injected thorotrast into the cervix uteri causing the nodes in the pelvis to become visible. In 1955, Servelle reported that under certain circumstances indirect lymphography was possible by means of subcutaneous injection of thorotrast. Most attempts to visualize lymphatic channels and nodes by injecting contrast media subcutaneously did not yield any results (Montanini 1935, Arnulf 1955, Collette 1955, Leenhardt and Colin 1957, and Gergely 1958).

Because it takes so long for the contrast fluid to enter the lymphatic channels and lymph nodes, the indirect method appeared to have no practical application – in spite of several positive results.

12

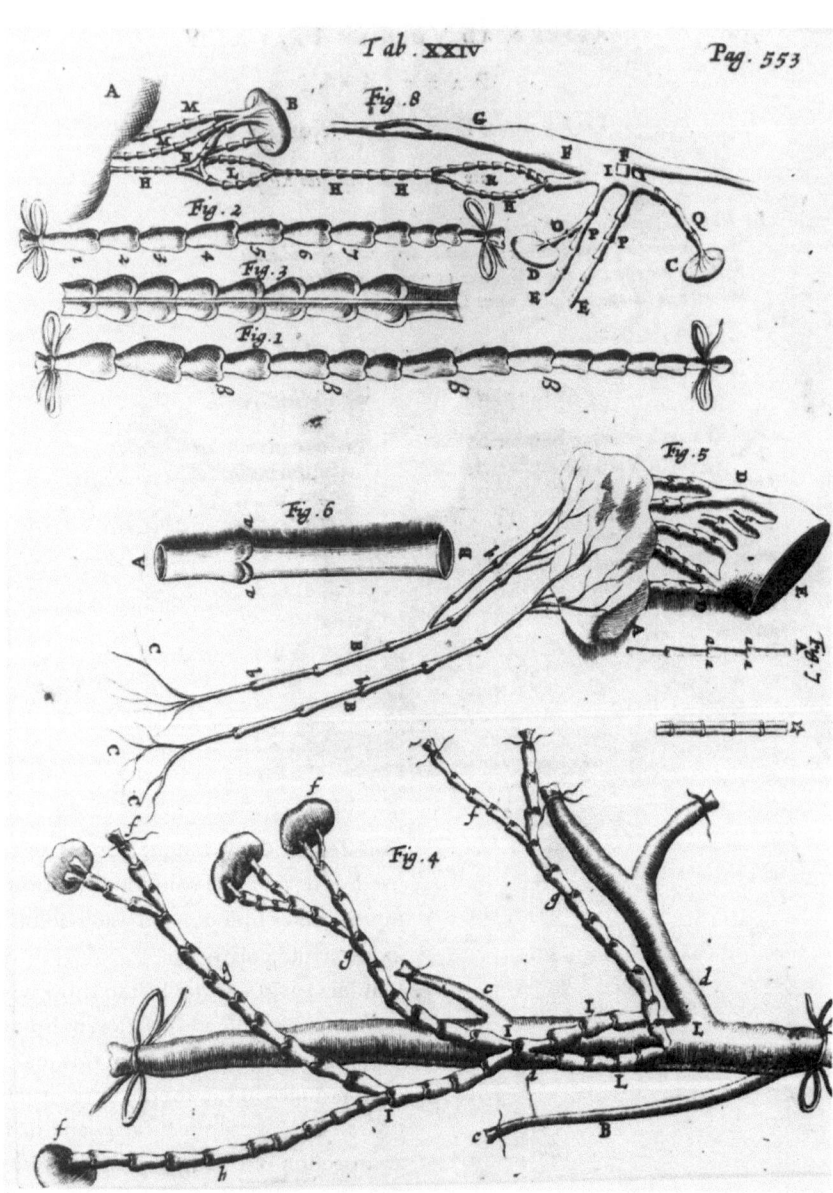

fig. 5 Drawing of lymph vessels by Jan Swammerdam. From the book "Joannis Veslingii
Syntagma Anatomicum Commentario atque
Appendice". Editor: G. Blasius, Amsterdam
(1666).

fig. 6 Lymphatic channels and lymph nodes
sketched by Antonius Nuck. From his book
"Adenographia Et Uteri Foemenei Anatome
Nova" (1692).

fig. 7 Enlargement of a lymph node from fig. 6.

fig. 8 Lymph vessels in the kidney of a dog.
Drawing from "Adenographia Et Uteri Foemenei Anatome Nova" by Antonius Nuck (1692).

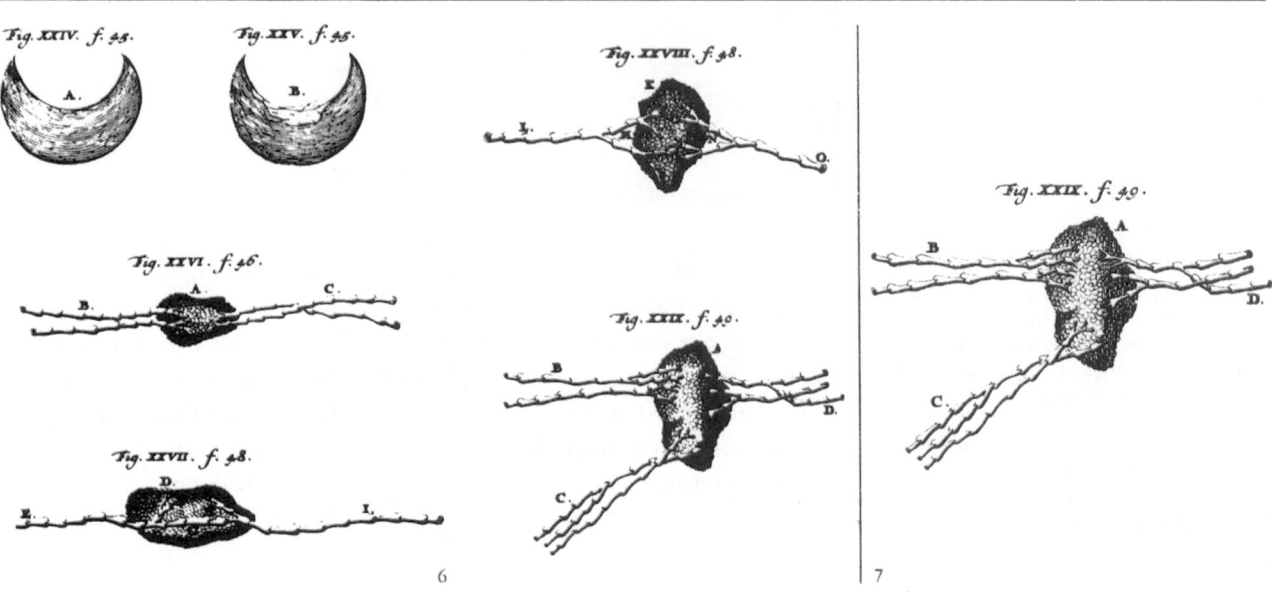

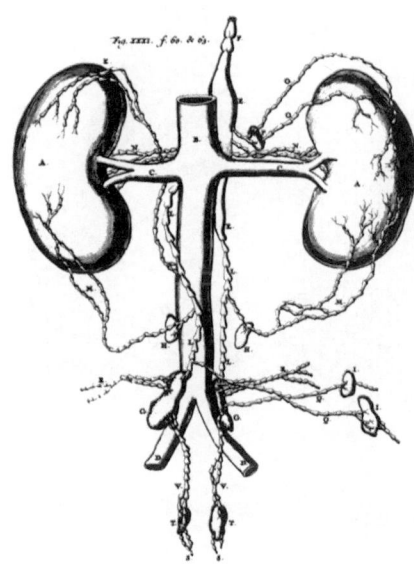

B *"The direct method"* Here the contrast fluid is injected directly into the lymphatic channels and nodes. Thorotrast, lipiodol, collargol, urografine and biligrafine were used as contrast media.

In 1931, Carvalho attempted to inject contrast fluid directly into the lymph nodes in man, without success however. Teneff and Stoppani (1934), Shdanow and Durmashkin (1938) and Servelle (1945) succeeded in visualizing the lymphatic channels and nodes in the pelvis by injecting thorotrast directly into the nodes in the inguinal region. In addition, Servelle (1945, 1947) injected the same contrast fluid percutaneously into varicose lymphatic vessels in several forms of lymphoedema.

As mentioned in the introduction, in 1952 Kinmonth introduced a revolutionary approach to these investigations. He injected patent blue violet (11% solution) subcutaneously.

As a result of the absorption of the blue tissue fluid, the subcutaneous lymph vessels became visible. This English publication caused renewed interest in the further exploration of the lymphatic system in man. The first studies involved the pathological changes in lymphoedema. Water-soluble solutions such as urografine and biligrafine were still in general use as contrast media. Thorotrast was abandoned because of marked toxicity and radioactivity.

The disadvantage of water-soluble contrast media was that the images were transient – disappearing soon after the injection. In addition, it was not possible to visualize the lymphatic channels and lymph nodes proximal to the pelvis since

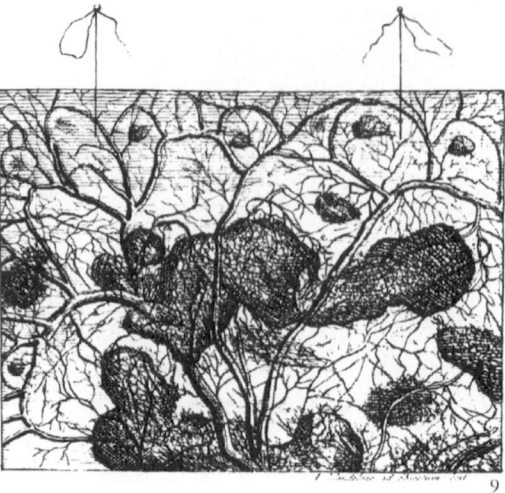

14

fig. 9 Lymph nodes in the mesenterium. Letter from Frederik Ruysch to Herman Boerhaave concerning "The origin of the nodes", Amsterdam (1722). From "Alle De Werken Van Frederik Ruysch", translated by Ysbrand Gijsbert Arlebout, Amsterdam, (1744).

fig. 10 Mesenterial lymph vessels. Illustration from the book "Prodrome D'un Ouvrage Sur Le Système Des Vaisseaux Lymphatiques" by Paul Mascagni, Sienne (1784).

the water-soluble contrast medium was highly diluted by lymph.

A significant advance was made in 1960-1961 when it was found that a direct injection of oily contrast medium made it possible to visualize the paralumbar and para-aortic lymphatics and lymph nodes as well as the thoracic duct (Rüttimann, Hreschchyshyn, Sheehan, Wallace, Malek, Belan and Picard). As of that time, interest in lymphography has increased considerably – which is evident from the overwhelming number of publications in this field today.

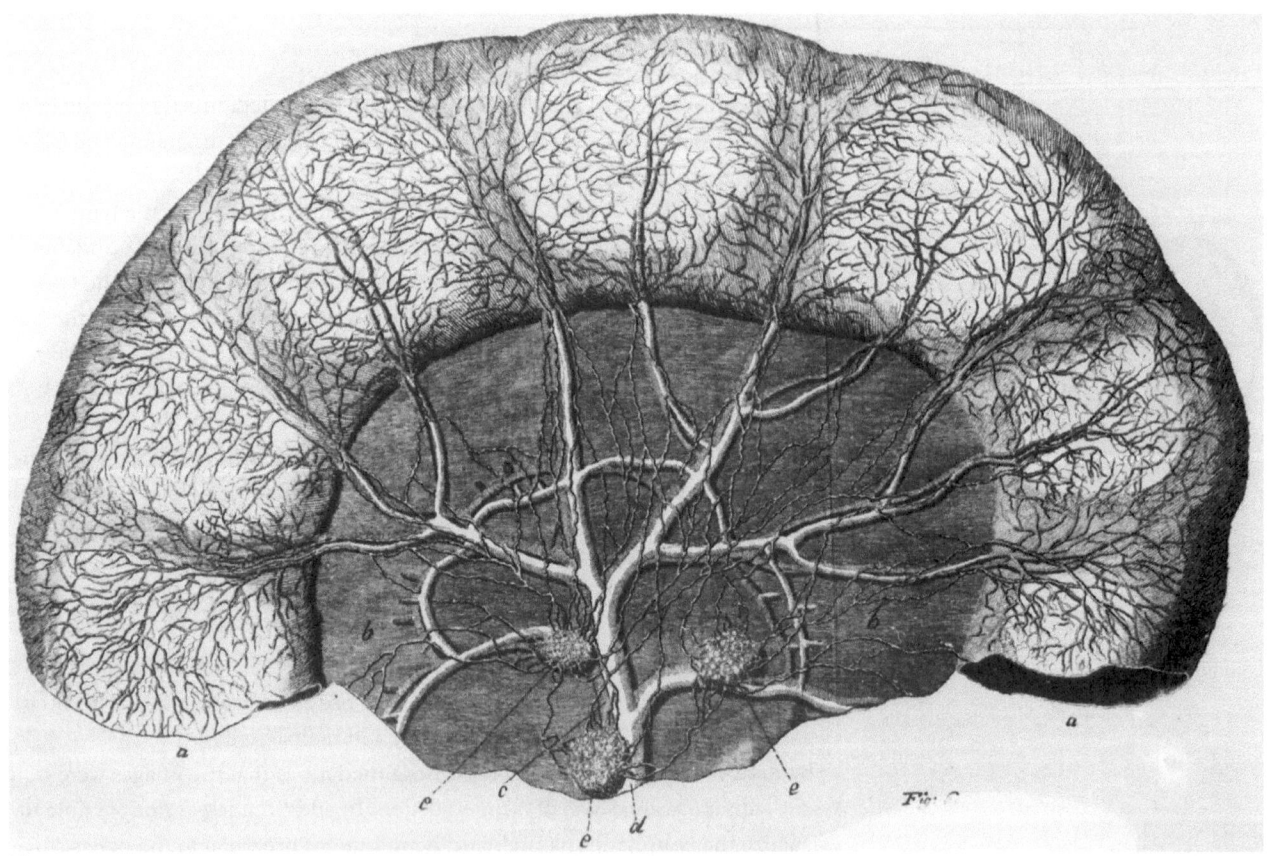

Anatomy

For the evaluation of lymphographic films, a thorough knowledge of the anatomy of the lymphatic system is essential. Only that anatomy which is pertinent to lymphography shall be discussed.

GENERAL ANATOMY OF NORMAL LYMPHATIC VESSELS

The lymphatic vessels stem from the fine, thin-walled lymphatic capillaries of the skin and subcutaneous fat tissue. Lymphatic capillaries vary in calibre but are generally larger than blood capillaries. They are lined by a thin membrane of endothelial cells with scalloped edges which mesh together. The capillaries form a dense network with blind branches. These lymphatic capillaries, which have no valves, open into the actual lymphatic vessels. The latter are not always larger than the lymphatic capillaries. As in the blood vessel, the walls consist of three layers: a tunica intima, a tunica media and a tunica adventitia. The lymphatic vessels do have valves which are a part of the tunica intima; they are grouped in pairs which close up whenever there is lymph backflow. The valves are so situated in the lymphatic vessel that lymph can only flow from the periphery to the centre. At the valves, the vessel is slightly dilated so that filled lymphatic vessels resemble a string of beads. In the smaller lymphatic vessels, the valves are approximately 2-3 mm. apart, in the large vessels 6-12 mm. and in the thoracic duct, 2-4 cm. Where lymphatic vessels drain into the large veins, there are always valves to keep the blood out.

The lymphatics, interrupted by regional lymph nodes, extend from all directions toward the centre of the body where they finally merge to form two large central lymphatic trunks: the thoracic duct (35-45 cm. long) which empties into the vena subclavia sinistra and the right lymphatic duct (1-1.5 cm. long) which opens into the vena subclavia dextra.

GENERAL ANATOMY OF THE NORMAL LYMPH NODE

The size of the normal lymph node varies between ½ and 2 cm.; it is oval, round or kidney-shaped and somewhat flattened. The lymph nodes are covered by an indistinctly defined capsule, which is in fact a thickening of the loosely meshed connective tissue surrounding the organ and often containing fat cells. A hilus can be discerned on the concave side, particularly of kidney-shaped lymph nodes. The thickening of the connective tissue at the hilus is clearly visible. From this connective tissue as well as from the capsule, dense strands of connective tissue penetrate the lymph node and extend to the hilus, forming the so-called trabeculae which carry the afferent and efferent blood vessels. With the exception of the capsule and the trabeculae, the organ is made up of reticular connective tissue. The latter forms a loosely meshed network with local dense areas. Under the capsule, these finely meshed areas are more or less globular in shape; toward the centre near the hilus, they are cord-like. As a result of

16

these different forms, a cortex and a medulla can be distinguished within the lymph node. Immediately under the capsule is a rim of loosely meshed reticulum, the so-called subcapsular or marginal sinus. The finely meshed areas, where lymphocytes are retained, form the follicles or nodules.

The arteries, which penetrate the trabeculae via the hilus of the lymph node, exit as smaller branched arteries enveloped in a coat of finely meshed reticular

fig. 11 Cross-section of a normal lymph node (22x).

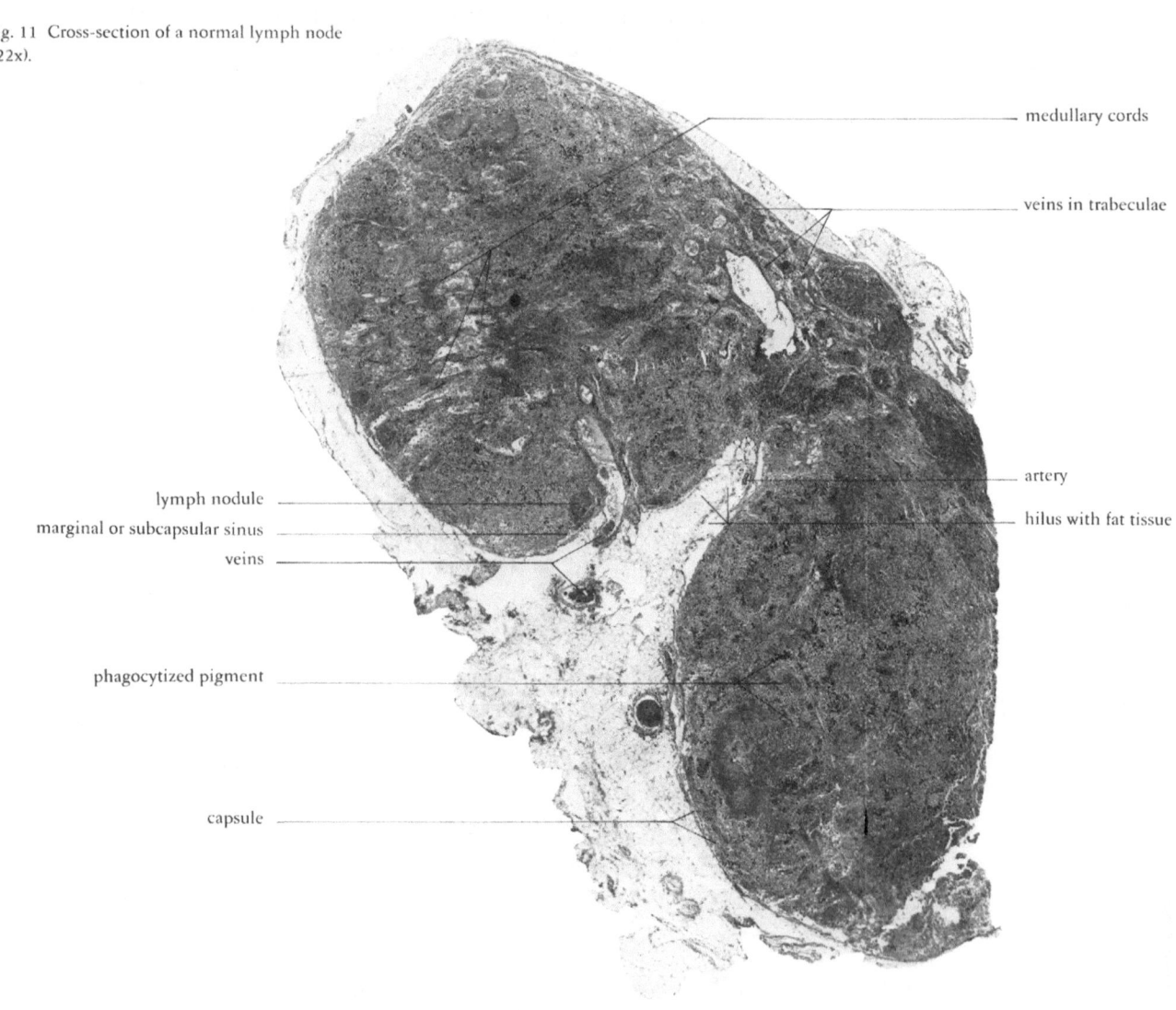

medullary cords

veins in trabeculae

artery

hilus with fat tissue

lymph nodule

marginal or subcapsular sinus

veins

phagocytized pigment

capsule

connective tissue. Capillaries are usually found throughout the periphery of the lymph node.

The afferent lymphatic vessels enter the lymph node on the convex side. The valves in these vessels determine the direction of flow of lymph. The lymph flows through the loosely meshed reticulum from the subcapsular sinus and leaves the lymph node by way of the hilus.

The cells of the loosely meshed reticulum can, as part of the so-called reticulo-endothelial system, become phagocytic and therefore contribute to the filtration of lymph. On the other hand, small lymphocytes are formed in the lymph nodes and added to the lymph flow. In addition to the small lymphocytes, there are also lymphoblasts, macrophages and plasma cells in the lymph node. Any granulocytes in the node usually enter via the blood.

The foregoing general outline of the anatomy of the lymphatics and lymph nodes shall be followed by a more detailed description of the anatomy of the lymphatic system insofar as it is pertinent to lymphography.

LOWER EXTREMITIES

In the lower extremities, we can differentiate between a *superficial* (subdivided into an *anterior* and *posterior*) and a *deep* lymphatic system. For lymphography, the anterior superficial system is the most important since the superficial as well as deep inguinal and subinguinal lymph nodes are filled by this system.

Anterior superficial system

a The Medial Channels stem from the lymphatic capillaries of the skin and subcutaneous fat tissue in the region of the first and second toes. They follow the course of the vena saphena magna. The number of channels is variable, usually 1-4. Above the knee, they fan out and for the most part empty into the superficial subinguinal lymph nodes (4-5); these nodes lie in the region of the fossa ovalis. A few of the medial lymphatics enter directly into the superficial inguinal lymph nodes (5-6) which are situated near the inguinal ligament, the superior inguinal lymph nodes and the inferior inguinal lymph nodes underneath the ligament.

b The Lateral Channels stem from the area between the third and fifth toes. They first extend upwards along the lateral side of the lower leg and then across the tibia. They are somewhat farther apart than the medial channels and are more numerous. Above the knee, they parallel the medial group and therefore also empty into the subinguinal nodes.

Posterior superficial system

This system stems from the lymphatic capillaries and subcutaneous fat tissue along the lateral edge of the foot and heel. This group includes only a few channels which converge in the upper two-thirds of the calf to form one channel which follows the course of the vena saphena parva. In the popliteal region, the lymphatic channels pass through 1 or 2 lymph nodes: the superficial popliteal lymph nodes which surround the arteria et vena poplitea. They subsequently drain into the deep popliteal lymph nodes (2-3). The channels of the deep system also open into the deep popliteal lymph nodes. Together the lymphatic channels follow the course of the vasa femoralia, pass through the femoral lymph nodes (1-4) and finally drain into the deep subinguinal and inguinal lymph nodes. These deep nodes in the groin are found under the fascia lata in the iliopectineal fossa. The uppermost lymph node is usually missing. The efferent vessels from the superficial nodes in the groin also drain into the deep inguinal and subinguinal nodes.

Deep system

This group stems from the lymphatic capillaries in bone marrow, bone, periosteum, nerves, fasciae, bands and capsules as well as muscle and fat tissue. The channels of this group follow the course of the arteries of the lower leg and, in contrast to the superficial system, pass through various lymph nodes.

INGUINAL REGION

In addition to the lymphatic channels of the leg described above, the lymphatics of the external genitals also drain into the superficial and deep nodes in the groin – as do the lymphatic channels from the posterior upper thigh, the gluteal region, one channel from the corpus uteri via the round ligament of the uterus and those from the pelvic wall up to the navel. Thus the superficial lymphatics of the entire lower part of the body converge at the nodes in the groin. Some of the deep lymphatic vessels from the abdominal wall, particularly around the navel, drain into the deep inguinal and subinguinal nodes. It should also be mentioned that numerous anastomoses exist between the superficial and deep groups of lymph nodes in the inguinal region; they should be regarded as a functional unit.

PELVIS

The lymph nodes in the pelvis are grouped around arteries and are therefore named accordingly. Thus the most important groups of lymph nodes to be distinguished are those around the (1) arteria iliaca externa et communis, (2) arteria hypogastrica and (3) arteria sacralis.

1 Iliac Lymph Nodes lie on both sides of the arteria et vena iliaca externa et communis. They are subdivided into:

a. (medial and lateral) external or inferior iliac lymph nodes extend along the

fig. 12 Diagram (anteroposterior) of the lymph node groups as projected on the lymphogram: (a) paralumbar and para-aortic lymph nodes, (b) common iliac lymph nodes, (c) external iliac lymph nodes and (d) inguinal and subinguinal lymph nodes.

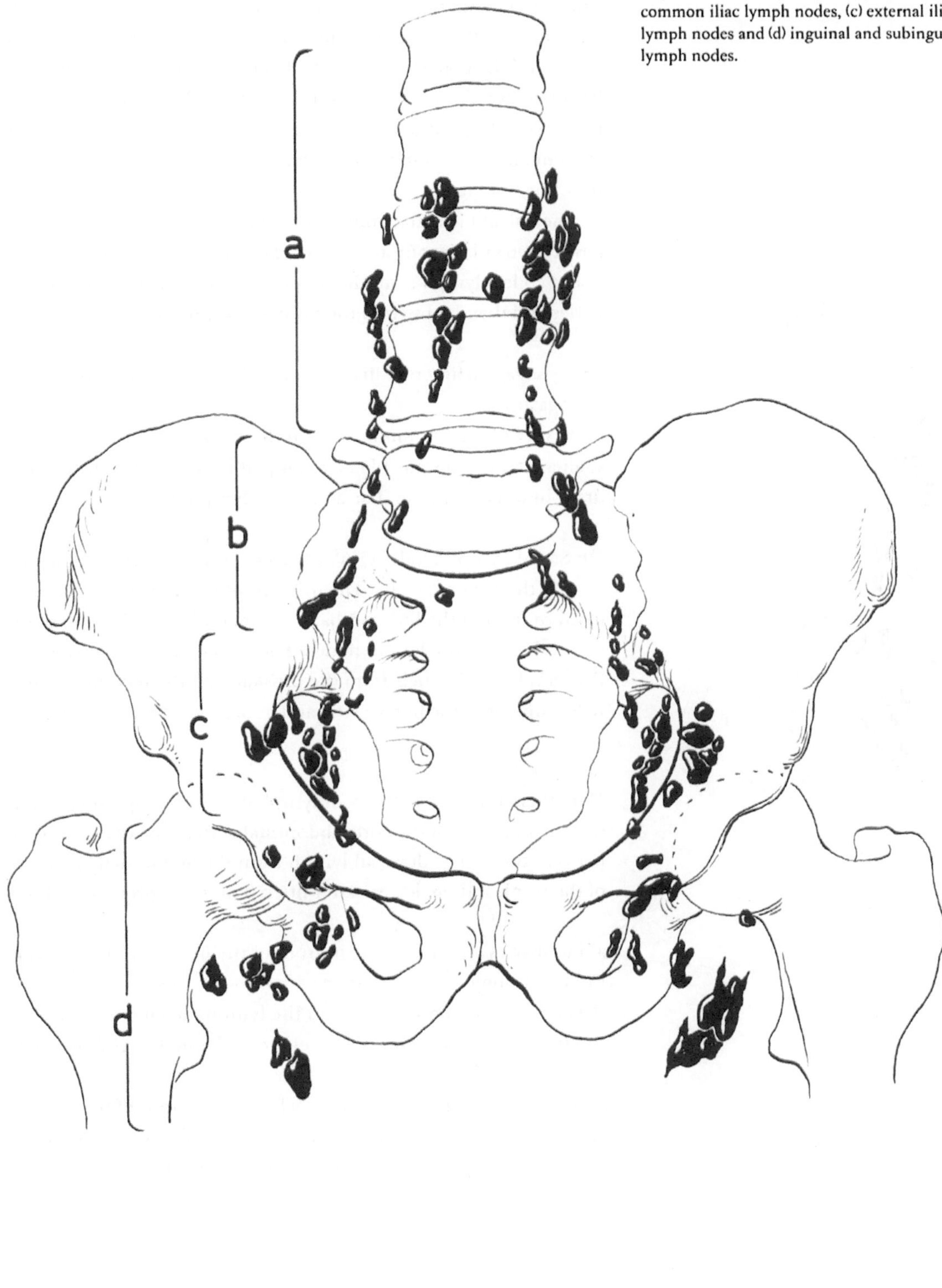

19

12

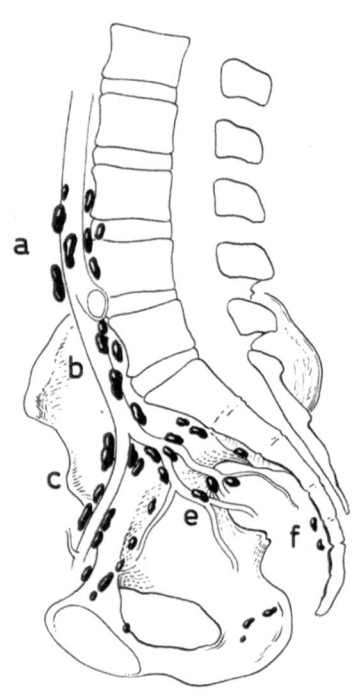

13

course of the arteria et vena iliaca externa (6-8). The lateral external iliac lymph nodes can again be subdivided into a superficial and a deep group of nodes, whereby the superficial are found on the ventral side and the deep on the dorsal side of the A. iliaca externa. The lowermost external iliac lymph nodes, which lie around the femoral ring, are called the medial and lateral suprafemoral lymph nodes. They collect lymph from the abdominal wall and the lower extremities via the deep and superficial lymph nodes in the groin; they also drain the efferent channels from the bladder, vagina and uterus as well as one channel from the testicles.

b. (medial and lateral) common or superior iliac lymph nodes lie along the arteria et vena iliaca communis (4-6). The efferent channels from the iliac lymph nodes collect lymph from the hypogastric, inguinal and subinguinal lymph nodes and then empty into the lumbar lymph nodes.

II Hypogastric (internal iliac) Lymph Nodes (9-12) lie along the arteria et vena hypogastrica.
They vary greatly in number. All of these lymph nodes receive lymph from the vagina, uterus, prostate, bladder and part of the penis. The efferent channels drain into the common iliac and aortic lymph nodes.

III Sacral Lymph Nodes (5-6), which are found in the middle of the sacrum, lie around the arteria sacralis. The uppermost of these lymph nodes, which are located in front of the fifth lumbar vertebra under the division of the aorta, are called the subaortic lymph nodes. The sacral lymph nodes are connected with the lymphatic channels from the prostate and the rectum. Their efferent channels empty into the hypogastric and aortic lymph nodes.

ABDOMEN
Here there is a large network of lymphatics and lymph nodes situated in front of and along side of the aorta abdominalis, the vena cava inferior and the lumbar vertebrae. They drain all lymph from the abdominal organs, the lower part of the trunk and the lower extremities. These lymph nodes fall into two groups:

a Lumbar Lymph Nodes lie in front of the lumbar vertebral column, and behind and along side of the aorta abdominalis. They are closely connected with the aortic lymph nodes and drain the lymphatic channels which run parallel to the arteria iliaca communis. The efferent channels form the two lumbar trunks.

b Aortic Lymph Nodes are those which lie in front of the aorta abdominalis and the vena cava inferior. Because of the topographical location and their connection with the abdominal organs, the aortic lymph nodes can be divided into

fig. 13 Diagram (lateral) of the lymph node groups as projected on the lymphogram: (a) paralumbar and para-aortic lymph nodes, (b) common iliac lymph nodes, (c) external iliac lymph nodes, (e) hypogastric lymph nodes and (f) sacral lymph nodes.

fig. 14 Diagram (oblique) of the lymph node groups as projected on the lymphogram: (a) paralumbar and para-aortic lymph nodes, (b) common iliac lymph nodes, (c) external iliac lymph nodes, (d) inguinal and subinguinal lymph nodes and (e) hypogastric lymph nodes.

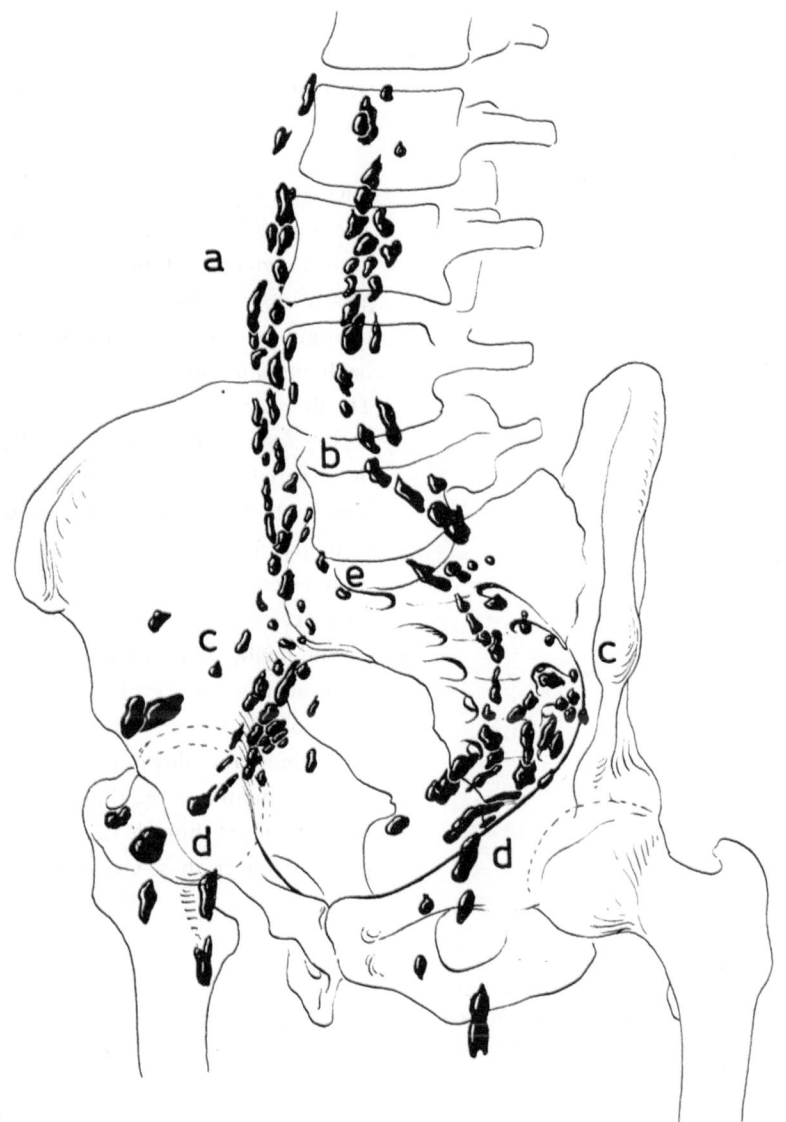

14

two groups: an upper and a lower group. The upper group is situated at the origin of the arteria coeliaca and the superior mesenterium. The lymph vessels from the diaphragm, liver, stomach, spleen, pancreas, duodenum, small intestine and the proximal part of the colon to the transverse colon pass through this group. The lower group, located at the origin of the arteria renalis and the inferior mesenterium receive the efferent channels from the hypogastric and sacral lymph nodes as well as the lymphatics from the kidneys, adrenals, testicles (one

22

vessel however drains into the inferior iliac lymph nodes), the upper part of the uterus, vagina, uterine tubes, ovaries and descending colon. The lymph exits through one vessel: the intestinal lymphatic trunk which in turn empties into the left lumbar trunk.

THORACIC DUCT

The thoracic duct is approximately 35-45 cm. long. It begins at the 1st or 2nd lumbar vertebra and includes a dilated part, the cysterna chyli, which varies greatly in shape. The cysterna chyli is formed by two afferent lymphatic vessels: the right and left lumbar trunks, the left trunk having merged with the intestinal lymphatic trunk.

The thoracic duct (the calibre varies between 0.5 and 1.7 cm.) enters the thorax via the aortic hiatus through the diaphragm and then continues upward in front of the vertebral column (usually slightly to the right of the median line) with the aorta to the left and the vena azygos to the right. At the 4th and 5th thoracic vertebrae, it deviates and runs along the left side of the thoracic vertebral column, extends upwards to the 6th cervical vertebra, twists to the left behind the arteria carotis communis and the vena jugularis interna over the arteria subclavia and finally curves downwards to the left to open into the upper side of the vena subclavia sinistra. The last part of the thoracic duct is somewhat distended. The thoracic duct has valves; where it enters the vena subclavia, the valve prevents blood from flowing out of the vein into the duct. Most of the lymphatic channels drain into the thoracic duct, except for those draining the right side of the head, neck, thoracic cage, right arm, right lung, right side of the heart and part of the liver; these channels drain into the right lymphatic trunk.

fig. 15 Opening of the thoracic duct into the vena subclavia sinistra: 1. thoracic duct, 2. subclavian trunk, 3. jugular trunk, 4. lymphatic channels and nodes of the jugular plexis and 5. vena subclavia.

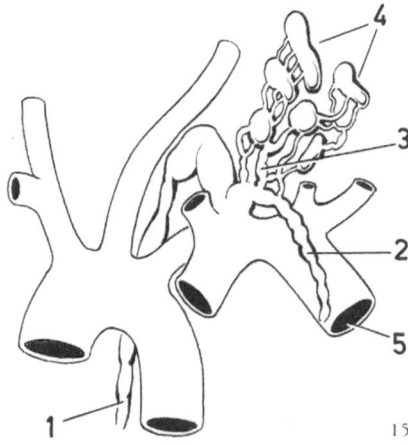

15

RIGHT LYMPHATIC TRUNK

In contrast to the thoracic duct, the right lymphatic trunk is short, 1-2 cm. at the most, with a diameter of 0.2 cm. It is located in the right side of the neck and empties into the vena subclavia dextra. Valves regulate the flow at the junction.

UPPER EXTREMITIES

As in the leg, the lymphatics of the arm also form a superficial and a deep network.

The *superficial* lymphatic channels, which stem from the lymphatic capillaries of the skin and subcutaneous fat tissue of the 3rd, 4th and 5th fingers and the ulnar regions of the hand and forearm, form a highly developed, dense network in the fingers and hand. In general, the superficial lymphatics in the forearm and upper arm follow the course of the superficial veins. Lymphatic channels from the hand run via the wrist to the forearm, extend upwards on the dorsal side in parallel and finally join the channels on the ventral side. The channels on the volar side of the wrist extend along the forearm to the cubital region. From there, they run on the medial side of the upper arm and drain into the superficial group of axillary lymph nodes. The channels on the lateral side of the wrist, which stem from the thumb and index finger as well as the radial portion of the hand and forearm, follow the course of the vena cephalica in the forearm to the insertion of the deltoid muscle; there most of them cross to the medial side to enter the superficial group of axillary lymph nodes. One single channel continues to follow the vena cephalica and sometimes drains into the superficial brachial lymph nodes between the deltoid muscle and the pectoralis major muscle; it ends in the subclavicular nodes.

The channels on the medial side of the wrist, which stem from the 3rd, 4th and 5th fingers, follow the course of the vena basilica. Where they penetrate the fascia together with the vena basilica, one or two channels pass through a few superficial lymph nodes, the so-called superficial cubital lymph nodes. Together with the lymphatics of the deep system, they continue to follow the course of the vena basilica and finally drain into the deep axillary nodes. Most channels of the medial group however remain subcutaneous, deviate from the course of the vena basilica and open directly into the superficial lymph nodes.

The Deep Lymphatic Channels, which like those in the lower extremities are less important for lymphography, follow the large veins of the hand and arm; we can therefore distinguish between a radial, ulnar and intermediate group. They are fewer in number and drain into the deep axillary lymph nodes. Their course is interrupted by several lymph nodes: the deep cubital lymph nodes in the elbow and several deep brachial lymph nodes in the upper arm.

AXILLARY REGION

The axillary lymph nodes are found in the fat of the axilla and surround the large blood vessels. They vary in size and number (11-38) and can be subdivided into various groups, which cannot be sharply defined on the lymphogram. There are *deep* and *superficial* axillary lymph nodes. The superficial axillary lymph nodes lie in front of the fascia in the fat tissue of the axilla. They drain the superficial lymphatic channels of the arm, shoulder girdle, chest and mammae. Their efferent channels pass through the deep axillary lymph nodes, which lie along the vessels and nerves of the axillary and subclavicular regions. These nodes can be subdivided into 7 groups:

1 pectoral lymph nodes (3-6): under or behind the pectoralis major muscle.
2 subscapular lymph nodes (1-5): near the nerves and arteries bearing the same name, at the 5th rib.
3 brachial lymph nodes (1-6): behind the vasa axillaria.
4 subpectoral lymph nodes (2-3): under the pectoralis major muscle, on the medial side of the vasa axillaria, at the 2nd and 3rd ribs.
5 intermediate lymph nodes (2-6): near the long thoracic nerve, in particular at the origin of the vasa thoracalia longa. They are connected with all other axillary lymph nodes.
6 subclavicular and supraclavicular lymph nodes (1-11): between the upper edge of the pectoralis minor muscle and the clavicle, above and to the medial side of the vena subclavia. The efferent vessels of these nodes penetrate the coracoclavicular fascia, anastomose with the supraclavicular lymph nodes and then empty into the subclavian trunk.
7 deltoideopectoral lymph node (1): in the deltoideopectoral sulcus. The efferent vessels enter the subclavian trunk.

All axillary lymph nodes are interconnected by lymphatics. The brachial and intermediate lymph nodes receive lymph from the arm; the pectoral lymph nodes drain the lymph from the side of the chest wall, mammae and abdomen. The subscapular lymph nodes receive lymph from the region of the shoulder blade, upper arm and back of the neck. The deltoideopectoral lymph node drains lymph from the subcutaneous lymph vessels of the upper arm.

SUBCLAVICULAR AND SUPRACLAVICULAR REGION

On the lymphogram, the subclavicular and supraclavicular lymph nodes are found above and below the clavicle; they receive lymph from the axillary lymph nodes and one single vessel from the upper extremities as well as the mammae, sternoclavicular articulation and the vessels leading from the muscles and bones of the shoulder girdle. Their efferent channels drain into the subclavian trunk, which opens into the thoracic duct to the left and joins the jugular trunk at the right to form the right lymphatic trunk.

Insofar as pertinent to lymphography, data for lymph nodes (position, origin and drainage) are listed in table I.

Table I

Lymph node	location	origin	drainage
superficial subinguinal	superficial in the region of the fossa ovalis	medial and lateral channels of the superficial system of the lower extremities; external genitals, gluteal region, pelvic wall, corpus uteri (via round ligament of the uterus)	iliac lymph nodes (one leads to deep subinguinal lymph nodes and superficial inguinal lymph nodes)
deep subinguinal	under fascia lata in the iliopectineal fossa	efferent vessels of the preceding	iliac lymph nodes
superficial inguinal	above and below the inguinal ligament	efferent vessels of the preceding	iliac lymph nodes
iliac	both sides of the arteria et vena iliaca externa et communis	efferent vessels of the subinguinal, inguinal and hypogastric lymph nodes; bladder, vagina, uterus as well as one vessel from testicles	lumbar lymph nodes
hypogastric	along the arteria et vena hypogastrica	efferent vessels from the vagina, uterus, prostate, bladder and part of penis	common iliac and aortic lymph nodes
sacral	around the arteria et vena sacralis	efferent vessels from the prostate and rectum	hypogastric and aortic lymph nodes
lumbar	at the lumbar vertebral column, behind and on both sides of the aorta abdominalis	efferent vessels from the iliac lymph nodes	lumbar trunks
aortic	in front of the aorta abdominalis and vena cava inferior	efferent vessels from the sacral and hypogastric lymph nodes as well as kidneys, adrenals, testicles, uterus, vagina, uterine tubes, ovaries, diaphragm, liver, stomach, spleen, pancreas, duodenum, jejunum, ileum and colon	intestinal lymphatic trunk, which enters the left lumbar trunk
axillary	in front of the fascia in fat tissue of the axilla	efferent vessels from the arm, mamma, shoulder, back of neck, chest wall and abdominal wall (above navel)	subclavicular and supraclavicular lymph nodes
subclavicular and supraclavicular	above and below clavicle	efferent vessels of preceding, as well as mamma, sternoclavicular articulation, shoulder girdle and one single efferent vessel from upper arm	subclavian trunk

Technique

A special technique is required for the visualization of the lymphatics and lymph nodes. Two methods of approach are available:

A the indirect method
B the direct method

A   The indirect method
For this method, the contrast medium is injected into body cavities or soft tissue and is absorbed by the efferent lymphatic channels. The interval between injection and the appearance of contrast medium in the lymphatic system is so long that this method has little practical value. In addition absorption is insufficient so that the lymphatics and lymph nodes are only partially filled with contrast medium; a total survey cannot therefore be obtained. The best contrast medium for the indirect method is thorotrast, which is however only suitable for use in animals and cadavers because of its toxicity and radioactivity. This approach is therefore totally useless in man.

B   The direct method
Here the contrast medium is injected directly into a lymph vessel or node. Kinmonth developed the first clinical method for visualizing the lymphatics of the lower extremities in man. He injected patent blue violet (11%) subcutaneously into the dorsum of the foot. The blue tissue fluid entered the lymphatics which because of their colouring could then be isolated for a direct injection of contrast medium.

The technique for lymphography as routine examination must satisfy several criteria, namely:
1   The technique must be simple to ensure fast and accurate work. The surgico-technical part (up to and including preparation for the injection) may not take too long.
2   The instrumentarium must be as simple as possible; this means that such instruments as a magnifying lens or binoculars should be superfluous.
3   It is imperative that work be carried out under asceptic conditions to prevent infections of the wound.
4   The entire examination must be executed by one person.

Because this examination is time-consuming and thus unpleasant for the patient, the above is important since it will reduce the chance of failure or prolongation of the examination.

The following procedures shall be discussed:

I   The examination technique when the contrast medium is injected via the lower extremities.

II   The examination technique when the contrast medium is injected via the upper extremities.

Both techniques include the following steps:

A   The surgico-technical part of the examination, to be subdivided into:

1   preparation of the patient

2   injection of dye

3   isolation of a lymphatic vessel

4   puncture of a lymphatic vessel

5   injection of contrast fluid

6   treatment of the wound

B   The roentgenological examination, to be subdivided into:

1   lymphograms

2   lymphadenograms

3   tomograms (if necessary)

4   chest films

I   THE EXAMINATION TECHNIQUE WHEN THE CONTRAST MEDIUM IS INJECTED VIA THE LOWER EXTREMITIES

A   SURGICO-TECHNICAL PART OF THE EXAMINATION

1   *Preparation of the patient.* For a lymphographic examination, the patient need not be admitted to hospital; the procedure can be carried out quite easily in the outpatient clinic. Fasting is not required; the patient may consume a light meal shortly beforehand without any objection.

Furthermore, coffee, tea or broth may be taken during the examination. It goes without saying that the patient should assume a comfortable position from the beginning since he must remain supine during the entire examination. It is also recommended that he or she be distracted by providing reading material. Total immobilization is not necessary. The use of sedatives is superfluous, although it is recommended for very young patients.

2   *Injection of dye.* Beforehand the entire foot (between the toes as well) must be washed with spiritus saponatus, alcohol (70%) and ether. To visualize the lymphatic channels of the anterior superficial system, the dye patent blue violet is injected into the distal part of the dorsum of the foot between metatarsal bones I

and II (½ cc.), III and IV (¼ cc.) and IV and V (¼ cc.), partly intradermally and partly subcutaneously. Since these injections are painful, it is recommended that 1% novocain be added to the blue dye in a ratio of 1:3. The total amount of dye required for both feet is 2 cc.

For visualization of the lymphatics of the posterior superficial system, ¼ cc. blue dye is injected below the ankle at the edge of the heel. A lymphographic examination must always be carried out bilaterally. At the site of injection, a blue spot ± 1 cm. across will develop; these spots are massaged for several minutes to enhance absorption of the dye into the efferent lymphatic channels. The lymphatics become visible as fine, light blue lines (figs. 16, 48). Several remarks on patent blue violet are in order.

It belongs to the triphenylmethane series (molecular weight 515.6). An 11% solution is used because this dye in this low concentration will pass on through the venous system. The dye is excreted by the kidneys and colours the urine blue for 24 hours. After the injection, the skin over the entire body is bluish for one day. The blue spots on the feet disappear one-two weeks later.

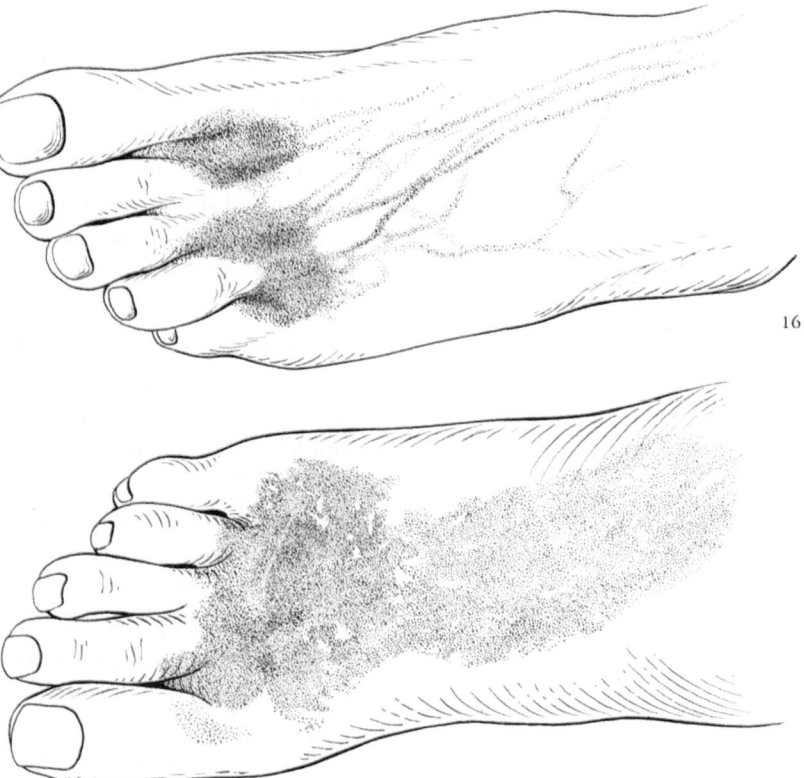

16

17

fig. 16 After the injection of patent blue violet, the subcutaneous lymphatic vessels usually become visible as fine, light blue lines.

fig. 17 In the event of lymphoedema, the lymphatics are usually not visible after injection with patent blue violet. The blue dye spreads out over a large area on the dorsum of the foot via the lymphatic capillaries in the skin.

3   *Isolation of a lymphatic vessel.* It is necessary to work under aseptic conditions during this part of the examination. After 1% novocain is injected as local anaesthetic, a 1-1½ cm. skin incision is made in the proximal part of the dorsum of the foot along the long axis directly above one of the blue lymphatic vessels. For the lymphatic channels of the posterior superficial system, the skin incision is made in back below the ankle in the same manner. A tiny forceps is subsequently used to carefully dissect the lymphatic vessel from the subcutaneous fat tissue (fig. 49). This is easily accomplished since the wall of the vessel is quite strong in comparison to its small diameter (0.2-0.8 mm.).
The vessel is clamped on the proximal side with a rubber-covered clamp (figs. 18, 50). The distal side of the foot is massaged to cause a slight local elevation of the pressure in the lymph vessel and therefore distension (fig. 19).
In some cases, such as lymphoedema of the extremities, the efferent lymphatics are not or barely visible. The blue dye spreads out through the lymphatic capillaries of the skin over a large part of the dorsal surface of the foot (fig. 17). The physiological flow of lymph is then disturbed. In such cases, a transverse incision about 2 cm. long should be made on the lateral side of the tendon of the extensor halucis longus in order to find a lymphatic vessel.

4   *Puncture of a lymphatic vessel.* This is the most difficult part of the technique. Should the lymphatic vessel be damaged during the puncture procedure (fig. 20) or the needle be retracted for any reason whatsoever, the advantage of the local distension is lost and the lymphatic vessel cannot be punctured. It is then necessary to find another lymphatic vessel and to repeat the entire procedure once again, which is not only time-consuming but also unpleasant for the patient. To avoid this, a forceps and a needle have been designed especially for this procedure.
The lymphatic vessel is stretched with the forceps, which has smoothly polished inner surfaces to prevent damage to the vessel. As small metal plate is attached to one of the tips of the forceps (fig. 21). The plate is slipped under the lymph vessel; thus when the vessel is subsequently stretched, it lies fixed on the plate (figs. 22, 51). Puncturing is now easier.
The puncture needle has two parts: a blunt hollow needle (0.5 mm. in diameter and 3.7 cm. long) and a sharply pointed stylet (4.5 cm long) with a diameter slightly less than that of the needle. Where the stylet locks into the needle, there is a small spring (fig. 23). The end of the stylet protrudes only 0.5 mm. beyond the needle. Before puncturing, the needle is held between the thumb and index finger and the end of the stylet is pressed down by the third finger thereby stretching the spring (fig. 52). The lymph vessel is now punctured by the slightly protruding, sharp point of the stylet (figs. 24, 53). As soon as the front blunt end of the needle reaches the vessel wall, a slight resistance is felt. The position

fig. 18 Special clamp (3.8 cm long) with rubber-covered tips.

fig. 19 With the clamp in position, the dorsum of the foot or hand is massaged in the proximal direction only; this causes distension of the lymphatic vessel to as much as 4 times its normal calibre.

fig. 20 Wrong method of puncturing. The lymph vessel can roll back and forth; furthermore there is the danger of perforation of the posterior wall of the lymph vessel.

fig. 21 Special forceps (11.7 cm long) with smoothly polished inner surfaces and small metal plate attached to one tip; this plate is slipped under the lymphatic vessel to protect and support it.

fig. 22 The lymph vessel is stretched between clamp and forceps; it then lies fixed on the plate and puncturing is easier.

fig. 23 Special puncture needle, consisting of two parts: a smooth, blunt hollow needle (3.7 cm. long and 0.5 mm. in diameter for the foot, 0.4 mm. for the hand) and a sharp pointed stylet (4.5 cm. long) with a small spring where the stylet locks into the needle.

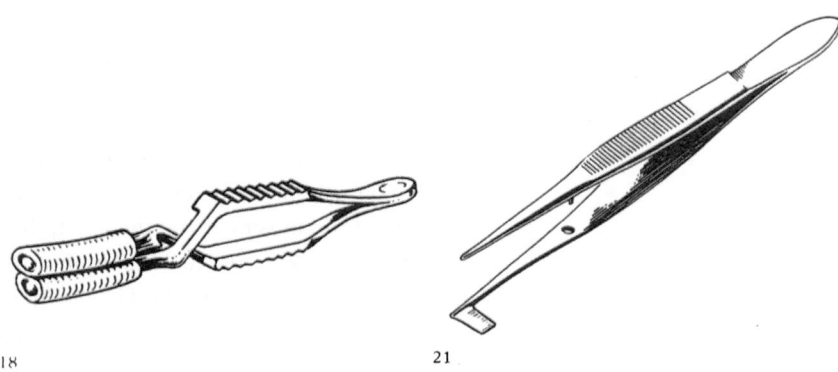

18   21

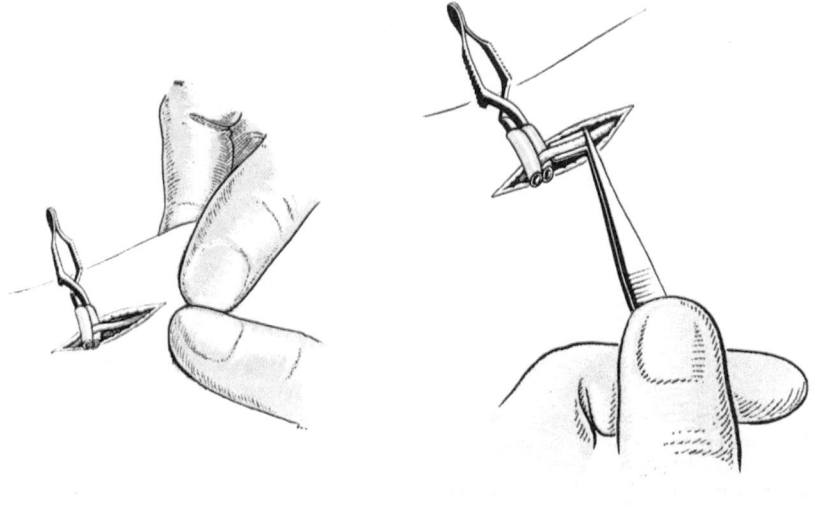

19   22

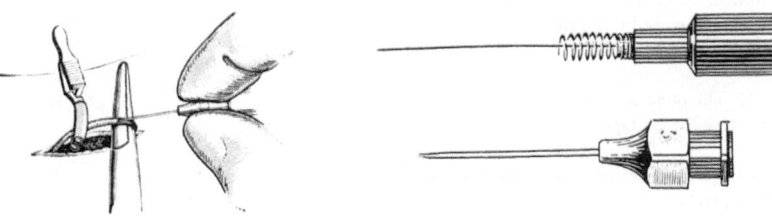

20   23

32

is now satisfactory and the protruding point of the stylet cannot yet have perforated the posterior vessel wall. The needle is now held in a horizontal position and is advanced, by rotating, several millimetres farther into the lymph vessel. The third finger releases the stylet, the spring is relaxed and the stylet shoots back (figs. 25, 54). The blunt hollow needle is slid a few millimetres farther into the lymph vessel (fig. 55). The clamp is removed and placed around the needle and the vessel to keep the needle from slipping (figs. 26, 56); it is subsequently

fig. 24 The needle is held in position between the thumb and the forefinger; the end of the stylet is pressed down by the third finger thus stretching the spring. The lymphatic vessel is punctured by the slightly protruding sharp point of the stylet.

fig. 25 By a rotating movement, the needle is advanced a few millimetres into the lymphatic vessel; then the third finger releases the stylet, the spring is relaxed and the stylet shoots back.

fig. 26 The blunt hollow needle is slid into the lymphatic vessel, the clamp is removed and replaced on the needle and the vessel to keep the needle from slipping.

fig. 27 The puncture needle and clamp are secured by adhesive tape.

fig. 28 Specially designed motor-driven injection apparatus.

fig. 29 The two upright conical rolls rotate in opposite directions; adjustment of the position of the intermediate disk causes a change in the rate of flow at any time during the injection.

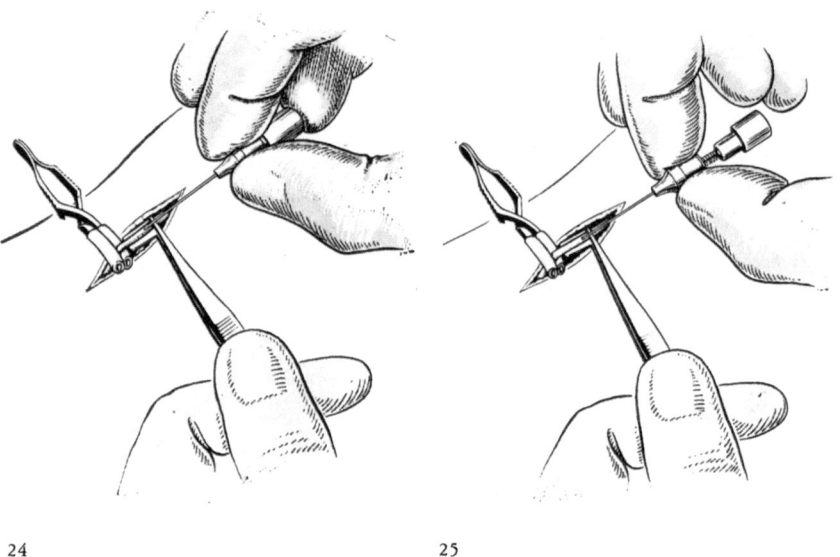

24   25

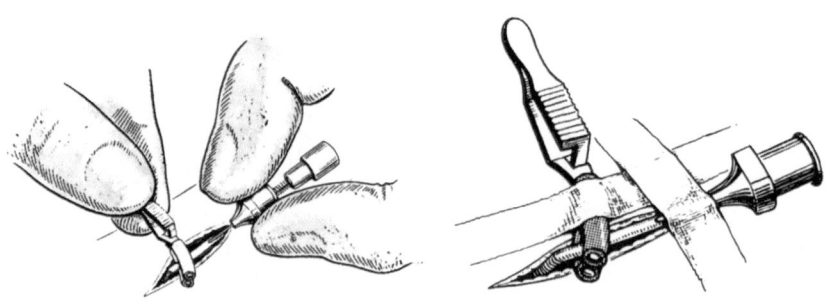

26   27

secured with adhesive (fig. 27). A polythene catheter connects the needle to a 10 ml. injection syringe with a Luer lock connection.

5 *Injection of the contrast fluid.* Lipiodol ultrafluid is used as contrast medium. Lipiodol ultrafluid consists of iodized ethylesters of fatty acids in poppyseed oil; the iodine content is 480 mg./ml. This offers better diagnostic possibilities than water-soluble solutions of contrast media. The disadvantage of water-soluble contrast media (e.g. urografine or pyelombrine) is that the images disappear quickly after the injection since these contrast fluids pass through the vessel wall within several minutes.

Furthermore it is not possible to visualize the lymphatics and lymph nodes proximal to the pelvis because the water-soluble contrast medium becomes highly diluted by lymph. Before injection, the lipiodol ultrafluid is warmed to body temperature. For the lower extremities, approximately 6-10 cc. contrast medium for each side or a maximum of 25 cc. is recommended. For children, ± ⅓ of this amount is used depending upon the age. The injection is constant and uninterrupted as a result of a specially designed motor-driven injection apparatus (fig. 28).

Two upright conical rolls are driven in opposite directions; the rate of injection can be changed smoothly from 1 cc. per 5 minutes to 1 cc. per 20 minutes by adjusting the position of the intermediate disk (fig. 29). It is essential that the rate of flow does not exceed 1 cc per 5 minutes (see chapter *complications*).

A safe rate is 1 cc. per 10 minutes. With this injection equipment, the injection can be given safely and still within the shortest possible time.

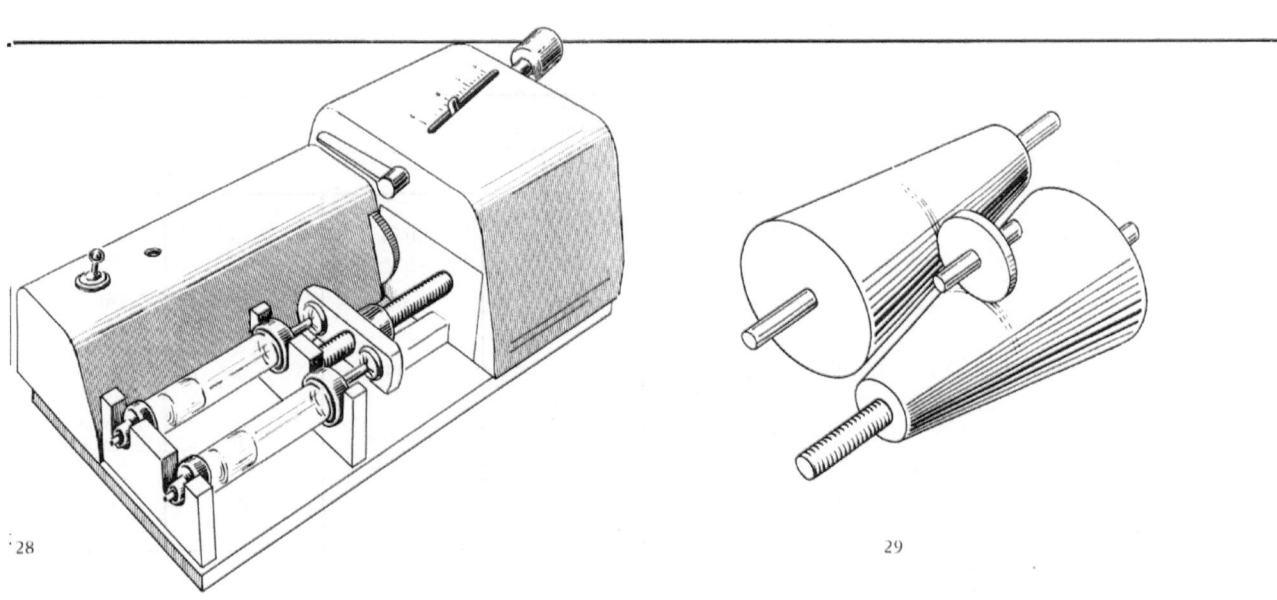

28   29

The procedure is as follows: at the beginning of the injection, the rate is set at 1 cc. per 10 minutes. The intermediate disk is adjusted to increase the rate; at the same time, the swelling of the lymph vessel proximal to the syringe is closely observed. The calibre of the vessel determines the increase in the rate of flow.

As soon as the swelling becomes too pronounced, the intermediate disk is turned back slightly and the resulting rate of flow is maintained for the rest of the injection (usually 1 cc. per 6 minutes). This equipment guarantees a slow rate of flow and a constant pressure. Another advantage is that a "slip" automatically occurs if the counterpressure in the lymphatic system becomes too high.

6 *Treatment of the wound.* After the injection, the small wounds in the dorsum of the foot are rinsed with cetrimide, sutured and painted with iodine. A pressure bandage is applied which can be replaced by an adhesive bandage two days later. The sutures can be removed one week later. A better and easier method is the application of tape strips which ensure continuous fixation of the wound edges. These strips can also be removed a week later.

B *ROENTGENOLOGICAL EXAMINATION*

The roentgenological examination includes taking *lymphograms, lymphadenograms, tomograms* (if necessary) and *chest films.* The lymphograms are made during the injection of contrast medium. The lymphatics contain no contrast medium within a few hours after the end of the injection; the lymphadenograms can be taken one or two days after the injection. If the lymph node architecture is not clearly defined, tomograms are also made (see also chapter *Supplementary Examination Methods).*

Table II

	Amount of contrast medium per injection	time	radiograms projection	film size (cm.)
ankles	½cc	5 min.	a.p.	24 × 30
lower legs	1½cc	15 min.	a.p.	30 × 40
thighs	3cc	30 min.	a.p.	30 × 40
pelvis and abdomen	10cc	100 min.	a.p. lat	30 × 40 30 × 40
thoracic duct	12cc	120 min.	a.p. lat	15 × 40 30 × 40

1   *Lymphograms.* The data for lymphograms are given in table II, assuming a bilateral rate of flow of 1 cc. contrast fluid per 10 minutes. Exposures: anteroposterior (a.p.) and/or lateral (lat.); film sizes: 24 × 30 cm., 15 × 40 cm. and 30 × 40 cm. Radiograms of the ankles are taken to avoid an intravenous injection (figs. 57, 58). In the event of an intravenous injection, drop-by-drop filling of the vessel is visible (fig. 385).

2   *Lymphadenograms.* For the lymphadenograms of the pelvis and abdomen, the following exposures are necessary: one anteroposterior and two oblique (if necessary also one lateral); film size: 30 × 40 cm.

3   *Tomograms.* Tomographic examination is adopted when the lymph node structure cannot be clearly defined on the lymphadenograms. The tomograms are made with linear blurring (even better images are obtained by cycloidal blurring), a focus-film distance of 1.50 m and an angle of 40′. The patient should lie in a prone position, if possible. For reference during the tomographic examination: the inguinal lymph nodes lie between 1 and 4 cm. deep, the iliac lymph nodes between 4 and 7 cm. and the para-aortic and para-lumbar lymph nodes between 7 and 11 cm. The distance between the various sections is ½ cm., ¼ cm. if necessary (figs. 86-104).

4   To complete the lymphographic examination, a *chest film* is made; of course a chest film made before the lymphographic examination must be available for comparison purposes (see also chapter *Complications).*

II THE EXAMINATION TECHNIQUE WHEN THE CONTRAST
    MEDIUM IS INJECTED VIA THE UPPER EXTREMITIES
    In general, the examination technique when the contrast medium is injected
    via the upper extremities parallels that described for the lower extremities.

A   *SURGICO-TECHNICAL PART OF THE EXAMINATION*

1   *Preparation of the patient.* Here the same criteria described for the lower extremities are also applicable.

2   *Injection of dye.* A small amount of patent blue violet is injected into the distal part of the dorsum of the hand between metacarpal bones II and III (½ cc.) and III and IV (¼ cc.), or proximal to the wrist joint and on the volar side of the forearm (¼ cc.).

3 *Isolation of the lymphatic vessel.* The method for the isolation of the lymphatic vessel is similar to that used for the lower extremities.

4 *Puncture of the lymphatic vessel.* The superficial lymphatics of hand and arm are smaller in calibre than those of the foot and have in comparison weaker walls. They tear easily during stretching and puncturing. One must therefore proceed carefully. The needle is thinner (0.4 mm. in diameter) than that used for the foot. The rest of the procedure is similar to that described for the lower extremities.

5 *Injection of the contrast fluid.* For the upper extremities, 5-7 cc. contrast fluid are injected. The rate of flow is ± 1 cc. per 15 minutes to prevent rupture of the vessel. The patient can remain supine if unilateral filling of the lymphatic system of the upper extremities is considered sufficient. For a bilateral examination, the patient should sit up before the two needles are connected to the syringes. The arms are brought close together in order to keep the distance to the injection equipment as short as possible.

6 *Treatment of the wound.* This is the same as described for the lower extremities.

B *THE ROENTGENOLOGICAL EXAMINATION*

As in the examination of the lower extremities, lymphograms, lymphadenograms, tomograms (if necessary) and a chest film should be made.

Table III

	Amount of contrast medium per injection	time	projection	radiograms	
				size	
				unilateral injection	bilateral injection
wrist(s) or forearm(s)	¼cc	±4 min.	a.p.	13 × 18	24 × 30
forearm(s) and upper arm(s)	2cc	30 min.	a.p.	15 × 40	30 × 40
shoulder(s)	5-7cc	75-100 min.	a.p.	24 × 30	2 × 34 × 30

1   *Lymphograms.* The data for lymphograms are given in table III for unilateral
    and bilateral injections. A rate of flow of 1 cc. contrast fluid per 15 minutes is as-
    sumed. The exposures are anteroposterior; film sizes: 13 × 18 cm., 24 × 30
    cm. and 15 × 40 cm.

2   *Lymphadenograms.* The lymphadenograms taken 24 to 48 hours later of the
    shoulder are: one anteroposterior exposure for unilateral filling and 2 anteropos-
    terior exposures for bilateral filling; film sizes: 24 × 30 cm. If the lymph nodes
    cannot be differentiated on the lymphadenogram, extra films can be made using
    radioscopy; the direction of exposure is chosen to ensure free projection of the
    lymph nodes.

3   *Tomograms.* These can be helpful when the internal architecture of the lymph
    nodes cannot be evaluated on the lymphadenogram.

4   As in the examination of the lower extremities, here too a *chest film* is made to
    complete the examination.

38

Normal lymphogram and lymphadenogram

For evaluation of a lymphogram, uniform and uninterrupted filling of the lymphatic system is essential. In addition to a general survey of the lymphatic system, the *lymphograms* offer in particular more information about the condition of the lymphatic channels. The *lymphadenograms* provide insight into the structure of the lymph node. The normal lymphogram and lymphadenogram shall be discussed with respect to (a) examination of the lower extremities, inguinal region, pelvis, abdomen and thoracic duct, and (b) examination of the upper extremities, axillary and subclavicular regions.

A *LOWER EXTREMITIES, INGUINAL REGION, PELVIS, ABDOMEN AND THORACIC DUCT*

LYMPHOGRAM

Lower extremities
A lymph vessel in the dorsum of the foot is injected with contrast fluid and the following lymph node groups of the *anterior superficial system* are filled: (a) the medial group, (b) the lateral group and (c) sometimes both groups. The *medial* channels are straight; they run in parallel and branch out in a proximal direction at the knee. It is possible that only one vessel will be filled; it too branches out proximally at the same location (fig. 59). About halfway up the lower leg, the *lateral* channels always curve over toward the medial side (fig. 60). The normal lymphatics of the lower extremities are thin and uniform in calibre; they differ in this respect from arteries and veins. These channels have many valves, which are irregularly spaced. On the lymphogram, the valves appear as small spheres of greater opacity; the contours are sharp. In the thigh, the vessels always run along the medial side; they are still of a uniform calibre (figs. 61, 62). The vessels are more numerous; the number of valves however is less than in the lower leg. The lymph vessels drain into the superficial subinguinal lymph nodes. Injection into a lymphatic vessel in back below the ankle fills the lymphatic channels of the *posterior superficial system*. Only one or two lymphatics become visible; in the popliteal region, they are interrupted by several lymph nodes (fig. 63). Subsequently after passing through the femoral lymph nodes, the channels empty into the deep nodes in the groin.

Inguinal region
The first group of lymph nodes are the superficial subinguinal lymph nodes. The vessels approach the convex side of the lymph nodes separately and empty lymph into the marginal sinus (figs. 30, 110). The sinuses of a lymph node are interconnected so that one afferent channel can fill a lymph node with contrast medium. The efferent channels leave the lymph node at the hilus; they are not

40 fig. 30 Lymphogram: normal lymph node with afferent and efferent lymphatic channels.

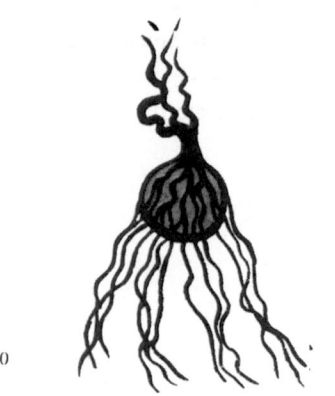

30

as numerous as the afferent channels. The afferent and efferent vessels can anastomose outside the lymph nodes. The lymphogram shows that most of the efferent channels lead directly to the lymph node groups in the pelvis; some of these channels pass through the deep subinguinal lymph nodes and others extend to the pelvis via the (inferior and superior) superficial inguinal lymph nodes. It should be noted that one single lymph vessel from the lower extremities can bypass the subinguinal lymph nodes and drain directly into the (inferior and superior) superficial inguinal lymph nodes or the deep subinguinal lymph nodes (figs. 64-67). After the subinguinal lymph nodes, the lymphatics change in appearance. The vessels are no longer straight; they run closer together, often twisting so that differentiation is difficult; the calibre becomes variable.
It is important that the lymphatics and lymph nodes in the inguinal region are seen as one functional unit, since numerous connecting vessels join the superficial and deep groups of lymph nodes together. Actually however, in 40% of the patients, the deep nodes in the groin are not filled by injection into the anterior superficial system only (figs. 68-73). When a precise evaluation of all of these regional lymph nodes is required, e.g. for melanoma of the extremities, it is essential that *both* the anterior and posterior superficial lymphatic systems be filled with contrast fluid.

Pelvis and Abdomen
In the pelvis, the lymphatic channels follow the course of the arteries and veins. They are interrupted by numerous lymph nodes which are named according to the blood vessels at that point. Near the arteria et vena iliaca externa et communis, the various lymphatics and lymph nodes resemble a string of beads. On the anteroposterior exposures (fig. 74), they lie close together making differentiation difficult; on the lateral exposures (fig. 75), the various bead-like chains are easier to observe. They form the medial, the superficial lateral and the deep lateral chains. Occasionally only two will be filled, probably as a result of anatomical changes in this region; it is difficult to determine which two channels they are. The lymph nodes around the arteria sacralis et hypogastrica (fig. 76) are seldom filled during injection of the contrast medium since the afferent channels do not stem from the inguinal lymph nodes. The lymph nodes of this group are sometimes visible on the lymphadenogram. The last lymph node group of the lymphatic system in the pelvis is the common iliac lymph nodes. In the abdomen, two groups of lymphatics and lymph nodes can be distinguished:

a   the paralumbar
b   the para-aortic

a   The paralumbar lymphatics and lymph nodes are a continuation of the
efferent channels from the common iliac lymph nodes. On the anteroposterior
exposures, they are visible on both sides of the lumbar vertebrae (fig. 74); on the
lateral films, they are found just in front of or partly on top of the lumbar vertebral column. Although the course of these vessels is normally straight, abnormalities are possible in some cases. At the 5th lumbar or 1st sacral vertebra, several channels may cross over to the other side. As a result, it is possible that a
unilateral injection will be sufficient to fill the right and left paralumbar lymph
node groups with contrast fluid (fig. 77). The paralumbar lymph vessels converge to form the right and left lumbar trunks (fig. 78).

b   The para-aortic lymphatics and lymph nodes lie in front of the aorta abdominalis and the vena cava inferior; they are a continuation of the efferent
lymphatic channels from the organs in the abdomen. The para-aortic lymphatic
channels are not always filled during injection of the contrast fluid. When visible during injection, they are seen on the anteroposterior exposure to extend
upwards approximately in the middle of the lumbar vertebral column (fig. 74).
The para-aortic lymphatics join to form the intestinal lymphatic trunk, which
in turn drains into the left lumbar trunk (fig. 78).

Thoracic duct
The right and left lumbar trunks merge to form the cysterna chyli (fig. 79),
which is in fact the beginning of the thoracic duct extending along the medial
line. On the lymphogram, the thoracic duct bends to the left at the 5th thoracic
vertebra and extends upward along side of the thoracic vertebral column. Three
or four cm. above the left clavicle, it turns sharply to the left and ends in the vena subclavia sinistra. Although the calibre of the thoracic duct is uniform, a
slight distension occurs just before it ends. There are also valves in the thoracic
duct; they may vary in number. Usually there is a single opening of the thoracic
duct into the vena subclavia sinistra (fig. 80); sometimes it is multiple (fig. 81).
Even more rare is a double-barrelled opening into the vena subclavia dextra as
well as the vena subclavia sinistra (fig. 83) or a right-sided opening into the vena
subclavia dextra (fig. 82).

LYMPHADENOGRAM

Inguinal region, pelvis and abdomen
The lymph nodes are more easily distinguished on the lymphadenogram. Their
size varies between ½ and 2½ cm; they are oval, round or kidney-shaped and
slightly flattened. One side shows an indentation which is in fact the hilus. The
lipiodol ultrafluid is collected in the reticular cells of the lymph node. The nor-

42

fig. 31 Lymphadenogram: normal, oval lymph node with intact marginal sinus and granular, uniform distribution of the contrast medium.

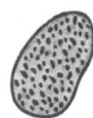

31

mal lymph nodes appear homogeneous and granular on the lymphadenogram. The marginal sinus is seen as a continuous line (figs. 31, 111).

It is important that anteroposterior (fig. 84), lateral and oblique (fig. 85) exposures are made of the inguinal region, the pelvis and the abdomen. Then comparison of the lymphadenograms will facilitate interpretation of the changes in internal structure and marginal sinus. In doubtful cases, tomograms may be helpful. It is odd that normal lymph nodes, which are usually rather small, can be discerned so clearly on several consecutive tomographic sections (figs. 86-104). The lymph nodes may remain visible on follow-up films for many weeks; they sometimes retain the contrast medium 6 months or longer.

B UPPER EXTREMITIES, AXILLARY AND SUBCLAVICULAR REGIONS

LYMPHOGRAMS

Upper extremities

A lymph vessel in the dorsum of the hand is injected with contrast fluid. The medial and lateral channels of the superficial lymphatic system are filled. Along the medial channels, several lymph nodes are visible above the elbow: the superficial cubital lymph nodes (fig. 106). Most of the lateral channels run alongside of the medial channels in the upper arm. Together they drain into the first lymph node group in the axilla: the superficial axillary lymph nodes. One single lateral vessel continues along the outside of the upper arm and opens directly into the lymph nodes below the clavicle: the subclavicular lymph nodes.

If a lymph vessel on the volar side of the forearm is injected with contrast fluid, then only one or two lymphatics become visible (fig. 107). They run straight along the medial side of the upper arm and also empty into the superficial axillary lymph nodes.

The normal channels are thin; they are smaller in calibre than those in the lower extremities. Valves are irregularly spaced.

Axillary and subclavicular regions

In contrast to the afferent channels, the efferent channels of the axillary lymph nodes follow a tortuous course. They are difficult to distinguish and pass through various lymph nodes (fig. 108), whereby it is practically impossible to determine which group of axillary lymph nodes is involved, to the subclavicular group. The lymph nodes above the clavicle, the supraclavicular lymph nodes, are almost never visible during injection.

LYMPHADENOGRAMS

Axillary and subclavicular regions

These films show that in general more lymph nodes are filled with contrast fluid than during the direct examination (fig. 109). The lymph nodes, which are seen to overlap, can still be differentiated from each other. In such a case, radioscopy can be used to determine that direction of exposure which will ensure free projection of the lymph nodes.

Eventually a tomographic examination can follow.

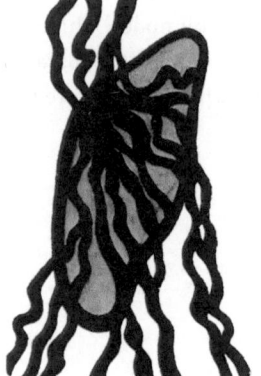

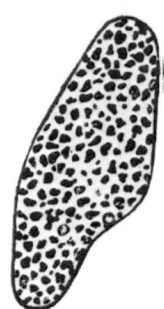

fig. 32 Acute inflammation; lymphogram.

fig. 33 Acute inflammation; lymphadenogram.

fig. 34 Chronic inflammation; lymphadeno-gram.

fig. 35 Hodgkin's disease, first type; lymphade-nogram.

fig. 36 Hodgkin's disease, second type; lym-phadenogram.

fig. 37 Hodgkin's disease, third type; lymphad-enogram.

fig. 38 Whipple's disease; lymphadenogram.

fig. 39 Reticulum cell sarcoma, first type; lym-phadenogram.

32   33

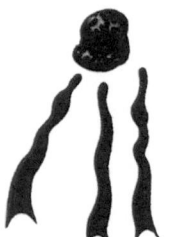

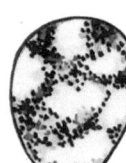

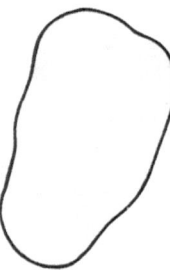

34   35   36

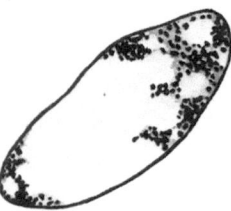

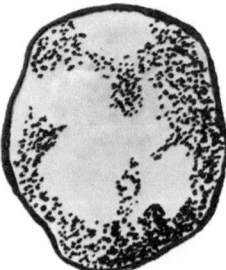

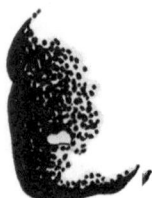

37   38   39

Indications and pathological lymphogram

In practice, the lymphographic examination is useful for:

I   Demonstration, differentiation and determination of the extent of (a) inflammatory changes in benign diseases and (b) lymphoreticular malignancies and metastatic carcinoma;

II   Demonstration and differentiation of primary and secondary lymphoedema of the extremities;

III   Demonstration of lesions and obstructions in the thoracic duct which cause chylothorax or chyloperitoneum, and establishment of the cause of chyluria;

IV   Assessment of the results of radiological, chemotherapeutical and surgical treatment of malignant diseases.

Only the healthy tissue in a lymph node absorbs contrast fluid; therefore the evaluation of pathological lymph nodes depends on the size and the appearance of the marginal sinus and internal structure as seen on the lymphadenogram. On the lymphograms, it is important to look for symmetry of the right and left sides, changes in course such as the presence of collaterals and phenomena resulting from lymphatic obstruction.

Ia   BENIGN DISEASES

The benign diseases can be divided into (1) acute inflammatory diseases, (2) chronic inflammatory diseases and (3) specific inflammatory diseases.

1   *Acute inflammatory diseases.* Lymph nodes involved by inflammatory diseases in conjunction with hypertrophic changes are enlarged. The afferent and efferent lymphatic vessels are dilated (figs. 32, 113). These lymph nodes are often found by chance in the inguinal or axillary regions. Their enlargement is the result of infections in the extremities. This should be considered during evaluation and differentiation of pathological lymph nodes in these regions.
These lymph nodes are also found in association with virus infections and near tumours (figs. 152, 153, 277, 278, 288, 348). The lymphadenogram reveals that in spite of the enlargement, the internal structure of the lymph nodes has remained normal. Furthermore, the marginal sinus is preserved (figs. 33, 114, 156).

2   *Chronic inflammatory diseases.* Lymph nodes affected by inflammatory diseases in conjunction with hypotrophic changes eventually become small and indis-

tinguishable. The marginal sinus is still intact but the nodal architecture can no longer be clearly recognized. On the lymphadenogram, the afferent channels are few in number and dilated (figs. 34, 116). In the case of lymphoedema of the lower extremities, for example, these lymph nodes are seen in the inguinal region.

3   *Specific inflammatory diseases.* Lymph nodes involved by an active specific inflammatory disease (tbc) show no characteristic phenomena (fig. 115). However, lymphography is not carried out in these patients. Old specific inflammations lead to the development of calcified lymph nodes which may or may not be enlarged. The lymph node tissue still functioning fills with contrast fluid and can be recognized as such (figs. 157-159).

Ib   MALIGNANT DISEASES

The malignant diseases can be separated into (1) lymphoreticular malignancies such as Hodgkin's disease, Brill-Symmers' disease, Whipple's disease, reticulum cell sarcoma, chronic leukaemia and lymphosarcoma, and (2) metastases such as carcinoma, seminoma and melanoma.

1 LYMPHORETICULAR MALIGNANCIES

Hodgkin's disease. The lymph nodes involved by Hodgkin's disease have various typical characteristics. The lymphograms show enlarged to greatly enlarged lymph nodes with dilated lymphatic channels (figs. 162, 166). Various types of pathological lymph nodes can be seen on the lymphadenogram, i.e. enlarged to greatly enlarged lymph nodes with in general an uninterrupted marginal sinus. Irregular filling defects are visible in the granular distribution of the contrast medium, giving the interior of the lymph node a moth-eaten appearance (figs. 35, 117, 163, 169, 170, 175, 354, 355). Another possibility is that the granular aspect has completely disappeared so that the internal nodal architecture appears lacy of foamy and the lymph node as a whole, ghost-like (figs. 36, 118, 165, 157, 169, 170, 176, 355). The marginal sinus remains intact. A combination of both forms in one lymph node is possible. Often the marginal sinus is locally indistinct (figs. 37, 119, 169, 170, 171, 173, 177-181, 355). The pathological-anatomical classifications of Hodgkin's disease, Hodgkin's sarcoma and paragranuloma cannot be distinguished as such lymphographically.

Brill-Symmers' disease. The pathologically changed lymph nodes cannot be distinguished from those due to Hodgkin's disease; they can become quite large (figs. 121, 139, 182-184).

fig. 40 Reticulum cell sarcoma, second type; lymphadenogram.

fig. 41 Chronic lymphatic leukaemia, first type; lymphadenogram.

fig. 42 Chronic lymphatic leukaemia, second type; lymphadenogram.

fig. 43 Lymphosarcoma, first type; lymphadenogram.

fig. 44 Lymphosarcoma, second type; lymphadenogram.

fig. 45 Metastases, first type; lymphadenogram.

fig. 46 Metastases, second type; lymphadenogram.

fig. 47 Metastases, third type; lymphadenogram.

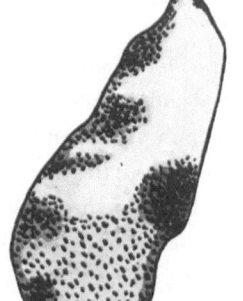

40

41

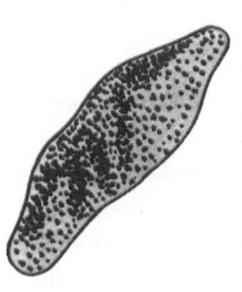

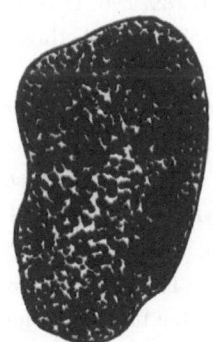

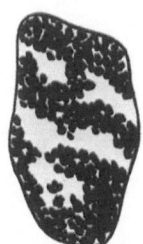

42

43

44

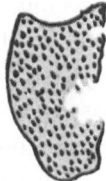

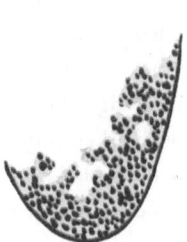

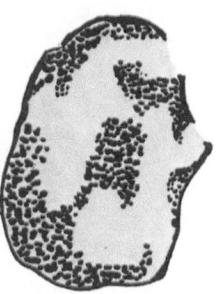

45

46

47

Whipple's disease. This syndrome is quite rare. Although benign histologically, the clinical course can appear malignant. The lymph nodes are enlarged to greatly enlarged; the marginal sinus is preserved for quite some time and also appears thickened. The internal structure is no longer recognizable as such (figs. 38, 121, 185).

Reticulum cell sarcoma. In general, the lymphograms show the lymph nodes to be enlarged and the afferent lymphatics dilated (fig. 186). Various types of pathological lymph nodes can be seen on the lymphadenogram. The lymph node is usually enlarged; the marginal sinus is interrupted and is only visible where the internal architecture of the lymph node appears granular. The contrast fluid collects in that section of the marginal sinus which is still intact (figs. 39, 122, 188, 190, 194, 195). It is also possible that the internal structure has become quite vague and no longer symmetrical while the granular appearance has become limited and very fine. To a large extent, the involved reticulum seems to have lost its ability to absorb contrast fluid.
In addition there are large areas without any granular structure at all; furthermore a considerable portion of the marginal sinus has disappeared (figs. 40, 123, 149-151, 189, 196, 197). The lymph nodes involved by reticulum cell sarcoma can closely resemble those affected by metastatic carcinoma.

Chronic lymphatic leukaemia. The lymphograms show large to very large lymph nodes, often enlarged along the long axis, with conspicuously sparse filling. As a result considerably less contrast fluid is needed to achieve filling of the pelvic, paralumbar and aortic lymph nodes, for instance. On the lymphadenogram, the lymph nodes are large to very large, often sausage-like along the long axis. The marginal sinus is generally preserved. The contrast distribution is granular, but blurs together in many places. Where the granular appearance is lost, the lymph nodes appear foamy (figs. 41, 124, 204-210). Another possibility is that the granular structure will take on the appearance of fine transverse stripes (figs. 42, 125, 204, 205, 208-210).

Lymphosarcoma. The pathological lymph nodes resemble those of chronic lymphatic leukaemia in many ways. The changes are however more pronounced and more massive. In the early stage, they resemble lymph nodes affected by inflammation (fig. 211). The lymph nodes can become very large. The lymphograms show marked filling of the lymph nodes with contrast medium; the lymphatics are distended (figs. 213, 215). On the lymphadenograms, the lymph nodes can be exceedingly large with in general an intact marginal sinus; the internal structure is gross and not symmetrical (figs. 43, 126, 211, 212, 214, 216-218). It is also possible that the contrast medium collects in some areas to form wide bands alternating with zones free of contrast fluid. (figs. 44, 127, 217, 218)

2 METASTASES

Lymph nodes infiltrated by metastatic *carcinoma, seminoma* or *melanoma* are
often enlarged. From the afferent vessels, malignant cells pass first into the
marginal sinus of the lymph node – where involvement begins. On the lymphograms, the lymph nodes may or may not be enlarged, the lymphatics may
or may not be distended. Obstruction of the efferent flow is possible; lymphatic
channels can arch outwards and collateral lymphatic channels might be present. On the lymphadenograms, various types can be differentiated according to
the advancement of the disease. The lymph nodes may or may not be enlarged.
The marginal sinus is interrupted in one or more places. The boundary between
the metastases and normal lymph node tissue is indistinct and irregular (figs. 45,
128, 305-309, 363). In the more advanced stages, there is probably only a small
amount of normal lymph node tissue left (figs. 46, 129, 225, 246, 301, 302, 346,
347). The involvement can also occur from within. The lymph node enlarges;
the internal structure disappears; the marginal sinus can be preserved for quite
some time (figs. 47, 130, 250, 292-294, 312-315, 327, 328, 330, 345). When the
lymph node is completely filled with carcinomatous tissue, it is no longer recognizable as such on the lymphadenogram; an abrupt discontinuity in the
lymphatic chain is then observed (figs. 132, 220, 224-227, 230, 275). In these
cases, the lymphograms are very important because displaced lymphatic channels can arch out around these interruptions (figs. 131, 219, 223, 276, 291). In
the event of lymphatic obstruction, the afferent lymphatics remain visible on
the lymphadenograms because of the resulting distension (figs. 222, 225, 273,
275).

In general, the basic types described above are correct as such. In practice however the structures of the various lymph nodes are sometimes very similar and
differentiation becomes difficult (figs. 133-141). This is quite understandable
since occasionally the pathological anatomist also has trouble establishing the
correct diagnosis for pathological lymph nodes. In particular, the early stages of
involvement by a malignant disease and considerable enlargement of the lymph
nodes (the marginal sinus is then almost always interrupted) can cause this type
of problem (figs. 172, 173, 205, 217, 218). The various types of nodal architecture are most easily recognized in the moderately enlarged lymph nodes. For
this reason, it is also necessary to have clinical data at hand. Special care is required for the interpretation of lymphograms taken of older individuals. Old
inflammations and degenerative processes can cause many misleading patterns
(fig. 112, 146, 147).
What type of cases are generally referred for lymphographic examination in a

routine practice? For lymphoreticular malignancies, the clinical diagnosis has usually been recognized; in these cases it is necessary to determine whether the retroperitoneal nodes are involved by malignant disease in order to initiate effective therapy (figs. 178-181, 183, 184, 191, 192, 208-210). Frequently on the other hand, the clinical diagnosis is not (yet) definite although a malignant reticulosis is suspected. The results of a lymphographic examination can be decisive.

For patients with carcinoma (seminoma, melanoma), it is essential to establish the presence of metastases and the extent of metastasizing with the greatest possible accuracy, for the determination of the correct therapy as well as prevention of useless procedures. For instance, often in cervical carcinoma, the clinically determined stage must be revised repeatedly after lymphographic examination (figs. 221, 222). It is practically impossible to demonstrate the spread of eventual metastasizing clinically – and this applies for all types of carcinoma.

In this respect, it is important that the clinician and the radiologist agree on the potentialities of a lymphographic examination so that patients are not referred after many therapeutic procedures and/or operations have been carried out, leaving lymphography only as a last resort (fig. 364).

II DEMONSTRATION AND DIFFERENTIATION OF PRIMARY AND SECONDARY LYMPHOEDEMA OF THE EXTREMITIES

Many classifications of lymphoedema of the extremities are known. One of the easiest to handle is separation into *idiopathic primary* and *secondary* lymphoedema. In primary lymphoedema of the extremities, neither clinical nor anamnestic causatory factors are known. The rare congenital familial type, Milroy disease is also included in this category. Primary lymphoedema usually develops in young individuals in the legs and is more frequent in woman than men. Sometimes it is unilateral and spreads to the other leg later, but both legs can also be affected simultaneously. *Congenital* abnormalities in the lymphatic system influence this type of lymphoedema.

In secondary lymphoedema, causatory factors can be shown. This type of lymphoedema can be the result of *inflammatory diseases, traumas, surgical removal of lymph nodes or radiation therapy;* it can also be caused by *tumour infiltration* into the lymph nodes. Before the diagnosis lymphoedema is established, whether idiopathic or secondary, the possibility of oedema of renal, cardiac or endocrinal origin must be ruled out.

Primary lymphoedema can be recognized on the lymphogram by the following pathological changes: *aplasia* (lack of lymphatic vessels), *hypoplasia* (decrease in the number of lymphatics: fig. 333) and *dilation and/or varices* (widening and/ or twisting course of the lymph vessels: fig. 334).

In secondary lymphoedema, the lymphatics undergo pathological changes which are visible on the lymphogram as: *numerous, small, irregular lymphatic channels in addition to normal ones* (figs. 335-340, 343, 348), *highly tortuous, sometimes varicose lymphatic channels* (figs. 336-340, 343, 349) and *retrograde filling with contrast fluid* of the lymphatic capillaries in the skin *(dermal back-flow)* (fig. 340).

In practice, there are actually four groups of patients with oedema:

a Patients with a clinical diagnosis of primary lymphoedema which is confirmed roentgenologically;

b Patients with a clinical diagnosis of primary lymphoedema whereby a secondary lymphoedema is demonstrated roentgenologically;

c Patients with a clinical diagnosis of primary lymphoedema whereby no abnormality of the lymphatic system is found roentgenologically;

d Patients with a clinical diagnosis of secondary lymphoedema which is confirmed roentgenologically.

a If the clinical diagnosis of primary lymphoedema is confirmed by lymphography, this implies that little can be done for the patient since no therapy is known at present for congenital causes. If lymphoedema develops in a young patient (and lymphoedema also occurs in the family), it is in fact useless to carry out lymphography which at the most will reveal only the extent of the disease – sometimes pertinent in employment and/or insurance questions.

b This group of patients is of course the most important. In these cases, a cause is demonstrated for which a therapy can be initiated. Lymphoedema in a mature person can be the first sign of a malignant disease characterized by tumour infiltration into lymph nodes (figs. 341-352).

c For these patients, a lymphographic examination is in fact superfluous. Actually the initial clinical examination of these patients should have been more thorough. It should be noted here that in the event of lymphoedema of the extremities, lymphographic examination should be preceded or followed by phlebography.

d For these patients, the primary purpose of lymphography is not to demonstrate the secondary lymphoedema but instead to establish the nature and extent of the disease responsible (figs. 353-365).

III DEMONSTRATION OF LESIONS AND OBSTRUCTIONS IN THE THORACIC DUCT WHICH CAN CAUSE CHYLOTHORAX OR CHYLO-PERITONEUM, AND ESTABLISHMENT OF THE CAUSE OF CHYLURIA

In the case of chyloperitoneum or chylothorax, the exact location of the lesion or obstruction in the thoracic duct (fig. 369) can be demonstrated and visualized by lymphographic examination. If in *chylothorax* due to a lesion or obstruction in the thoracic duct, collateral lymphatic channels do not form and lymph does not drain into the veins, then irrespective of the reason the effusion of chyle into the thorax will continue, leading ultimately to death. Only surgical intervention can save the patient – if the site of effusion is known.

The presence *of chyle in the urine* is the result of an abnormal anastomosis between the lymphatic system and the uropoietic system. The pyelolymphatic communication is due to an increase in pressure within the lymphatic system which causes the gracile lymph vessels around the renal calyces to tear. Chyluria is usually a symptom of Filaria bancrofti. The adult worms can cause attacks of lymphangitis and lymphadenitis. The wall of the lymph vessel shows proliferative inflammation; the tunica intima is festered and thrombi may sometimes form. On the lymphograms, extensive varicose lymphatic channels and distension of the lymphatics are seen (fig. 370). The development of chyluria is not dependent upon an obstruction in the thoracic duct. The lymphogram will reveal the pyelolymphatic communication (figs. 371-373) and demonstrate the severity and extent of the obstructing changes. In some cases, it will offer useful guidelines for surgery.

IV ASSESSMENT OF THE RESULTS OF RADIOLOGICAL, CHEMOTHER-APEUTICAL AND SURGICAL TREATMENT OF MALIGNANT DISEASES

The correct localization of pathological lymph nodes is particularly important. Since the oily contrast fluid is retained in the lymph nodes for many months, follow-up radiograms can be used to assess the results of radiation therapy or treatment with chemotherapeutics (figs. 178-181, 183, 184, 191, 192, 208-210). The presence or absence of metastasis in a lymph node can be essential in planning a surgical procedure.

Adding chlorophyll to the contrast fluid so that the lymphatics and lymph nodes become green, thereby simplifying the operation, has many drawbacks. Passage is impeded, the lymphograms are more difficult to evaluate, the lymph nodes develop marked inflammatory reactions and in practice the usefulness of the green colour is disappointing. Since it is in fact not easy to completely excise all lymph nodes in a specific area, it is wise to make survey films during or at the end of the operation rather than post-operatively (figs. 242, 243, 311, 326).

Selective supplementary examination methods

The conventional lymphographic examination does not always provide sufficient information concerning the location, type and architecture of normal and
pathological lymph nodes. The evaluation of involvement by metastases as well
as the differentiation of pathological lymph nodes is not always decisive on the
basis of lymphograms and lymphadenograms alone.

In the course of the development of any new method of examination, questions
are bound to arise; it is of course imperative that these problems be recognized
in time and that refined diagnostic procedures supplement them. This aspect
must be clearly recognized and the proper measures taken quickly; if not, the
number of faulty diagnoses will not remain within acceptable limits and some
indications will appear valid no longer. It goes without saying that the above-
mentioned criteria also apply for the lymphographic examination. The first step
is to recognize the most likely types of diagnostic problems. During the development of the lymphographic technique, the following problems were encountered:

1 matted lymph nodes
2 lymph nodes superimposed over parts of the skeleton or intestinal gasses
3 superposition of lymph nodes
4 very obese patients
5 empty area above a block or lymphatic obstruction in the lymphatic system
6 interruption in the lymph node chain
7 inadequate filling of lymph nodes with contrast fluid
8 lymph nodes outside the drainage area
9 lymph nodes which appear "irritated"
10 presence of fat and/or fibrosis in lymph nodes
11 presence of micrometastases in lymph nodes

Above all, it must be assumed that the radiologist is sufficiently experienced in
the evaluation of lymphograms and that the examination is executed compe-
tently. It should be noted here that a lymphographic examination must be carried out bilaterally at all times; a unilateral examination, for any reason whatsoever, must be considered a failure from a diagnostic point of view. The above-
mentioned problems encountered during the evaluation of lymphograms ne-
cessitated the introduction of selective supplementary examination methods in
order to arrive at the most reliable roentgenological diagnoses. For this purpose,
three methods are available:

A selective supplementary tomograms
B selective supplementary angiograms
C follow-up radiograms

Other supplementary examination methods such as *sterioscopic, subtraction* and *enlarged* radiograms do not offer a solution to the diagnostic problems in lymphography. The depth dimension of sterioscopic radiograms provides information about location; however there is not sufficient data as to the type, architecture and marginal sinus of the lymph nodes. Subtraction films can only be realized in incidental cases (figs. 157-159) but cannot be used as routine examination since it is impossible to take two exactly identical films before and after a lymphographic examination. Enlarged radiograms as supplementary examination also offer little clarification as to location and structure of the lymph nodes, not to mention the fact that it is exceptionally difficult technically to make good enlargements of the lymph nodes in the abdomen.

A Selective supplementary tomograms
A series of sections makes it possible to evaluate the lymph node in several planes. In this manner, further information becomes available concerning location, type, internal architecture and marginal sinus of normal and pathological lymph nodes. To establish the most reliable roentgenological diagnosis, it is essential to be able to interpret small changes in the internal structure and involvement of the marginal sinus. With this supplementary method of examination, small pathological changes can be found even in patients with an apparently normal lymphogram. On the other hand, presumed pathological changes are sometimes found to be the result of superposition of small and healthy lymph nodes (figs. 233-239). Thus in reference to the problems encountered in diagnostics, selective supplementary tomographic examination can be helpful in the event of (1) matted lymph nodes, (2) lymph nodes superimposed over parts of the skeleton or intestinal gasses, (3) superposition of lymph nodes and (4) very obese patients (figs. 172-176, 188-190, 194-197, 200, 201, 207, 227, 236-239, 247-249, 252, 259, 262, 293, 294, 296-298, 301, 302, 305-309, 313-315, 317-320, 322-324, 328, 330, 332, 345-347, 352, 359-361, 372).

B Selective supplementary angiograms
Supplementary angiographic examination includes cavography, phlebography, aortography and/or arteriography according to the method of Seldinger. Since lymph nodes are found around arteries and veins, they can if enlarged cause characteristic impressions in blood vessels. Since the location of the area requiring further study is known from the lymphogram, a supplementary angiographic examination can be directed to this region. One or two catheters are placed such that maximum filling and dilatation of the vessel in the suspect area is achieved. For phlebocavography, radiograms are made from two directions: anteroposterior and oblique for pelvic vessels and anteroposterior and lateral for the vena cava inferior. Aortography or selective arteriography can also be useful

in demonstrating pathological lymph node masses, particularly in the pelvis minor. A clearly recognizable indentation in an artery however must be expected at a later stage than compression of a vein. One advantage of arteriographic diagnosis is that evaluation is more reliable because compression cannot be confused with physiological narrowing as can occur in the venous system. Veins after all show physiological compression due to organs, arteries, tendons and bones.

In the event of diagnostic difficulties, a selective supplementary angiographic examination may aid in the further examination of (1) an empty area above a block or lymphatic obstruction in the lymphatic system, (2) interruption in the lymphatic chain, (3) inadequate filling of lymph nodes with contrast fluid and (4) lymph nodes outside the drainage area (figs. 202, 203, 228, 229, 231, 232, 253, 254, 260, 263, 264, 266, 268, 270, 271, 282, 285, 286, 289, 290, 299, 300, 342, 350).

C Follow-up radiograms

It is obvious that follow-up radiograms (for instance every 3 weeks) form an extremely reliable method from a diagnostic point of view. In practice, this method should only be used when the conventional examination in conjunction with the other supplementary methods offers no solution. The clinician cannot of course wait weeks or months for a diagnosis.

Sometimes the lymphatic system appears irritated on the lymphadenogram. This type of lymph node can for instance be due to inflammatory-like changes characterized by enlargement of the node. The lymph node may also appear disorderly and irregular or a combination of both types may occur (figs. 152, 153, 161, 277, 278, 288, 348). Roentgenologically there are no clear-cut indications of involvement by a malignant disease. Such nodes are seen near tumours or infections. From a diagnostic point of view, the important point is whether such an irritation should be considered a precursor or the initial stage of involvement by a malignant disease or a normal occurrence. A follow-up study of 200 patients with this type of lymph node showed that the appearance of irritated lymph nodes on the lymphogram was followed only in incidental cases by the development of malignant disease at a later date (figs. 154, 155). In most patients, the lymph nodes showed no changes at all on the follow-up radiograms. Post-operative pathological-anatomical studies of excised lymph nodes also revealed only an inflammatory reaction in these patients. Although in principle, this type of node can be considered normal roentgenologically, it is in the best interests of the patient to make follow-up studies when irritation has been seen – to intercept those few cases where malignant degeneration occurs.

The presence of fat or fibrosis in lymph nodes can cause diagnostic problems. In the centre of the lymph nodes, fat and connective tissue can be recognized as sharply defined, round filling defects; in the margin however they closely resemble involvement by metastatic carcinoma or reticulum cell sarcoma (figs. 112, 146-151). They frequently occur in the inguinal region, less frequently in the pelvis and rarely in the para-aortic and lumbar regions. In doubtful cases, follow-up films can be helpful.

Finally the last problem in diagnostics: the presence of *micrometastases* in lymph nodes. Micrometastases cannot of course be demonstrated by the conventional lymphographic examination nor by any of the supplementary examination methods. However this is true for all roentgenological examinations; only a pathological-anatomical examination can be decisive.
Table IV summarizes the diagnostic problems which can arise during lymphography, and the supplementary examination methods to be applied.

The above considerations lead to the question of whether these supplementary examination methods are necessary in general or only in incidental cases. Selective supplementary tomographic examination is time-consuming and selective supplementary angiographic examination is unpleasant for the patient. The clinician is not given an immediate guideline for eventual therapy if radiograms are made every three weeks. To answer the question then, it is necessary to differentiate between lymphographic examination for the demonstration of lymphoreticular malignancies on the one hand and metastatic carcinoma in lymph nodes on the other. In the event of lymphoreticular malignancies, the correct diagnosis has usually been recognized clinically and confirmed by histological studies. The involved lymph nodes almost always appear enlarged and usually are affected in groups. Then anteroposterior, lateral and/or oblique ra-

Table IV

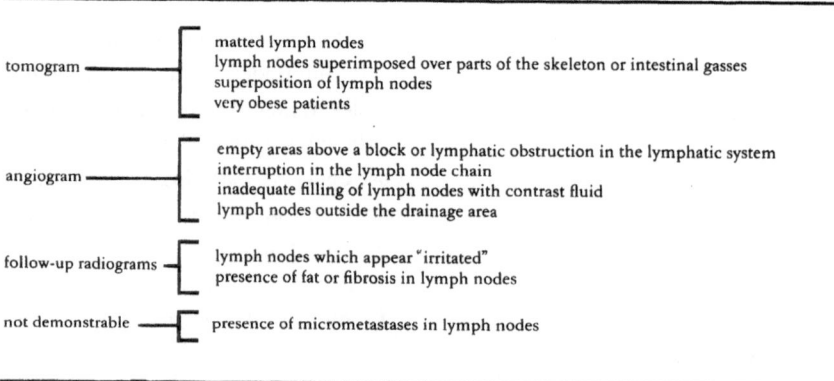

diograms are generally sufficient to pinpoint eventual localizations. Frequently however the clinical diagnosis is not definite although a malignant reticulosis is suspected. When pathological lymph nodes are found in such cases, it is essential to establish the correct diagnosis with reasonable certainty; selective supplementary examination methods are then usually indispensible. Examination for the presence of metastatic carcinoma is much more difficult; the lymph nodes are not necessarily enlarged and the metastases can be restricted macroscopically to one lymph node. Here it is important to determine as accurately as possible whether metastases are present as well as the extent of metastasizing – not only for the choice of therapy but also to prevent an unnecessary procedure. It goes without saying that selective supplementary examinations are essential in these cases. Furthermore it is not difficult to recognize large pathological lymph nodes but it is certainly not as easy to establish the correct diagnosis in doubtful cases or to declare a lymphogram normal. Of course a lymphographic examination is not presumed to be the equivalent of a pathological-anatomical examination since lymphography is not a microdiagnostic procedure. However the value of an examination depends directly upon whether faulty diagnoses remain within acceptable limits. In practice it has become clear that this is only possible if these selective supplementary methods of examination are used at the right time.

58

Complications

Only minor complications can develop after a lymphographic examination
with oily contrast fluid. The most common complication – one in three cases –
is fever, which generally does not last longer than several hours but can sometimes persist for a few days. Although the iodized oil flows through the thoracic
duct into the venous blood after lymphographic examination, serious phenomena due to oil emboli are rare. A light form, whereby fine stipples are seen in
the lung on the chest film, is not unusual; it persists one to three days although
the patient remains asymptomatic (fig. 373). The pulmonary capillaries can in
fact become blocked, but this obstruction is temporary and as a result, the sup-
ply and the breakdown of oil remain in equilibrium. It is obvious that such phenomena can be avoided to a large extent by restricting the amount of contrast
fluid injected. Another possibility is the accumulation of lipiodol in the lung
which is visible on the chest film as clearly defined, spherical opacities; this may
lead to the suspicion of pulmonary metastases (figs. 374-379). For this reason, it
is necessary to make a chest film at the end of the lymphographic examination
for comparison with one taken before lymphography.
Lymphatico-venous anastomoses can occur, not only in the event of an obstruction in the lymphatic system but also in older patients with a degenerative abnormality of the vessels as well as those known to have congenital anomalies
(figs. 380, 381). When such a lymphatico-venous anastomosis is found, the
examination should of course be discontinued to prevent the transport of too
much oily contrast medium to the lungs too quickly. If the contrast fluid is injected too rapidly, the lymph vessels or nodes may rupture which causes drainage impairment and therefore diagnostic problems (figs. 382-385).
Local complications may be wound infections, rarely lymphatic fistulas and
slow wound healing; the latter is seen mainly in patients with lymphoedema.
Although rare, a hypersensitivity reaction can develop after the injection of blue
dye; it is characterized by the spread of the dye over the entire body and blue,
swollen eyelids. These phenomena disappear after treatment with phenergan
and the lymphatic examination can then be continued.
Complications are more frequent when lymphography is carried out in the upper extremities after mamma amputation and excision of the axillary and subclavicular lymph nodes (figs. 386, 387). Fever, wound infections, a painful and
swollen arm, erysipelas-like infections, lymphoedema and ruptured vessels occur regularly. If there are no complications, there is good lymphatic drainage
via the collateral lymphatic channels in the axilla. It is also quite likely that not
only the lymphatic obstruction but in addition, the much smaller calibre of the
lymphatics in the arms is an important factor in the development of these complications – which are rare in the leg.
The only real contra-indication for the execution of a lymphographic examination is when the patient is in very poor general health.

Photographs

fig. 48 Visualization of lymph vessels after injection of dye.

fig. 49 Exposing the lymph vessel.

fig. 50 Clamp placed on proximal side of lymph vessel.

fig. 51 The small metal plate, attached to one of the tips of the forceps, has been slipped under the dilated lymph vessel. The vessel is then fixed by closing the forceps.

fig. 52 The needle is held between the thumb and the index finger. The third finger pushes the stylet into the vessel.

fig. 53 Puncture of the vessel. The point of the stylet protrudes from the needle.

fig. 54 After the lymph vessel has been punctured, the third finger releases the stylet, the spring is relaxed and the stylet shoots back.

fig. 55 When the stylet has retracted, the blunt hollow needle is pushed farther into the lymph vessel.

fig. 56 The clamp is removed and placed around the needle and the vessel. Finally it is secured with adhesive tape.

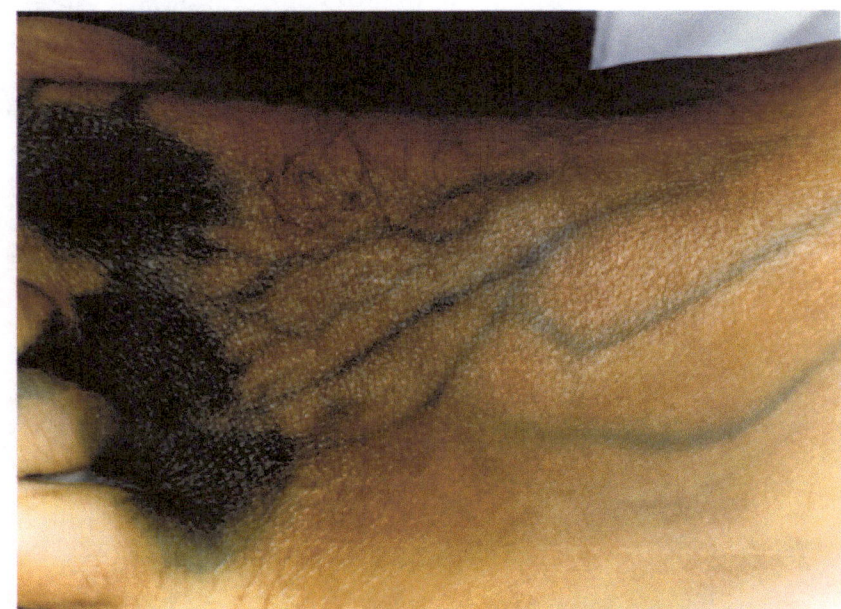

48

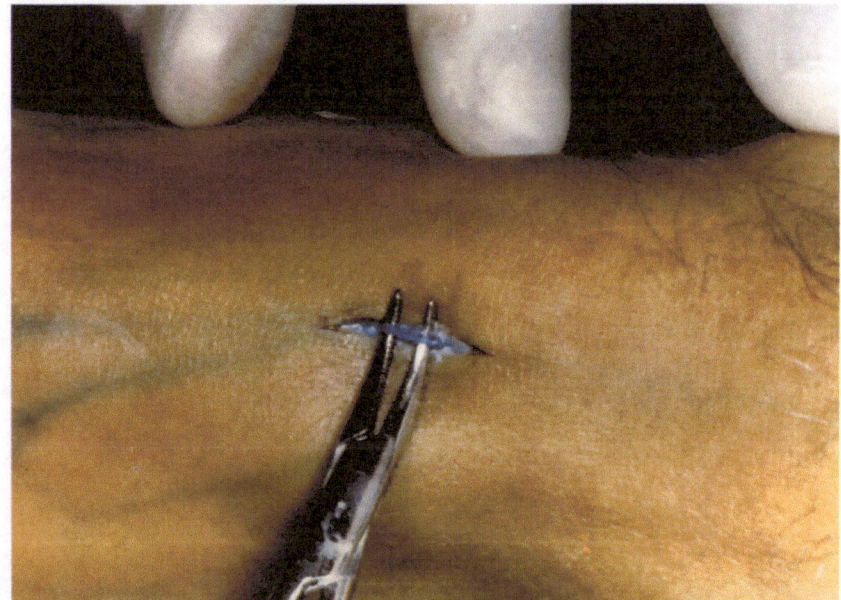

49

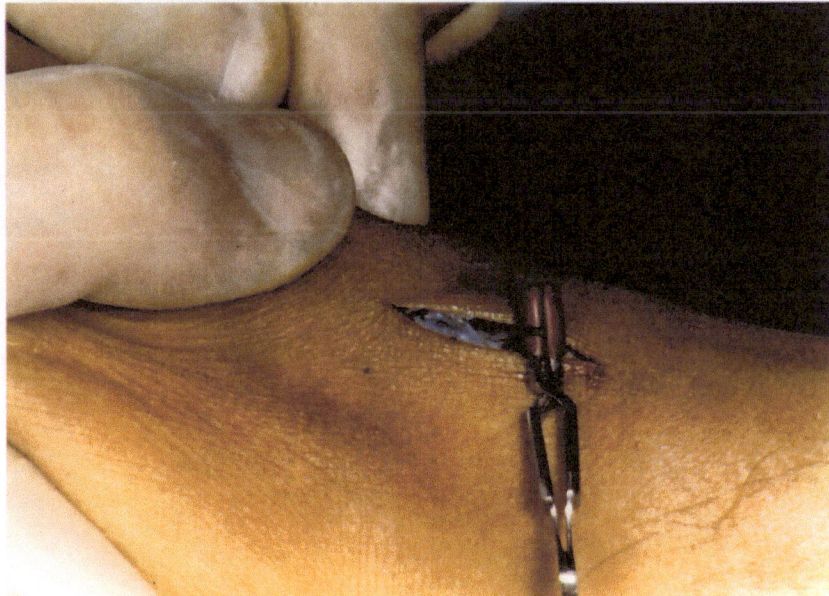

50

62

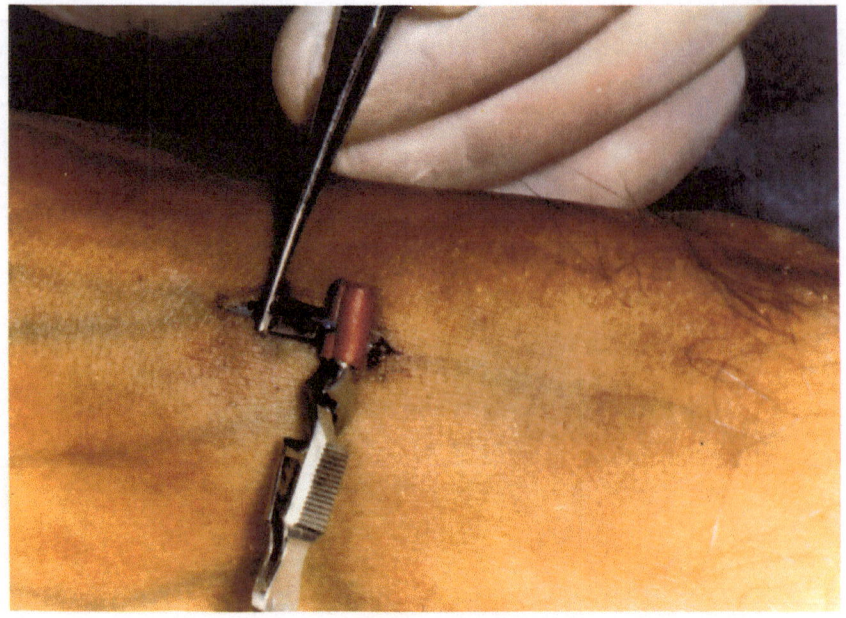

51

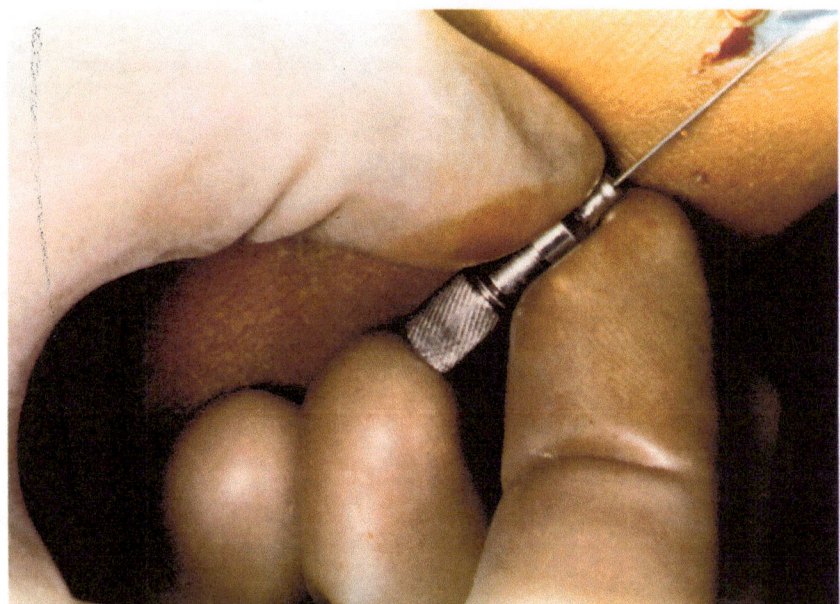

52

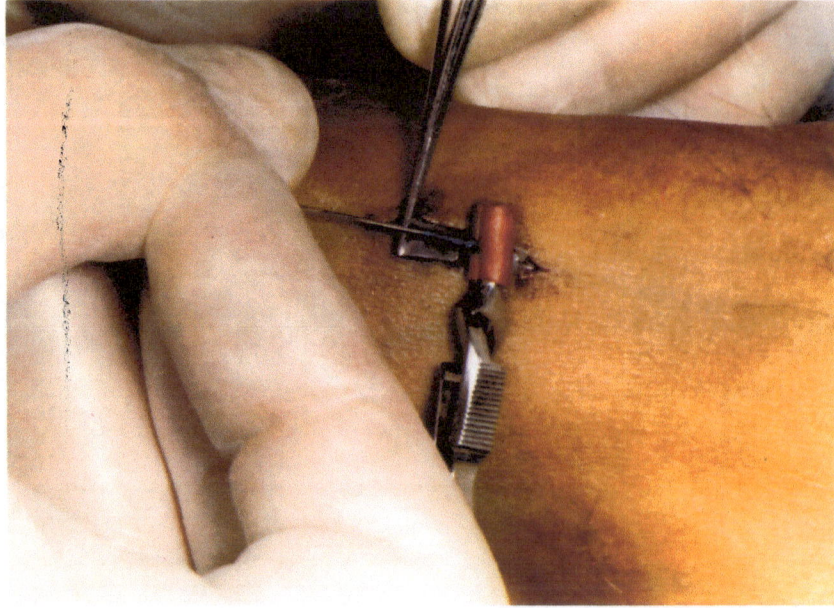

53

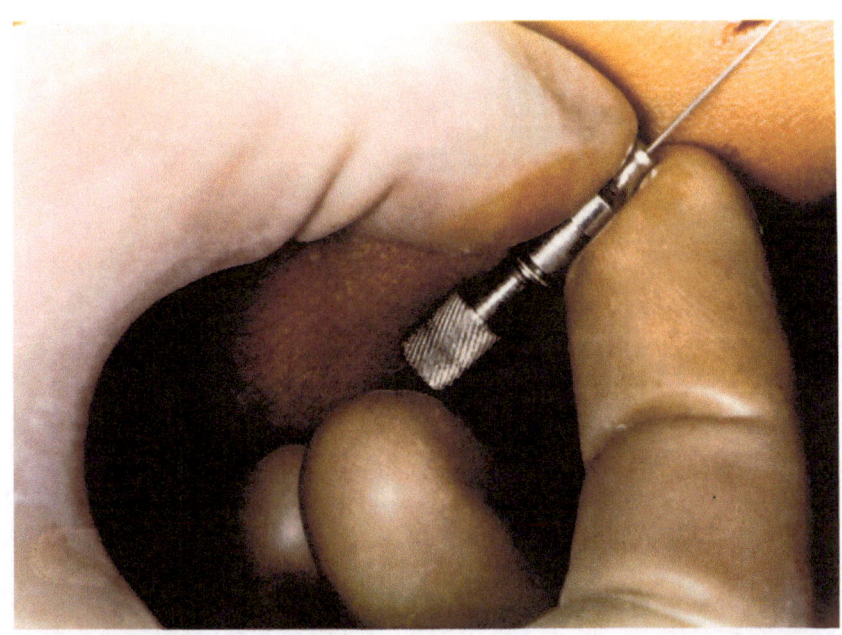

54

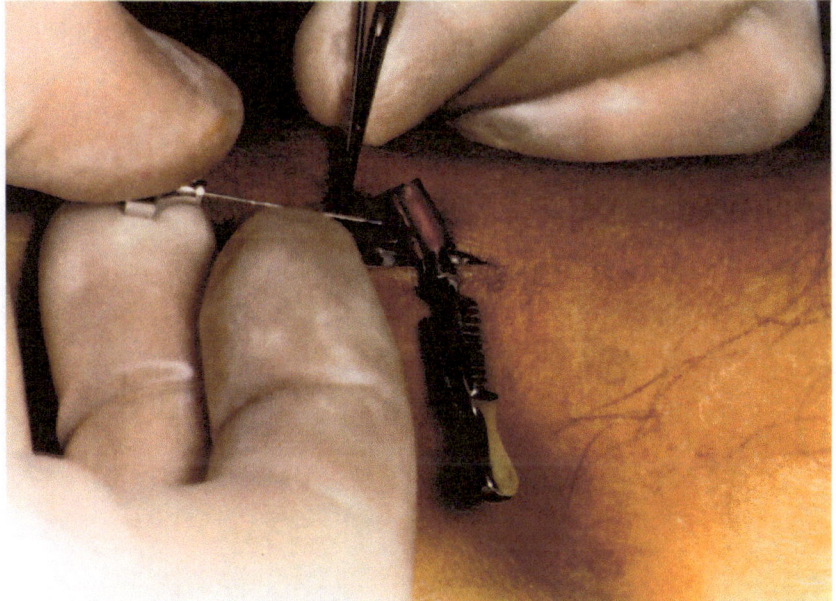

55

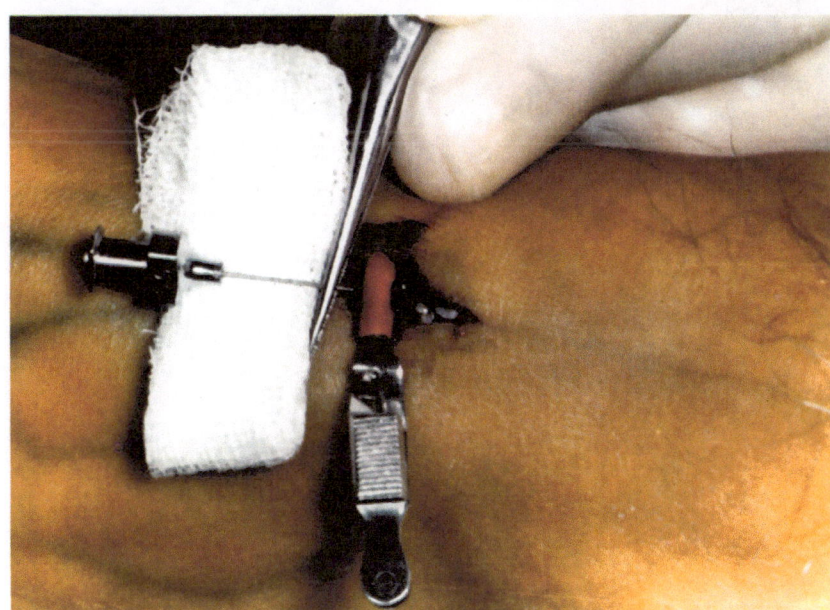

56

fig. 57 Puncture of a lymph vessel of the anterior superficial system on the dorsum of the foot.

fig. 58 Puncture of a lymph vessel of the posterior superficial system below the ankle.

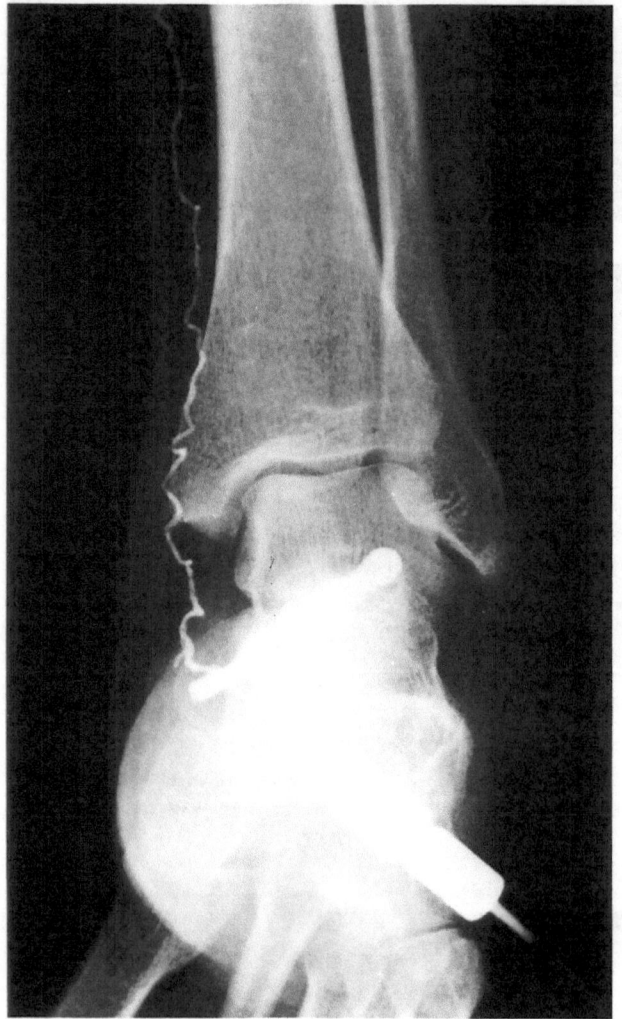

57

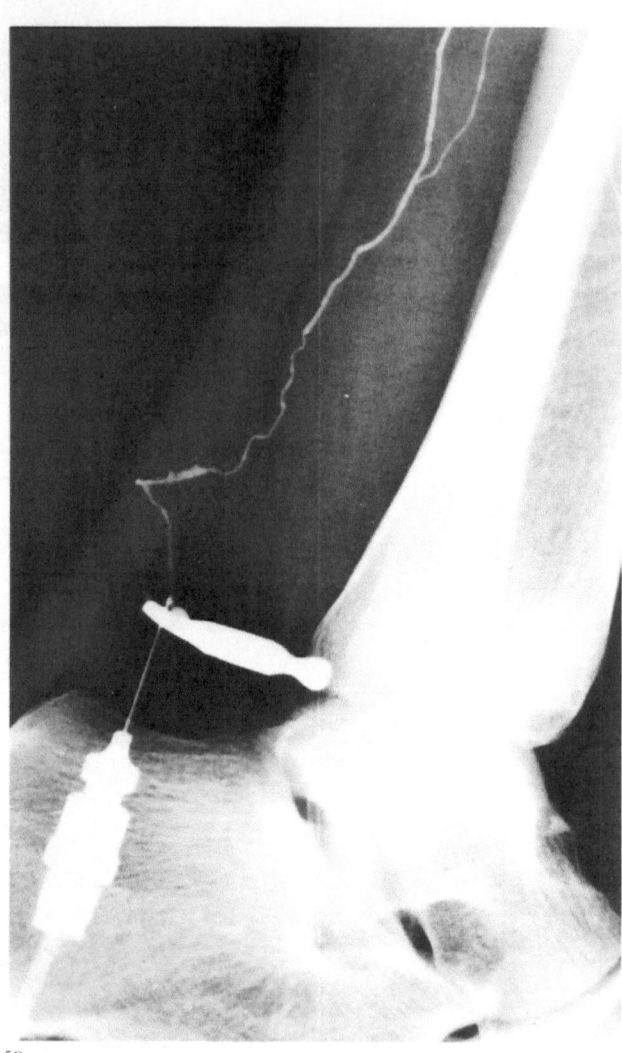

58

fig. 59 Normal lymphogram of the lower leg. Only one vessel of the anterior superficial system is filled; it branches out proximal to the knee.

fig. 60 Normal lymphogram of the lower leg. The lateral channels of the anterior superficial system are filled. Halfway up the lower leg, the channels cross over to the medial side. Valves are visible as irregularly spaced, spherical opacities.

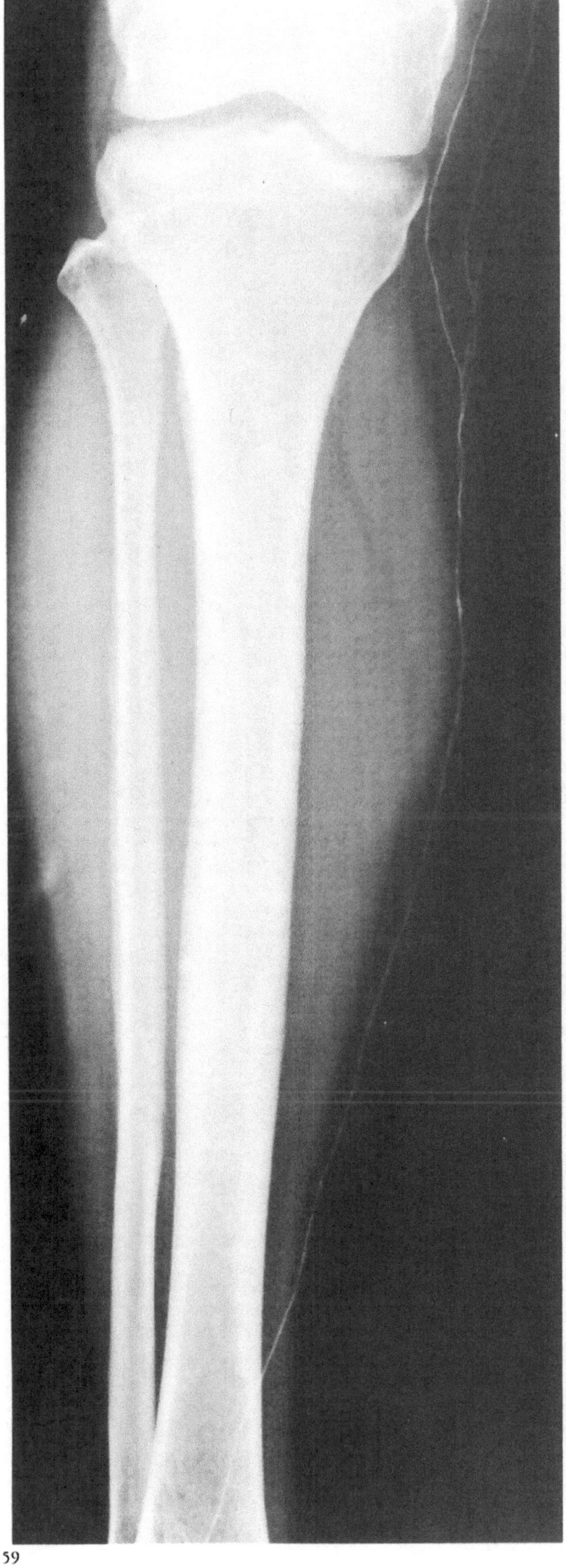

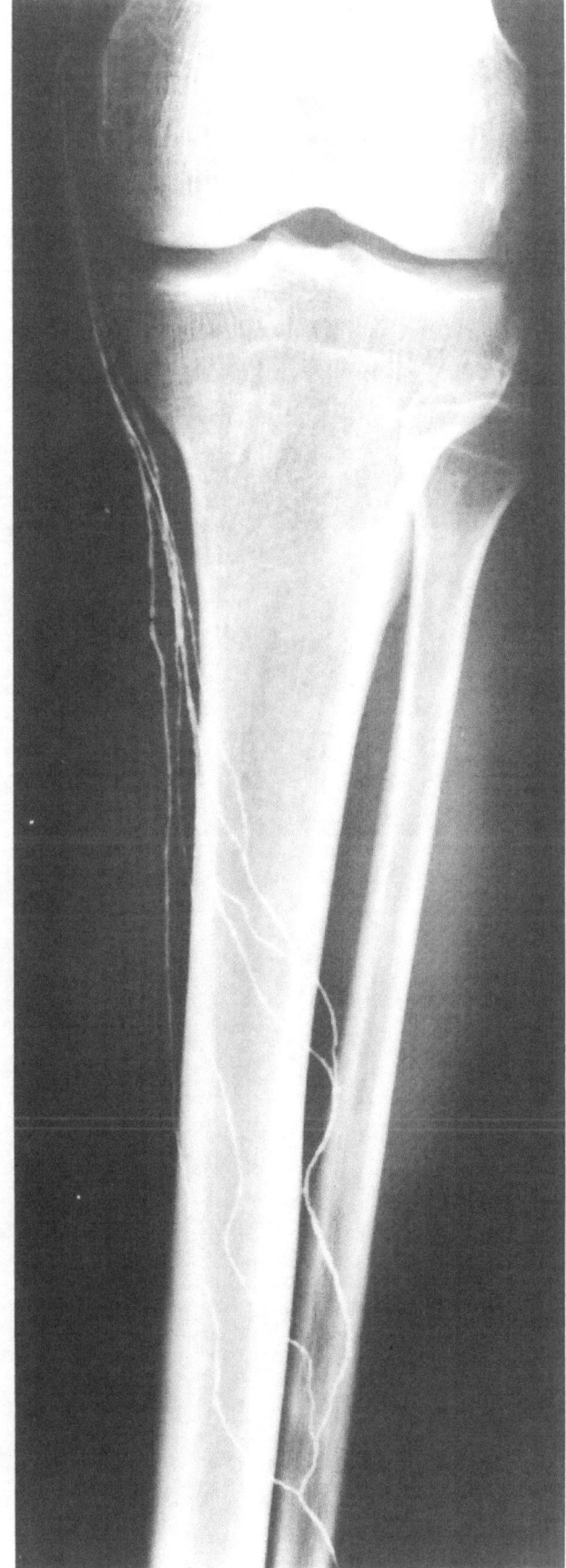

fig. 61 Normal lymphogram of the thigh. The
lymphatic channels are more numerous than in
the lower leg. The calibre remains uniform. The
lymphatic channels drain into the superficial
subinguinal lymph nodes.

fig. 62 Normal lymphogram of the thighs and
lower legs of a child. The medial channels of
the anterior superficial system are visible on
both sides.

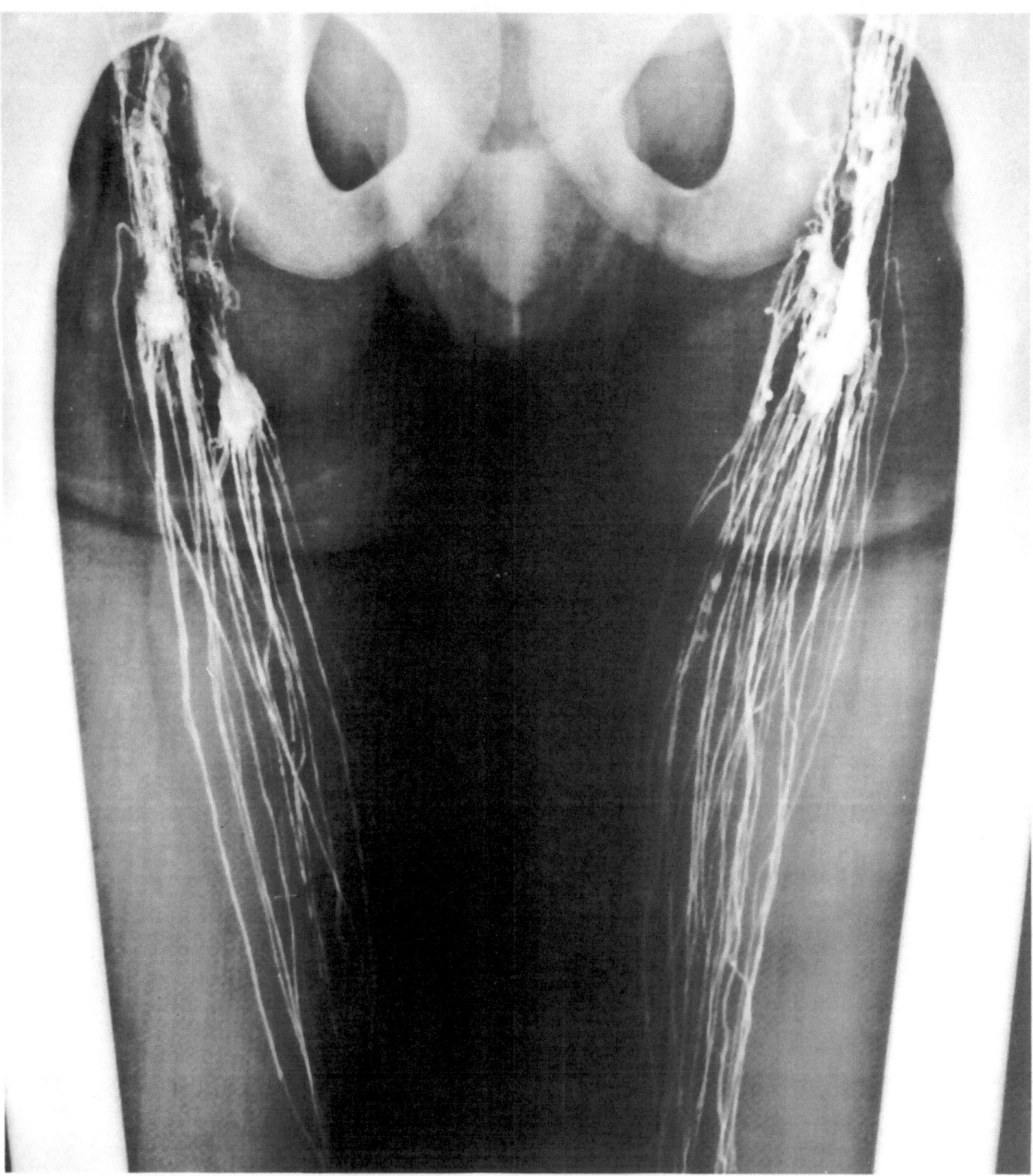

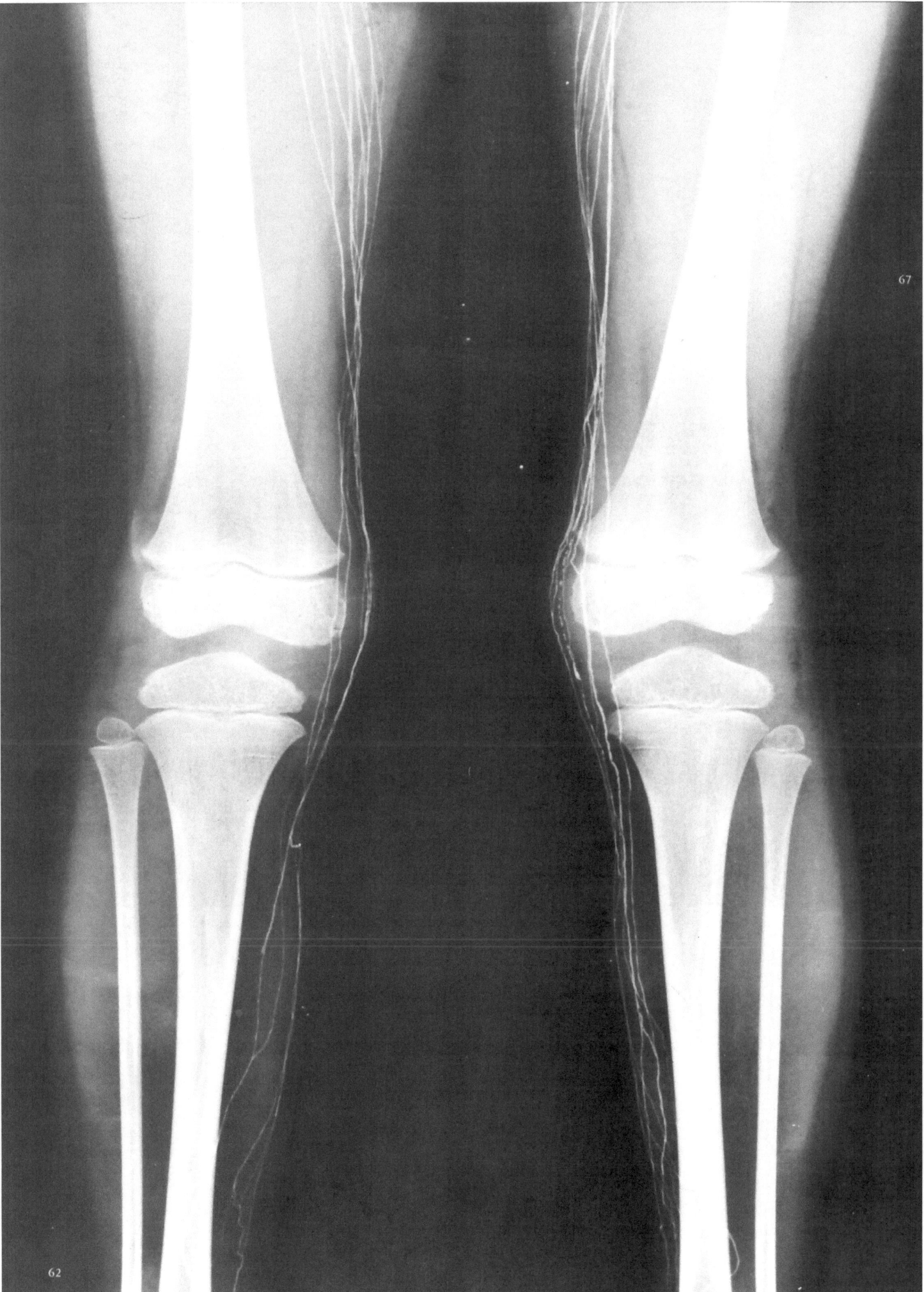

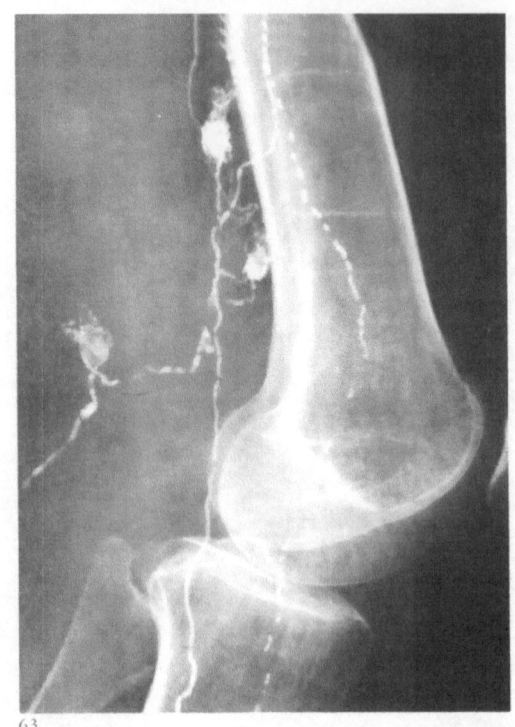

63

fig. 63 Normal lymphogram of the lymphatic channels of the posterior superficial system in the popliteal region. The channels pass through the deep and superficial popliteal lymph nodes.

fig. 64-67 Normal lymphograms of the inguinal region:
(1) superficial subinguinal lymph nodes, (2) deep subinguinal lymph nodes, (3) inferior superficial inguinal lymph nodes, and (4) superior superficial inguinal lymph nodes.

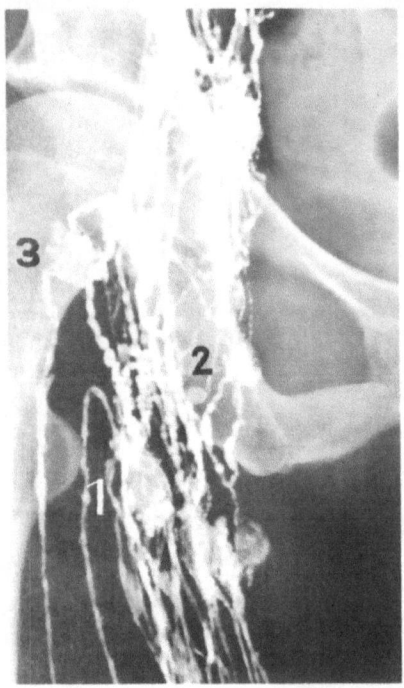

64

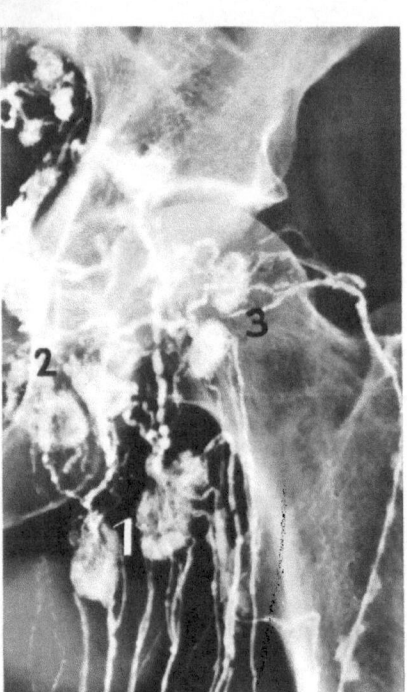

65

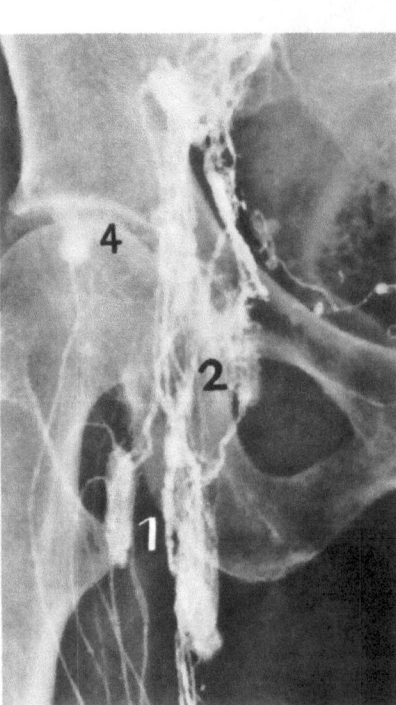

66

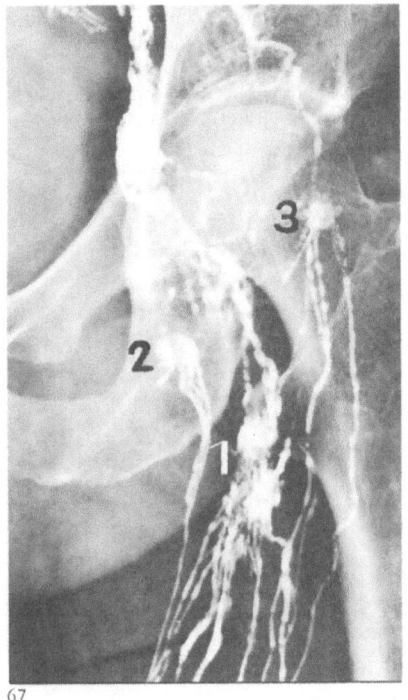

67

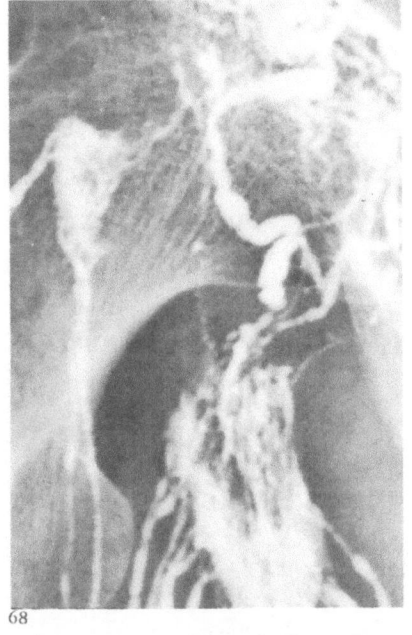

68

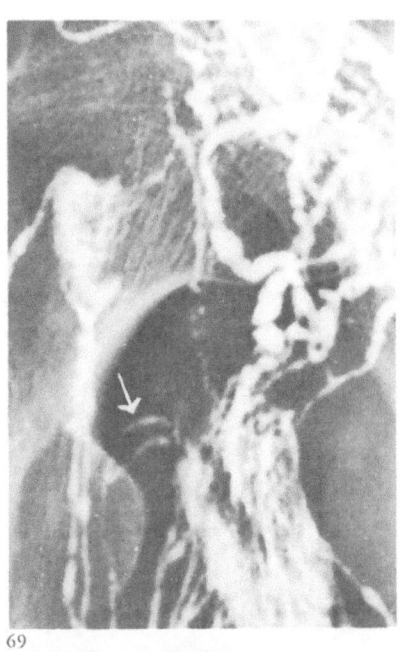

69

fig. 68-73 Normal lymphograms of the inguinal region. When the anterior superficial system
is injected with contrast medium (figs. 68, 70,
72), the deep lymph nodes in the groin are not
always filled. After subsequent filling of the posterior superficial system, the same lymph nodes
may still be seen (fig. 69 →) but other deep
nodes in the groin may also become visible (fig.
71 →). Sometimes the lymphatic channels of
the posterior superficial system pass directly to
the iliac lymph nodes (fig. 73 →).

Comment: Therefore for an exact evaluation of
all of these regional lymph nodes, as in melanosarcoma of the extremities for instance, both
the anterior and posterior superficial lymphatic
systems must be filled with contrast fluid.

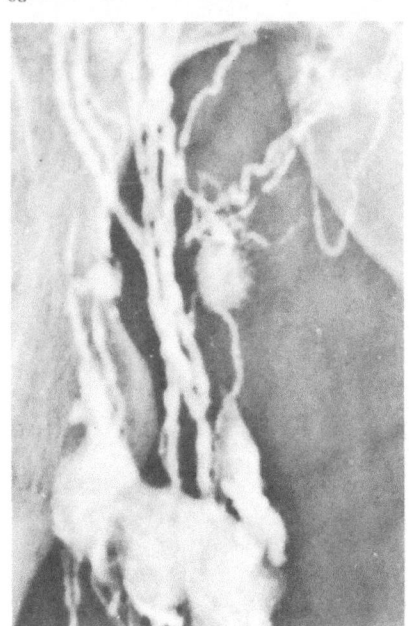

70

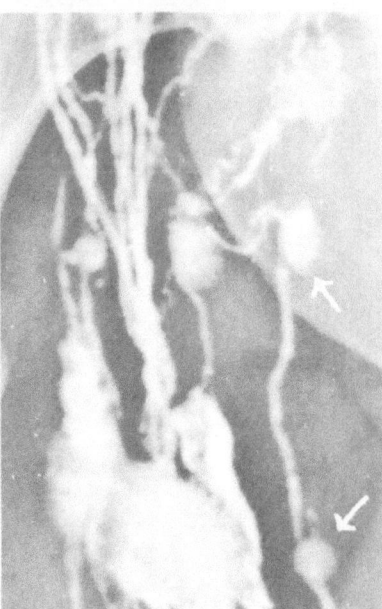

71

fig. 74 Normal lymphogram of the pelvis and abdomen. Lymphatic channels and nodes are grouped around the (1) arteria et vena iliaca externa, (2) arteria et vena iliaca communis, the (3) paralumbar region and (4) para-aortic region.

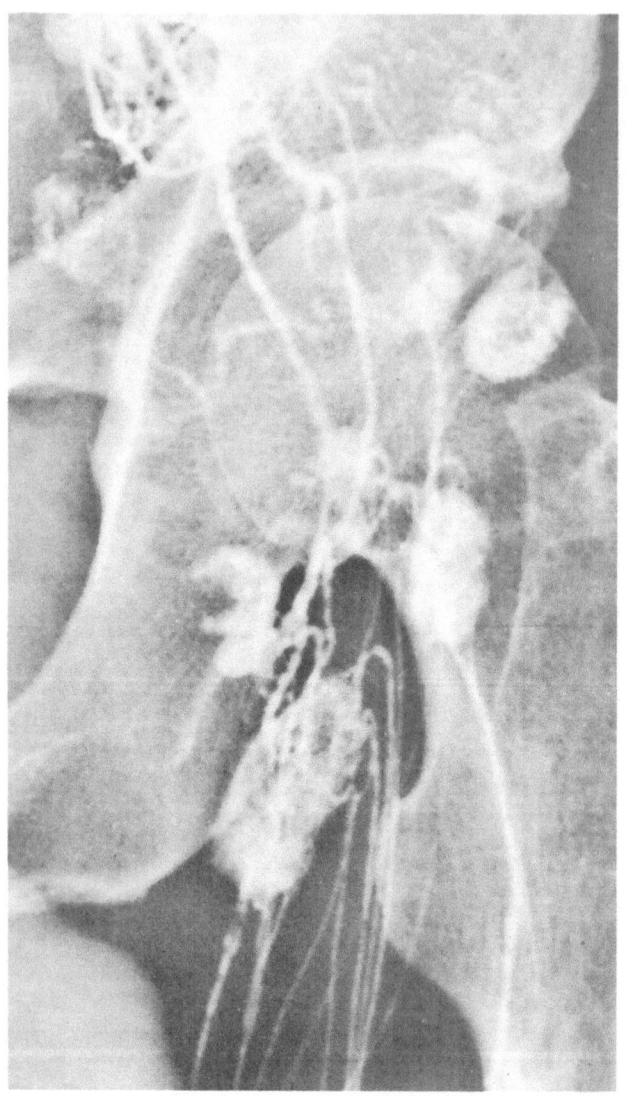

72

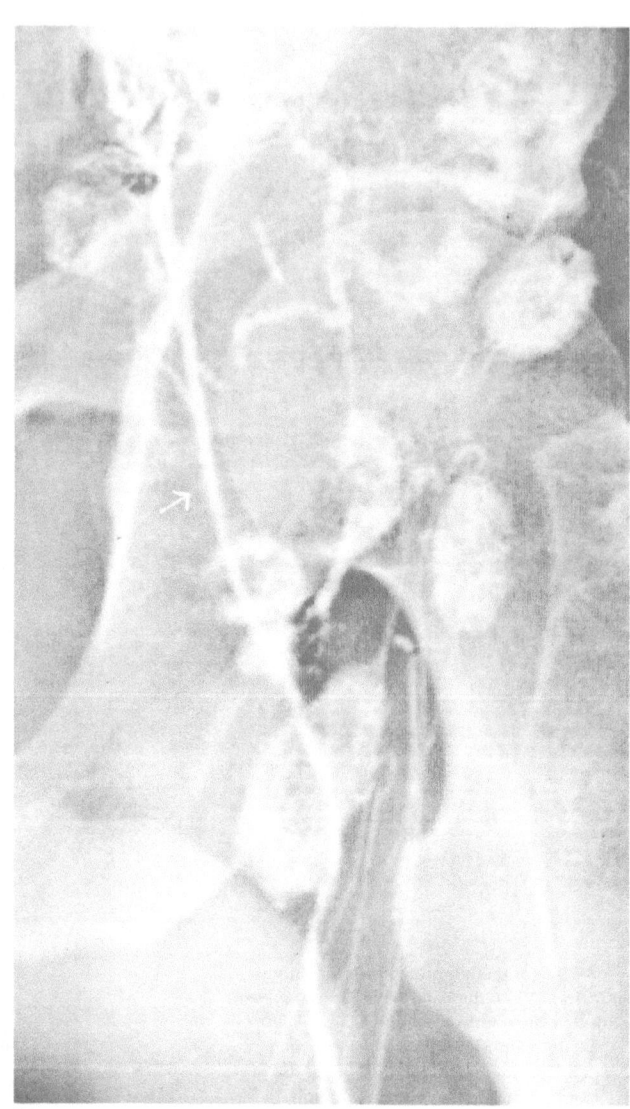

73

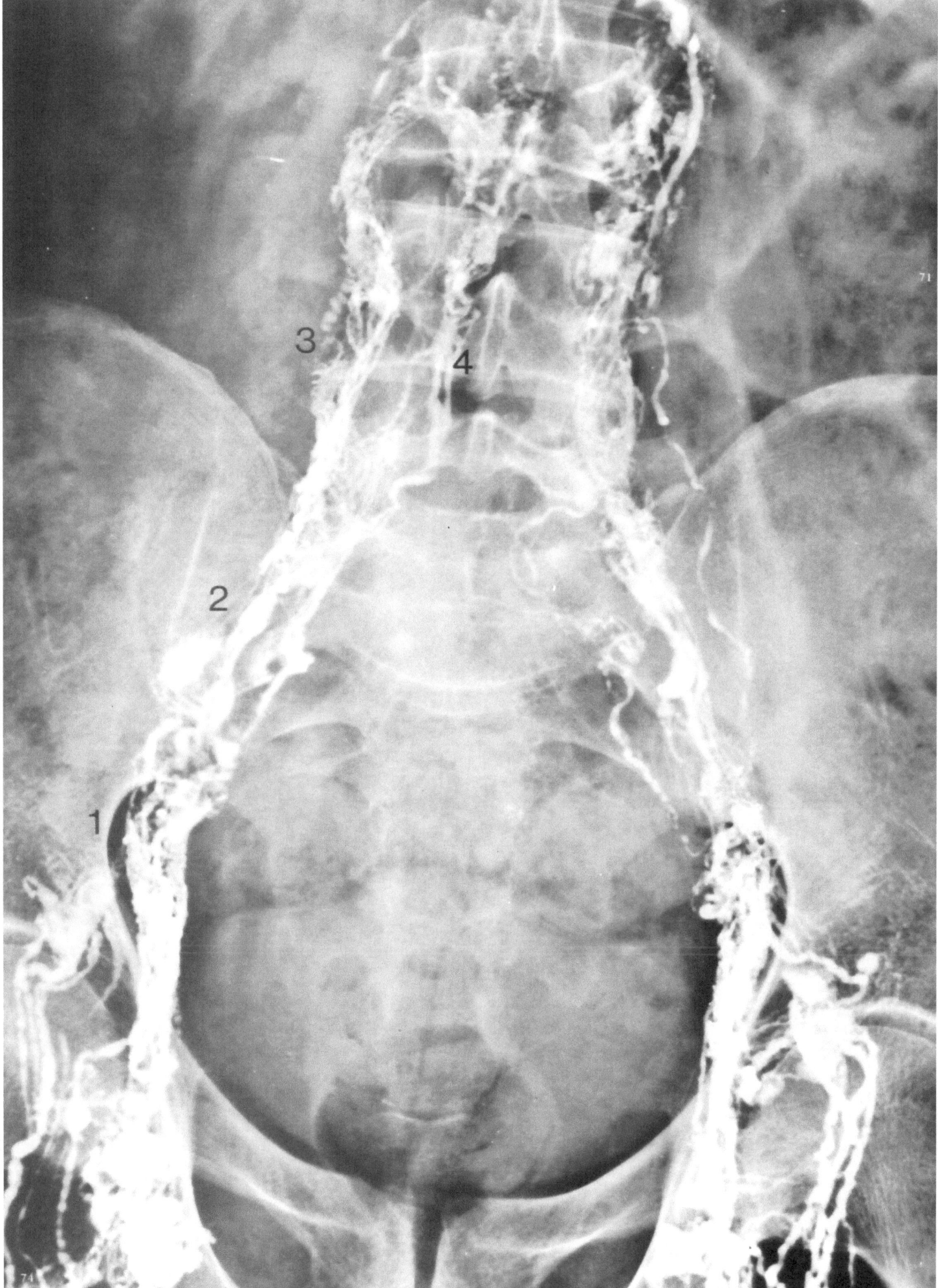

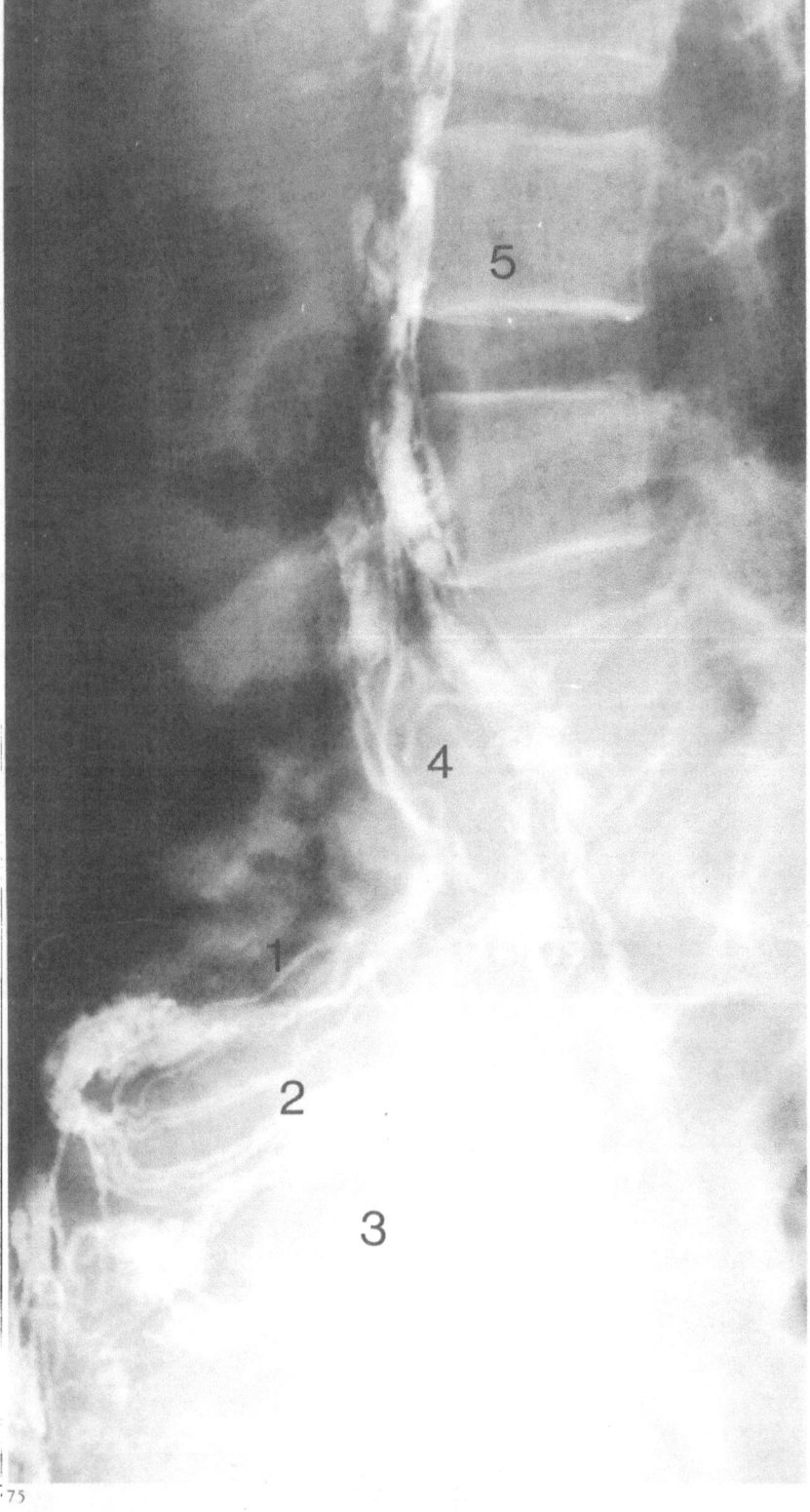

fig. 75 Normal lymphogram (lateral) of the pelvis and abdomen. Lymphatic channels and nodes around the arteria et vena iliaca externa: (1) the superficial chain, (2) the deep chain, (3) the medial chain, as well as (4) the lymphatic channels and nodes around the arteria et vena iliaca communis and (5) the paralumbar lymphatics and nodes.

fig. 76 Normal lymphogram (lateral) of the pelvis. Lymphatic channels around the arteria hypogastrica (→) are only rarely filled.

fig. 77 Normal lymphogram of right and left paralumbar lymphatic channels and nodes after unilateral filling.

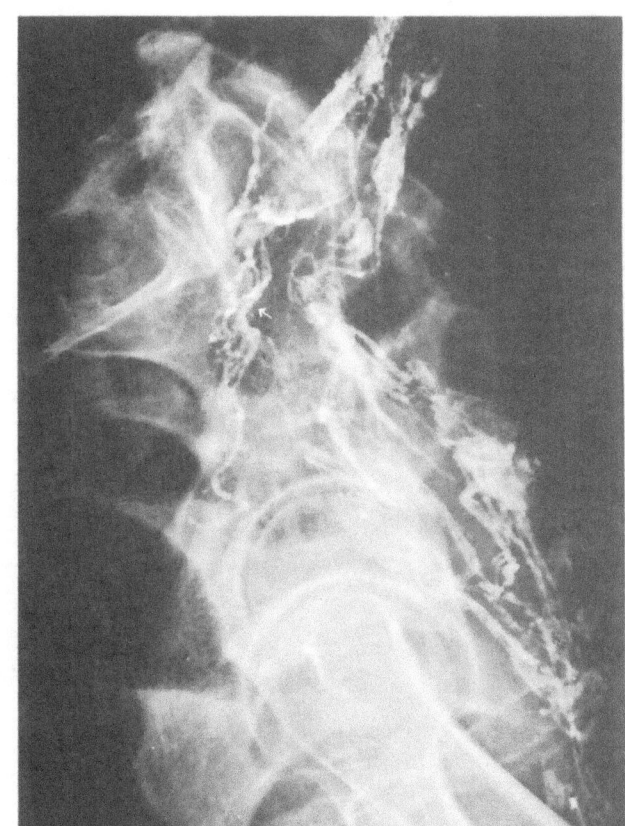

76

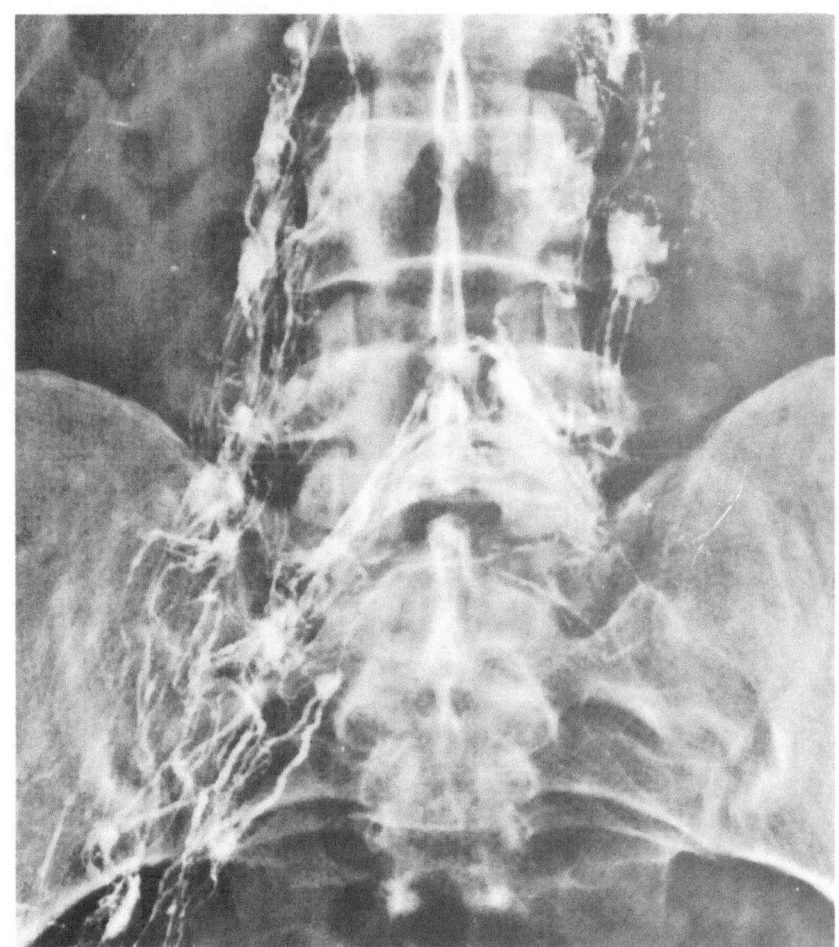

77

fig. 78 Normal lymphogram of the (1) left lumbar trunk, (2) right lumbar trunk, and (3) the intestinal trunk.

fig. 79 Normal lymphogram of the cysterna chyli (→) which becomes the thoracic duct.

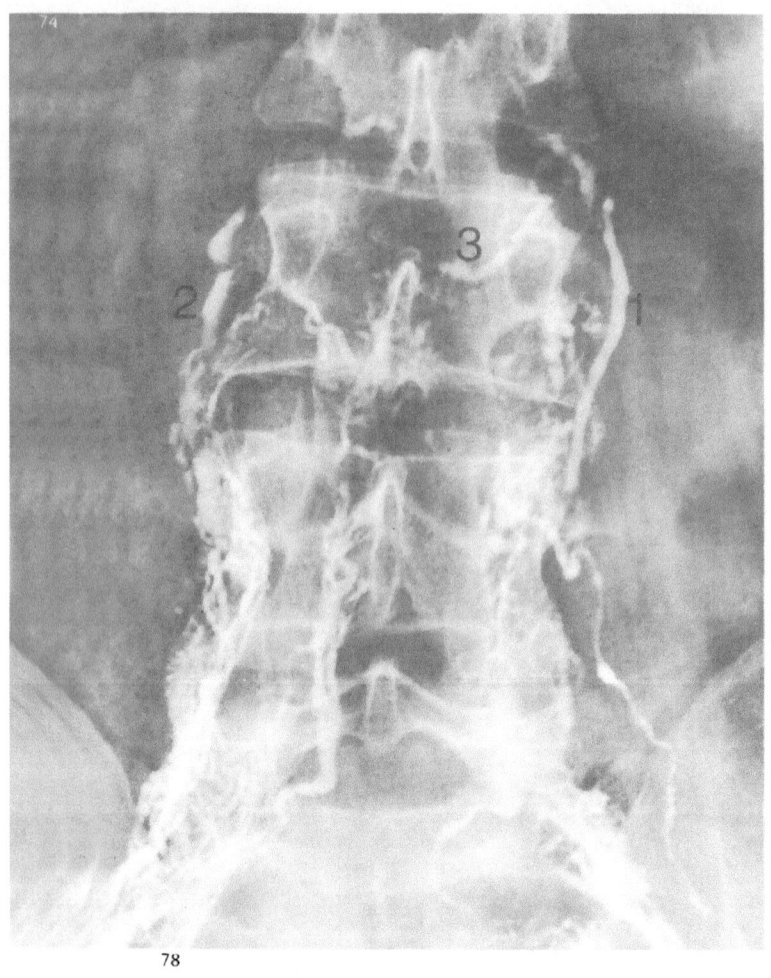

78

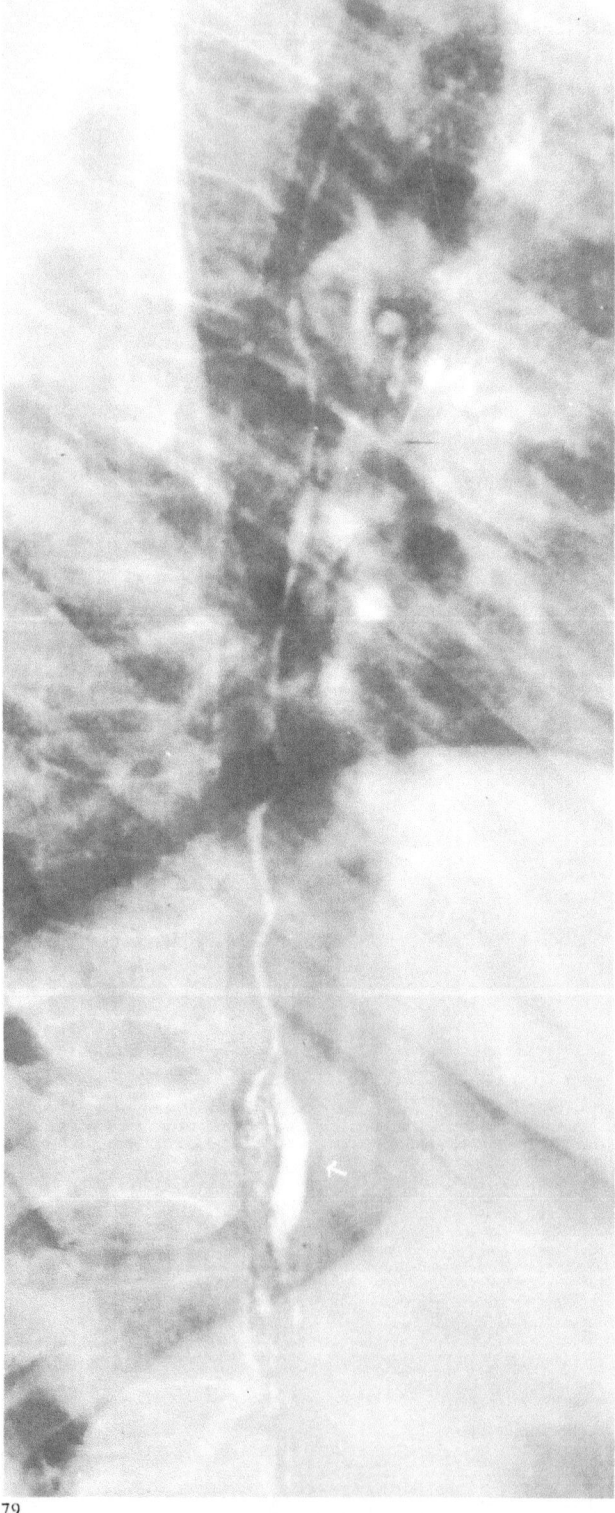

79

figs. 80-83 Normal lymphogram of the thoracic duct with left-sided single (fig. 80), left-sided multiple (fig. 81), right-sided (fig. 82) and double-barrelled (fig. 83) opening into the vena subclavia.

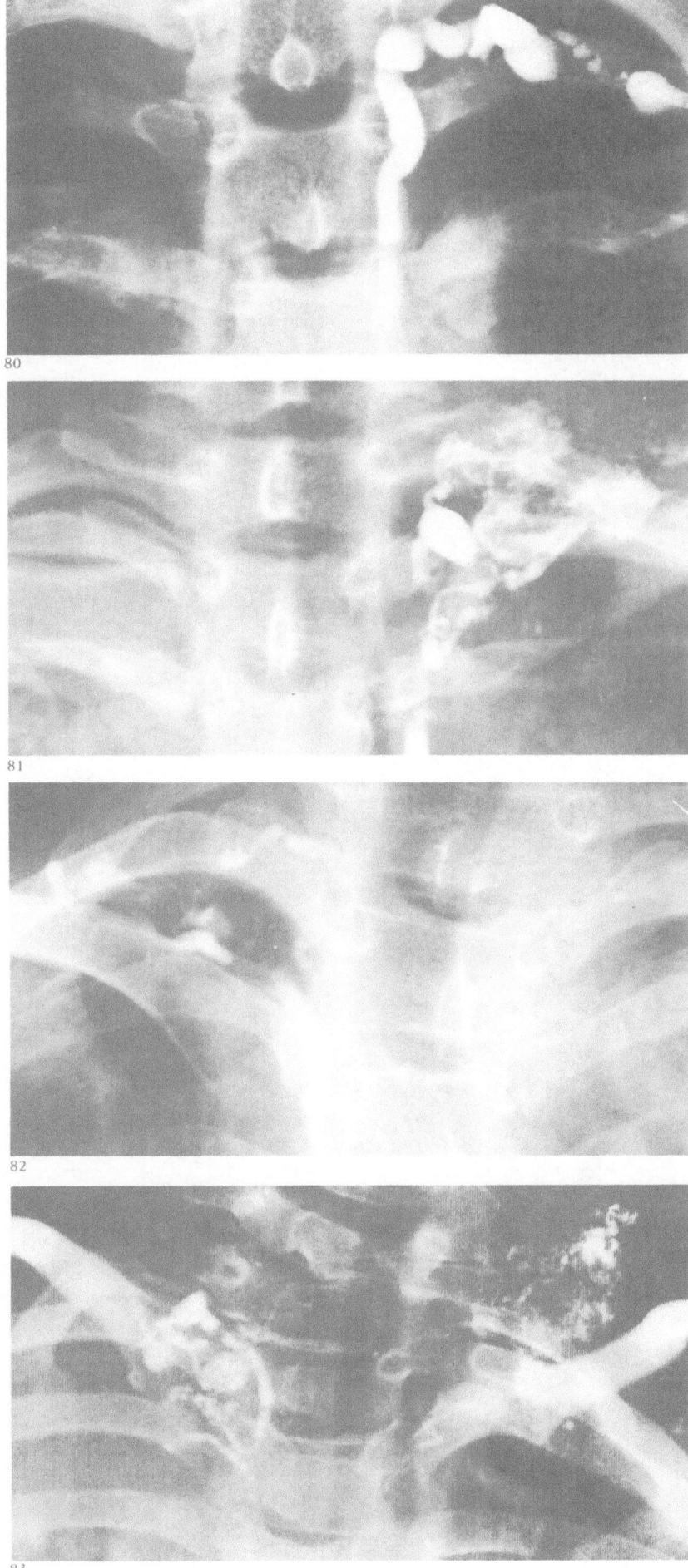

80

81

82

83

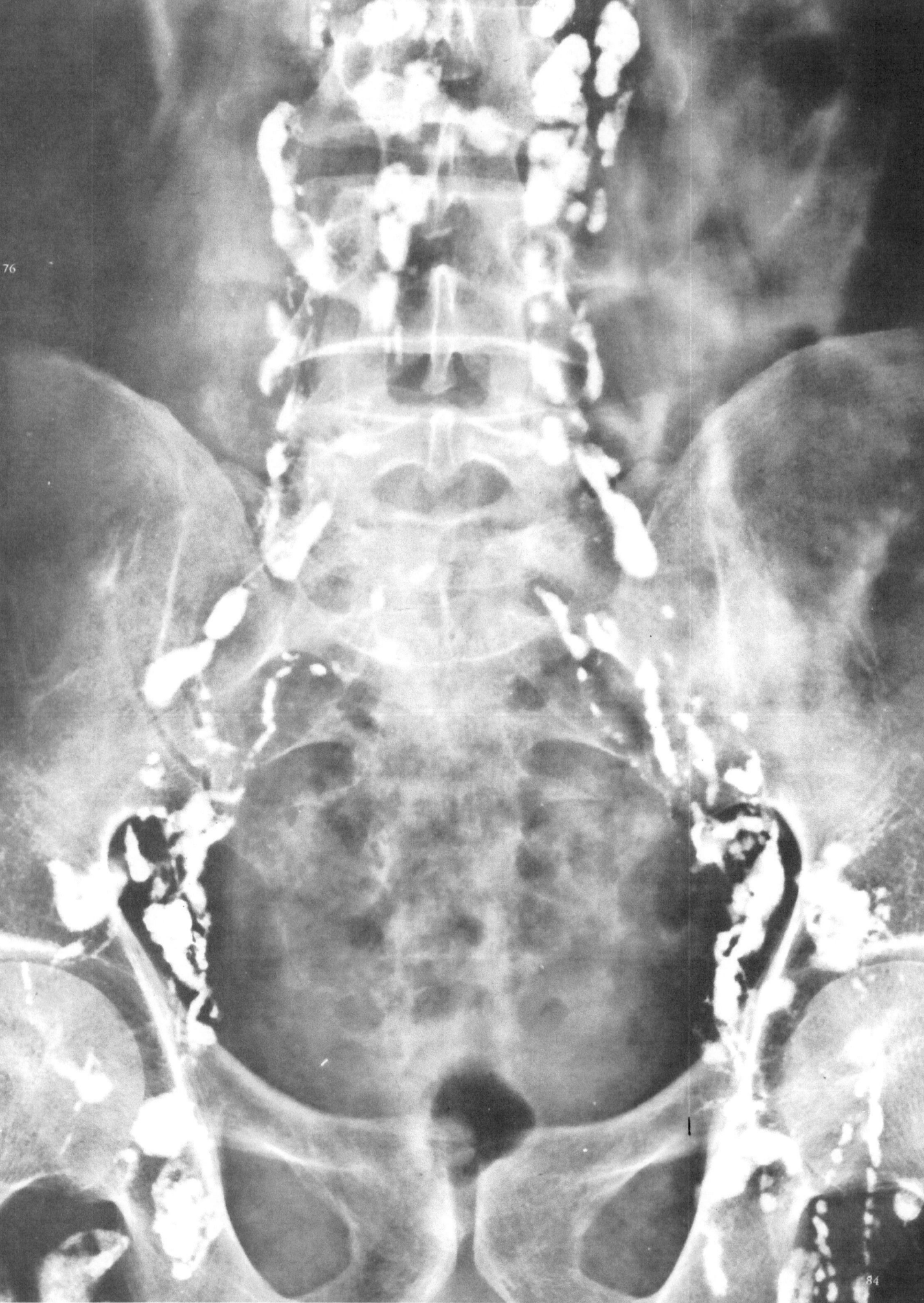

fig. 84 Normal lymphadenogram of the pelvis
and abdomen (anteroposterior).

fig. 85 Normal lymphadenogram of pelvis and
abdomen (oblique).

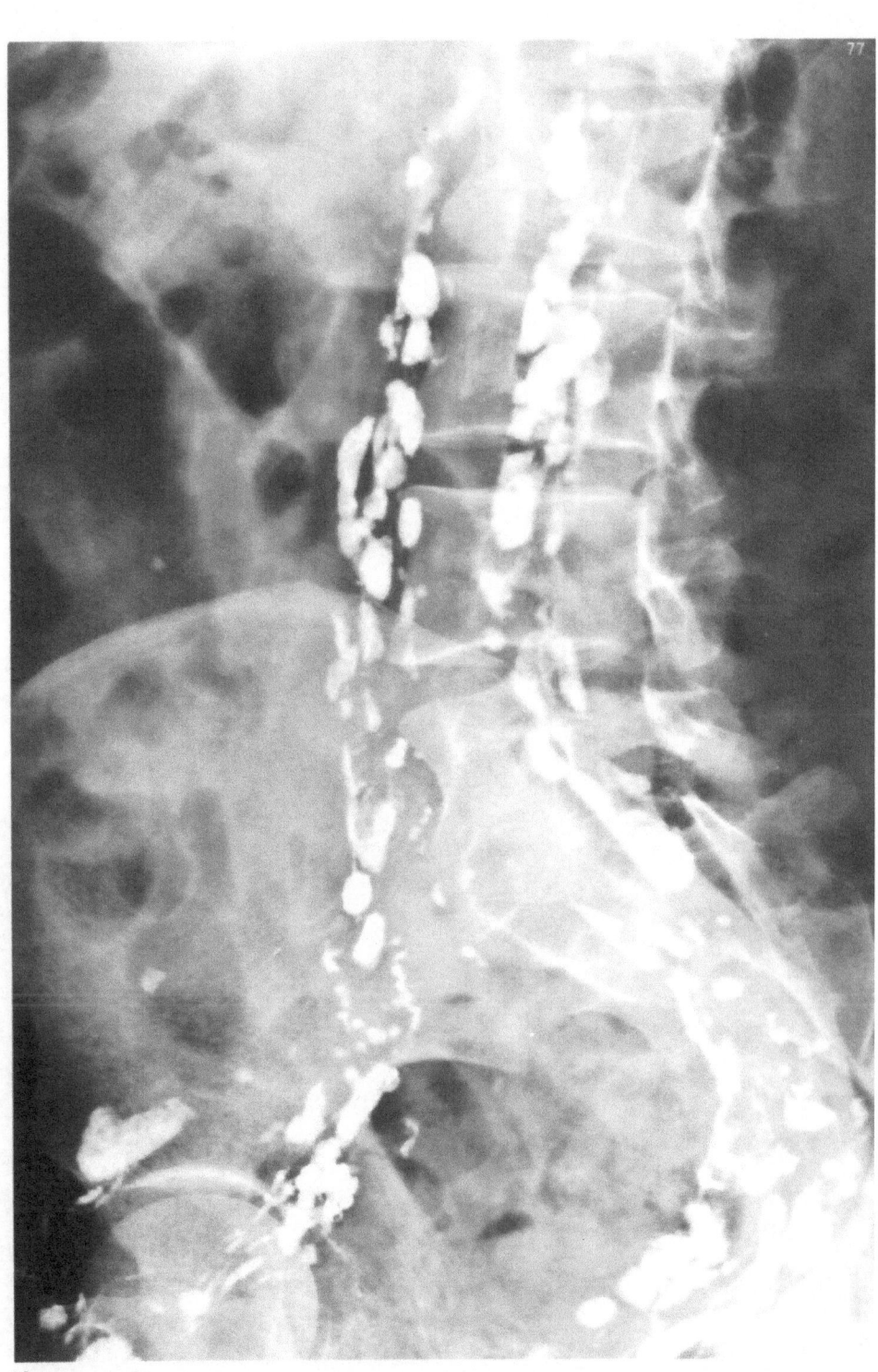

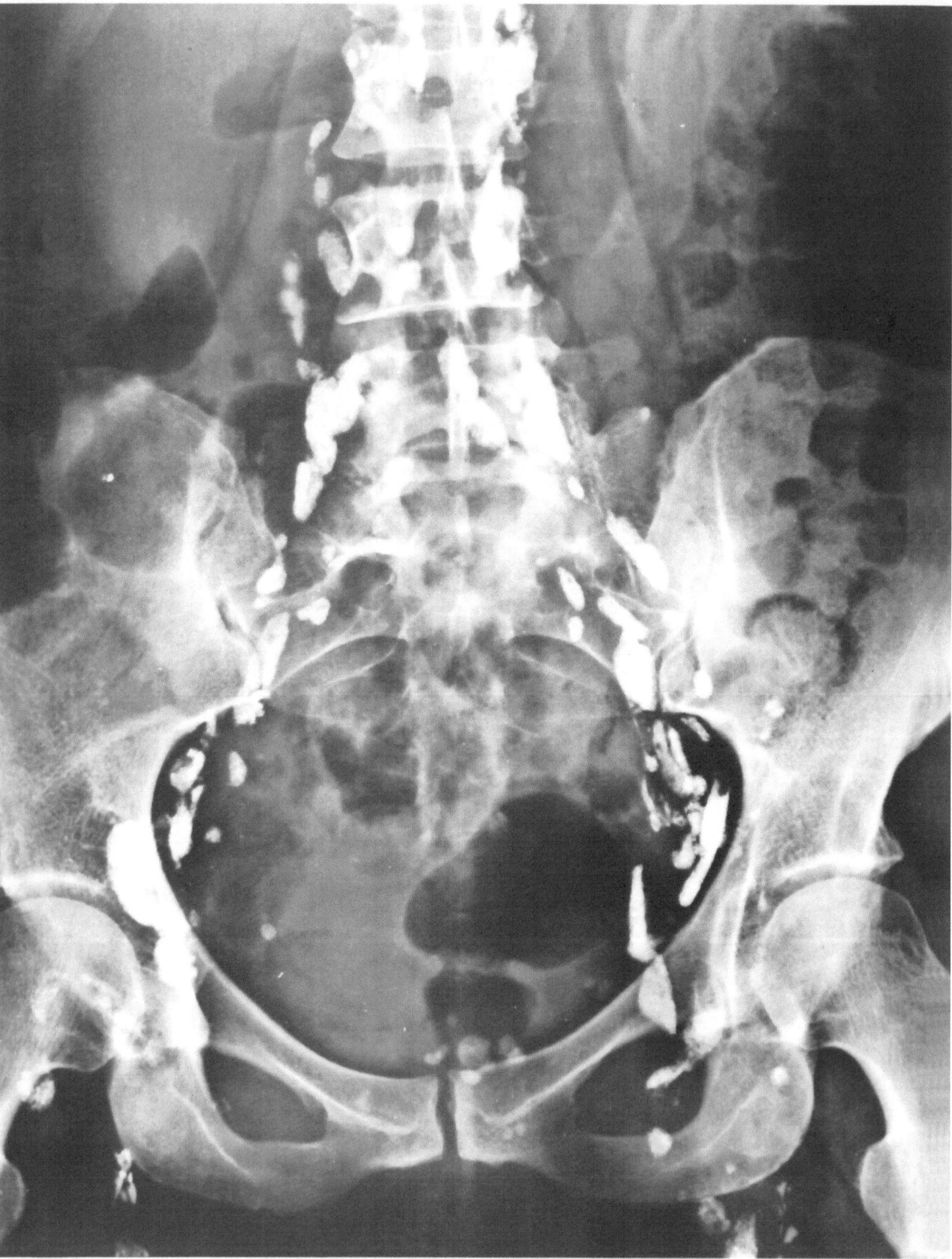

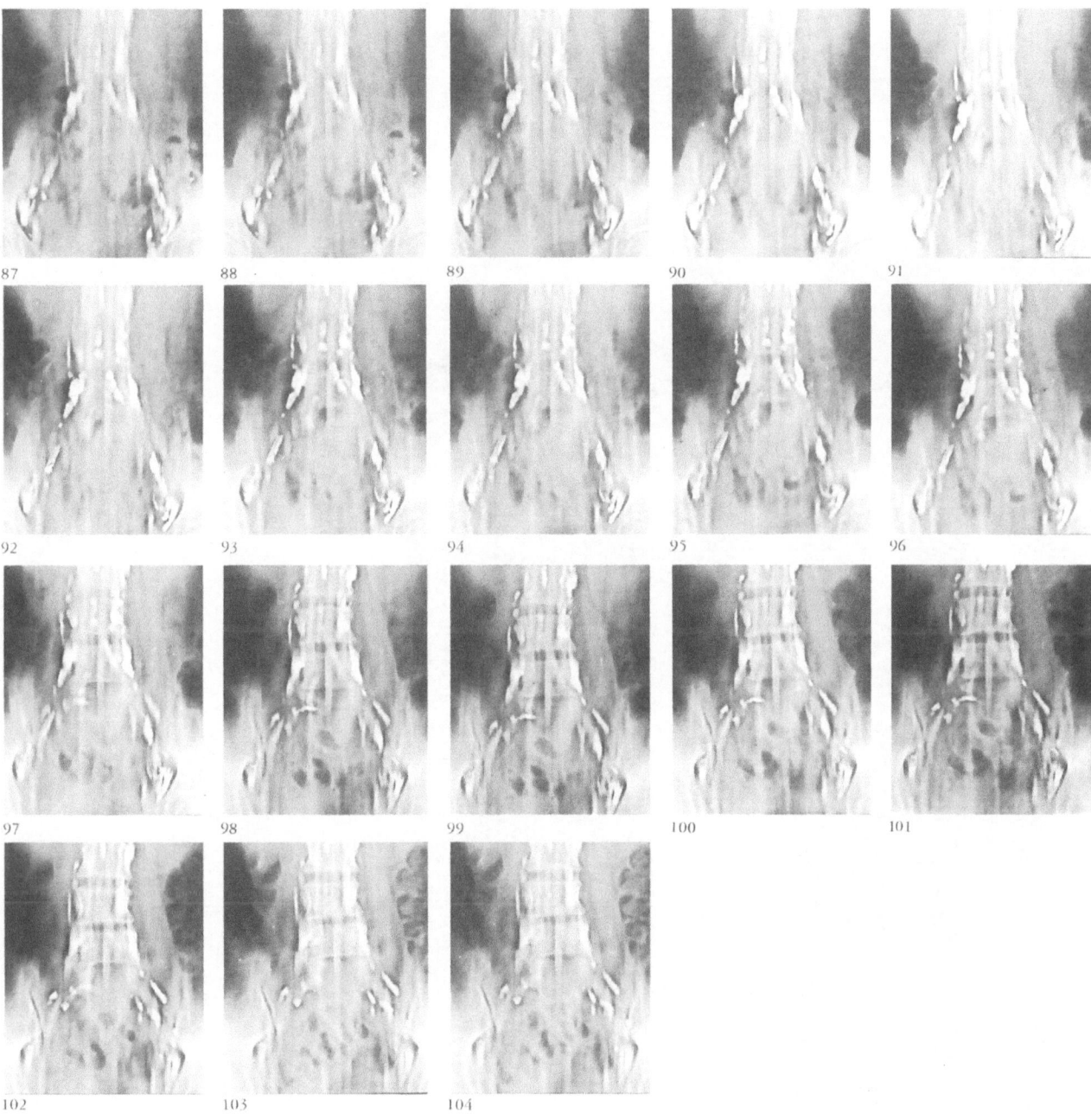

figs. 86-104 Normal lymphadenogram of the pelvis and abdomen with tomographic sections taken at ¼ cm. intervals from 6 to 10½ cm.

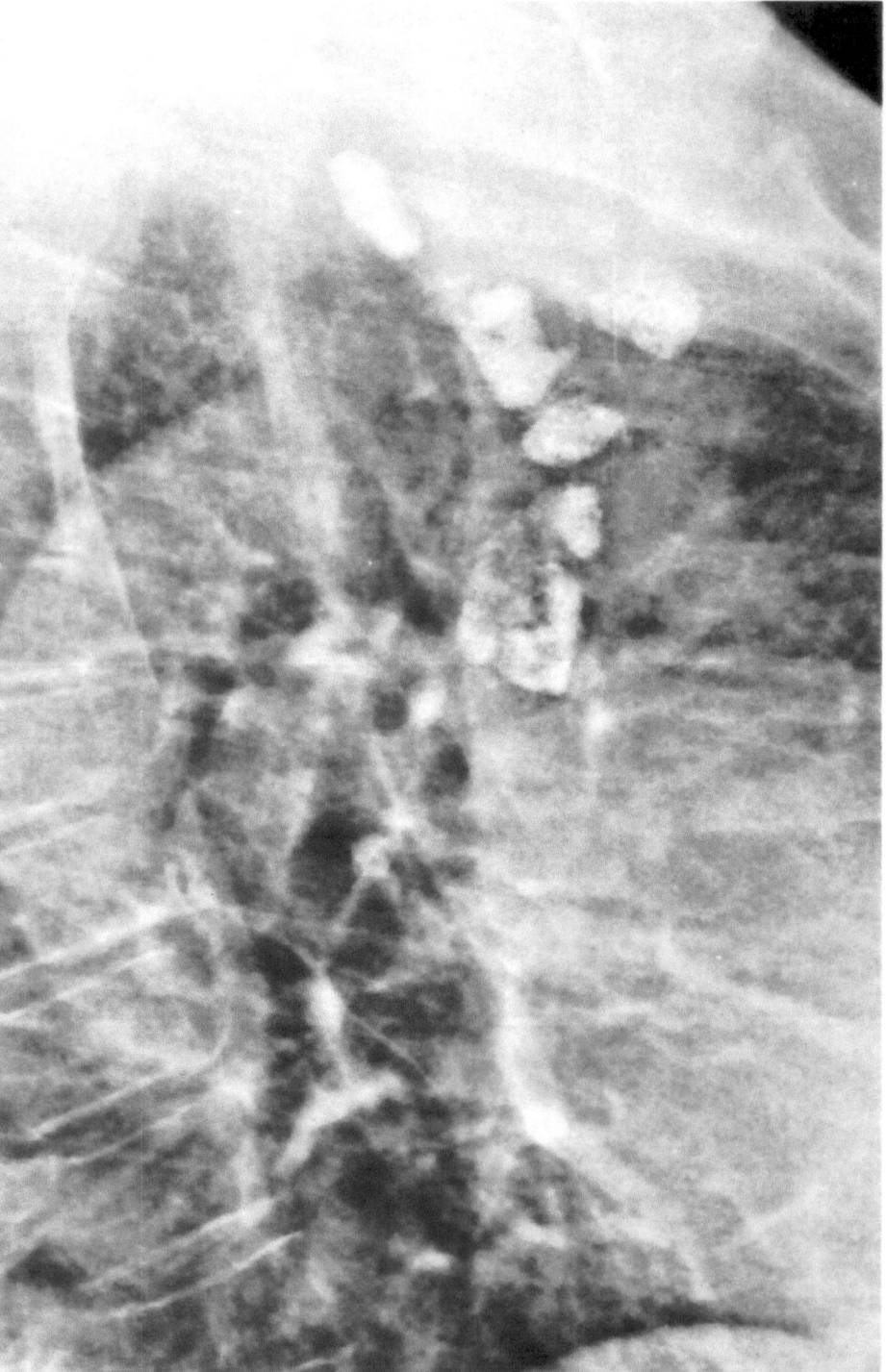

fig. 105 Normal lymphadenogram, lateral thorax exposure. Sometimes the mediastinal lymph nodes are filled via the thoracic duct.

figs. 106 and 107 Normal lymphogram of the arm. Lymphatic channels visible after injection of contrast fluid into a lymph vessel in the dorsum of the hand (fig. 106) and the volar side of the forearm (fig. 107).

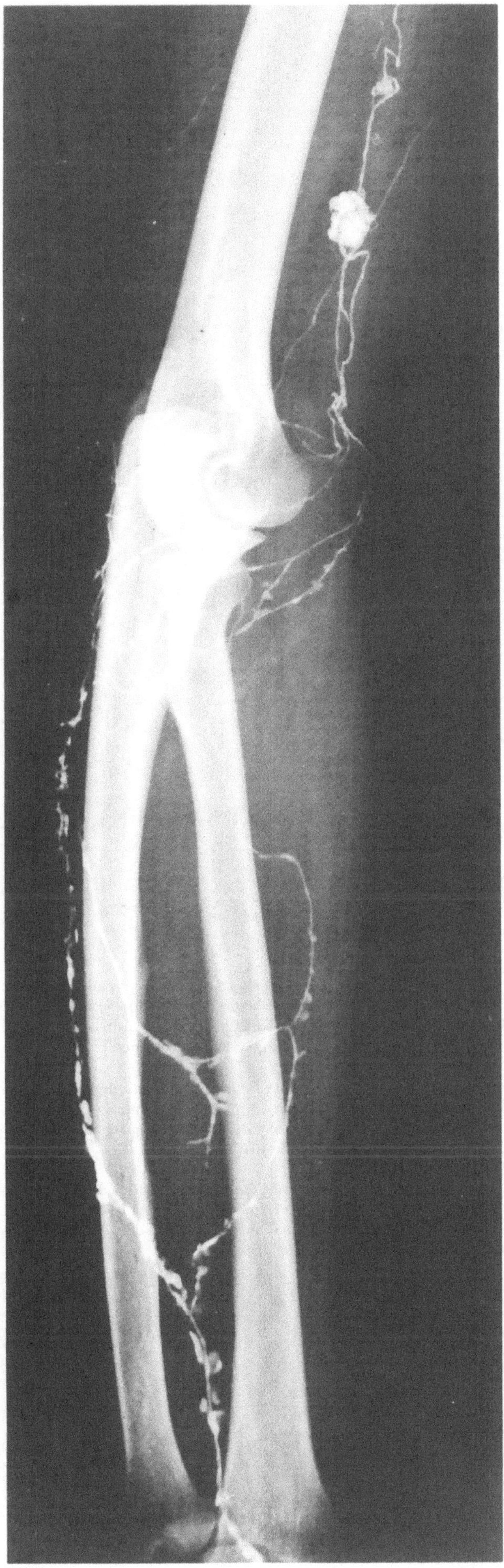

106

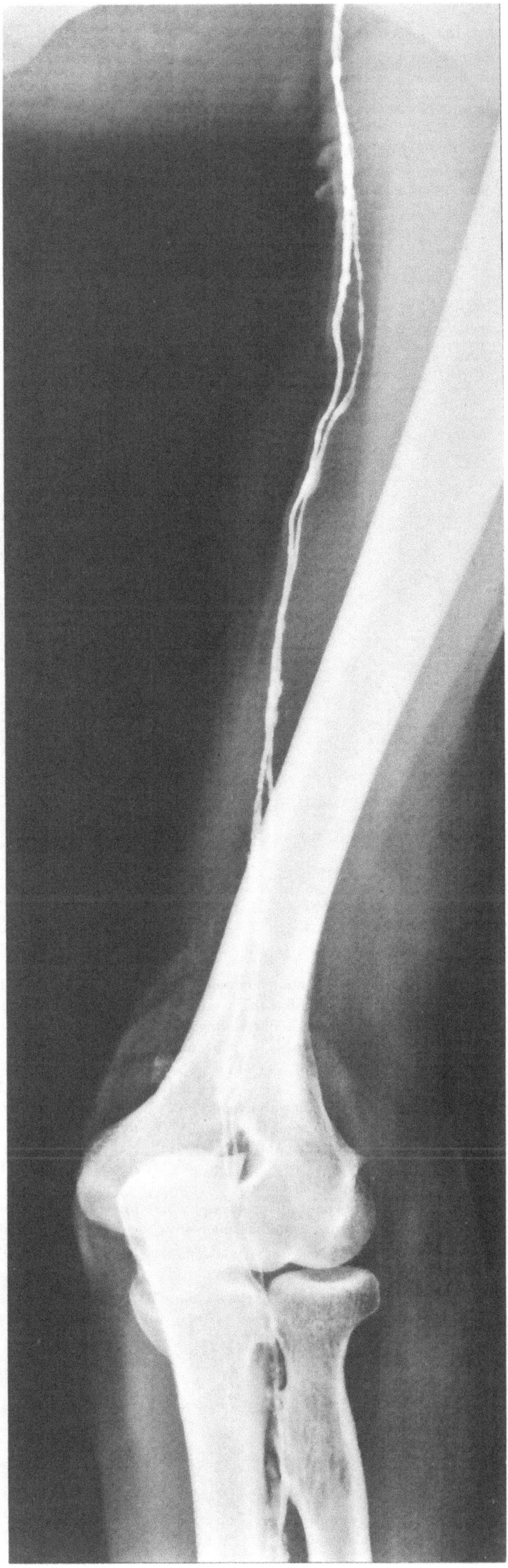

107

figs. 108 and 109 Normal lymphogram and lymphadenogram of the axillary and subclavicular regions.

fig. 110 Normal lymph node; lymphogram.

fig. 111 Normal lymph node; lymphadenogram. Internal structure with uniform, granular distribution, marginal sinus is intact.

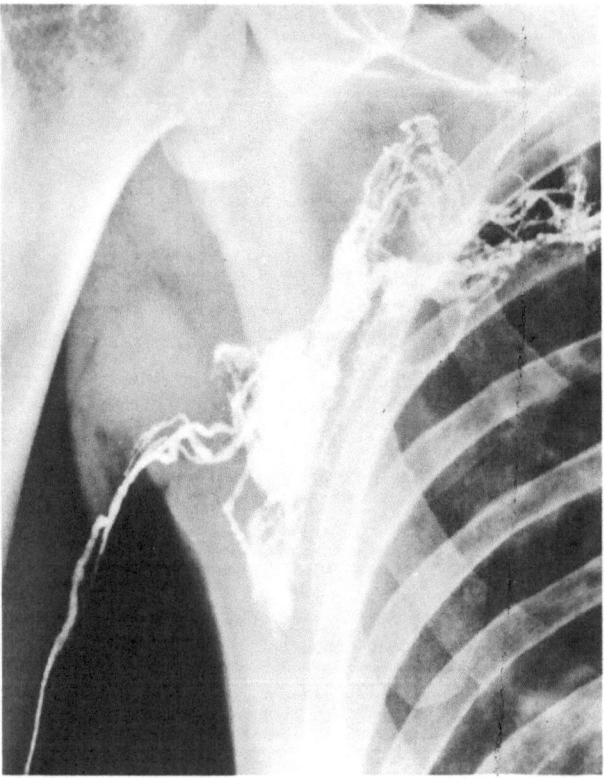

108

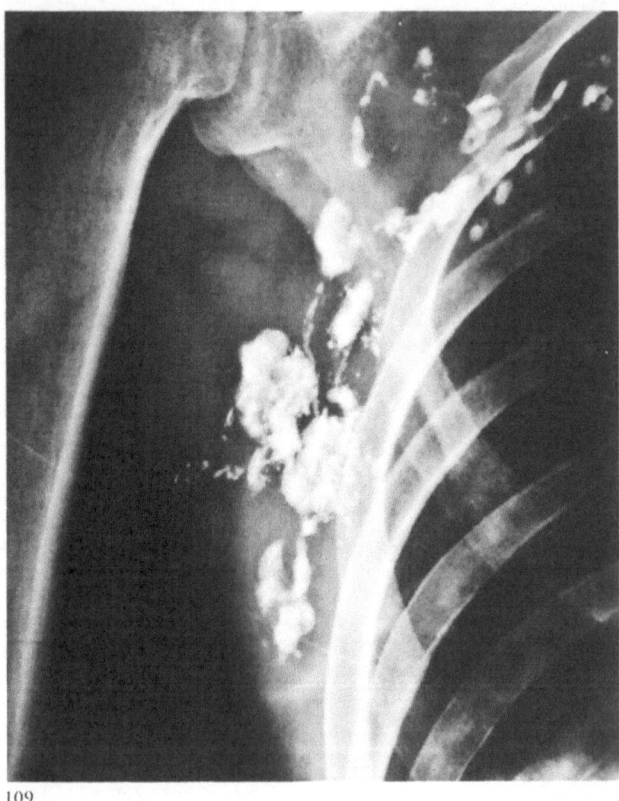

109

fig. 112 Fat and fibrosis in normal lymph nodes; lymphadenogram: visible in the middle of the lymph node as clearly defined filling defects, in the margin considerable similarity to metastatic carcinoma.

fig. 113 Acute inflammation with hypertrophic changes; lymphogram: enlarged lymph node with dilated afferent and efferent lymph vessels.

fig. 114 Acute inflammation with hypertrophic changes; lymphadenogram: enlarged lymph node, marginal sinus intact, internal structure symmetrical.

fig. 115 Acute specific inflammation (tuberculosis); lymphadenogram: lymph node enlarged, marginal sinus intact, filling defects in internal structure, no specific pattern.

fig. 116 Chronic inflammation with hypotrophic changes; lymphadenogram: lymph nodes greatly reduced in size, marginal sinus intact, internal architecture no longer clearly recognizable. Afferent lymph vessels still visible.

fig. 117 Hodgkin's disease; lymphadenogram: enlarged lymph node, marginal sinus intact, internal structure moth-eaten.

fig. 118 Hodgkin's disease; lymphadenogram: enlarged lymph node, marginal sinus intact, internal structure has foamy pattern giving the node a ghost-like appearance.

fig. 119 Hodgkin's disease; lymphadenogram: enlarged lymph node, marginal sinus locally blurred, internal structure partly mottled, partly a ghost-like appearance.

fig. 120 Brill-Symmers' disease; lymphadenogram: lymph nodes cannot be distinguished from those of Hodgkin's disease, can become quite large.

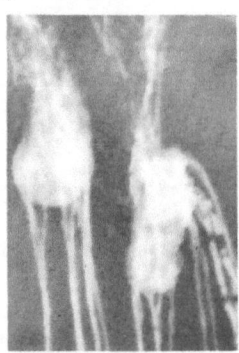

110

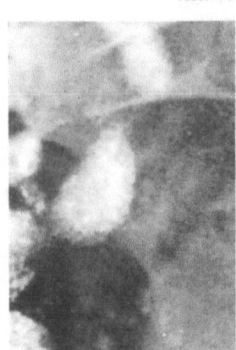

111

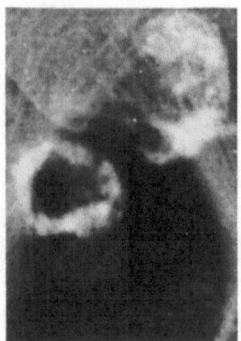

112

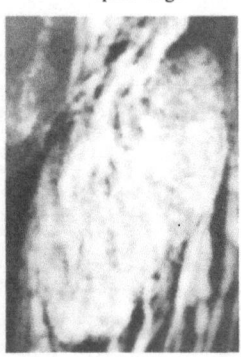

113

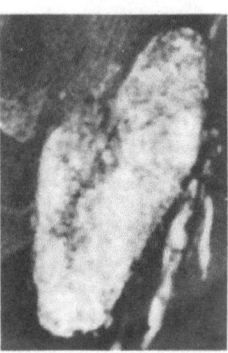

114

fig. 121 Whipple's disease; lymphadenogram: enlarged lymph node, marginal sinus intact and thickened, internal structure no longer clearly recognizable.

fig. 122 Reticulum cell sarcoma; lymphadenogram: enlarged lymph node, marginal sinus interrupted, contrast medium has collected in that part of the marginal sinus which is still intact.

fig. 123 Reticulum cell sarcoma; lymphadenogram: enlarged lymph node, marginal sinus interrupted, where present internal architecture is seen to be finely stippled, vague and asymmetric.

fig. 124 Chronic lymphatic leukaemia; lymphadenogram: lymph node enlarged along the long axis, marginal sinus intact, internal structure granular, merging in some places and appearing cystic in others.

fig. 125 Chronic lymphatic leukaemia; lymphadenogram: enlarged lymph node is elongated, marginal sinus intact; locally contrast medium is concentrated in transverse stripes.

fig. 126 Lymphosarcoma; lymphadenogram: enlarged lymph node, marginal sinus intact; internal architecture massive, gross and asymmetric.

fig. 127 Lymphosarcoma; lymphadenogram: lymph node enlarged, marginal sinus intact; contrast medium concentrated in broad, coarse bands.

fig. 128 Metastatic carcinoma; lymphadenogram: lymph node slightly enlarged, marginal sinus broken in two places, boundary between metastases and normal lymphatic tissue blurred and irregular.

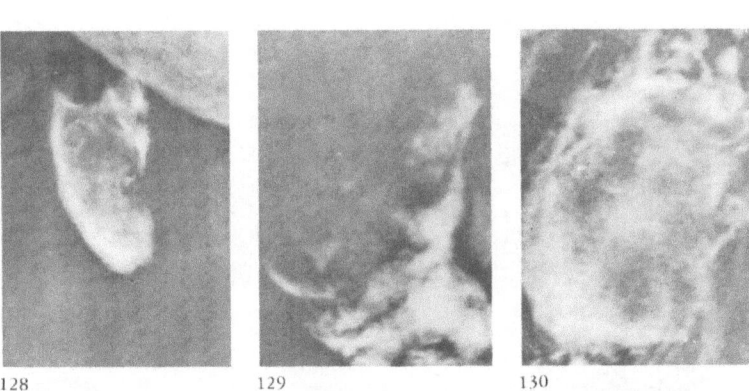

128   129   130

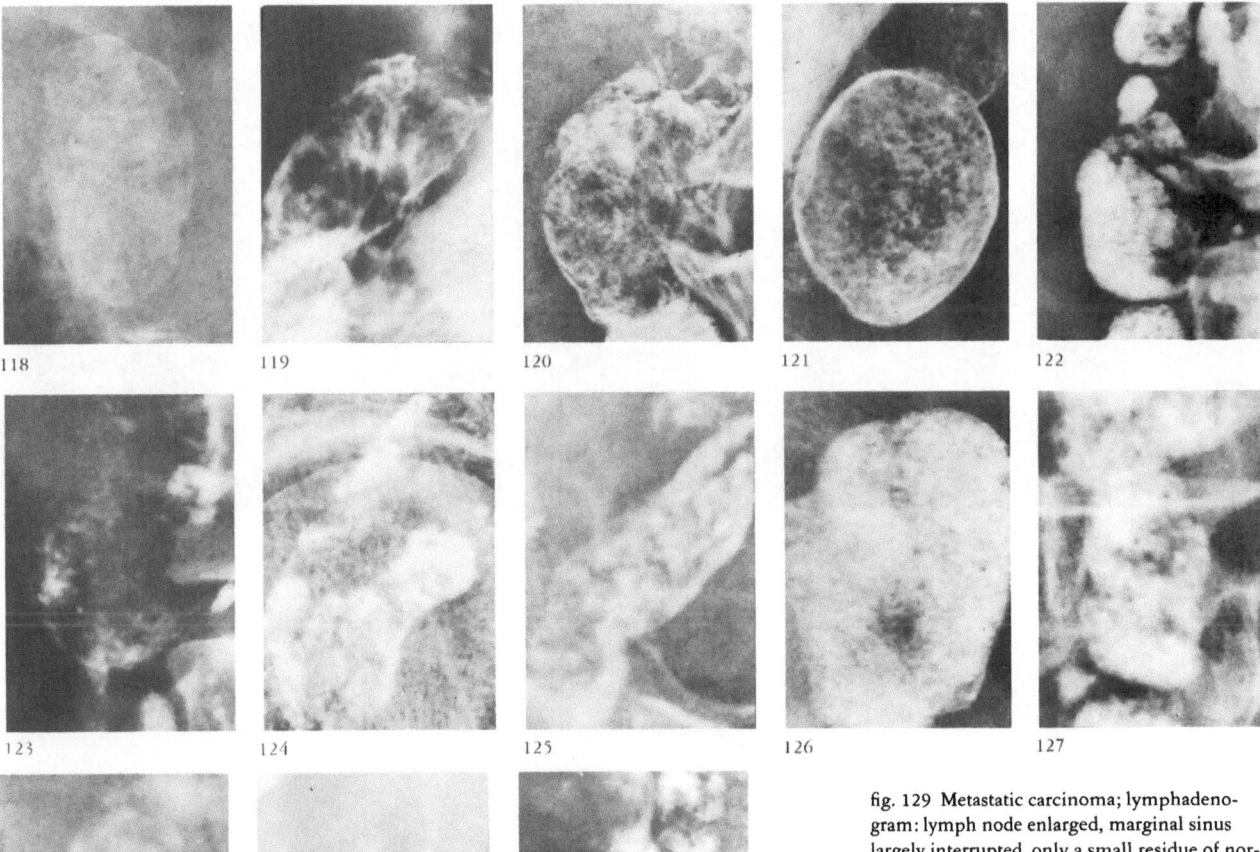

118   119   120   121   122

123   124   125   126   127

115   116   117

fig. 129 Metastatic carcinoma; lymphadenogram: lymph node enlarged, marginal sinus largely interrupted, only a small residue of normal lymphatic tissue still present.

fig. 130 Metastatic carcinoma; lymphadenogram: lymph node enlarged, marginal sinus interrupted locally, internal structure has disappeared for the most part.

figs. 131 and 132 Metastatic carcinoma (corpus uteri); lymphogram (fig. 131) and lymphadenogram (fig. 132): on the right the lymphatic drainage channels in the pelvis have arched out around the pathological lymph nodes which have not absorbed the contrast medium, these lymph nodes have been completely filled with carcinoma and are consequently no longer visible thus causing an interruption in the lymph node chain.

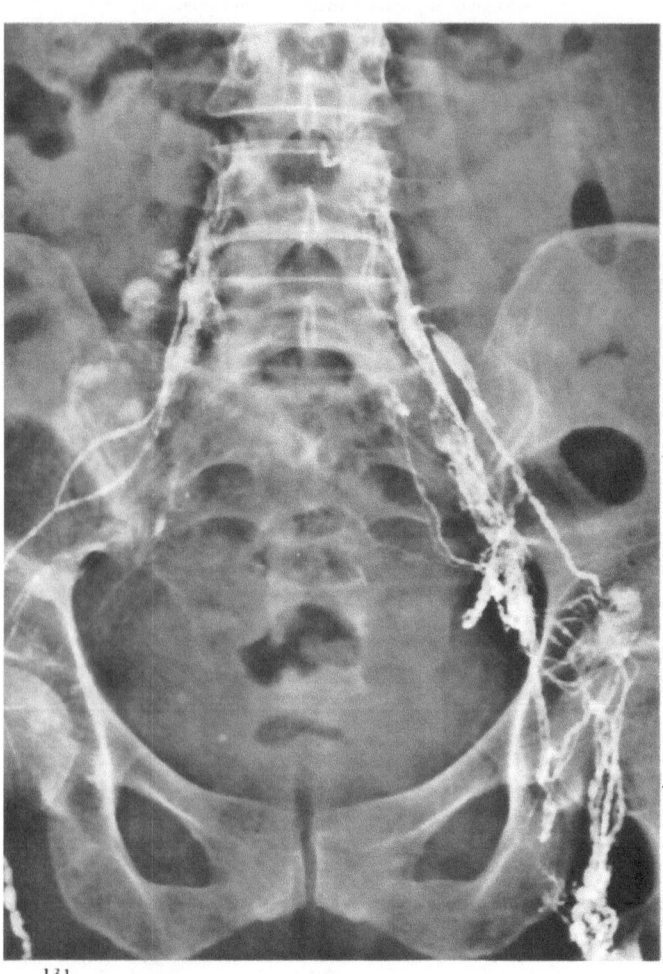

131

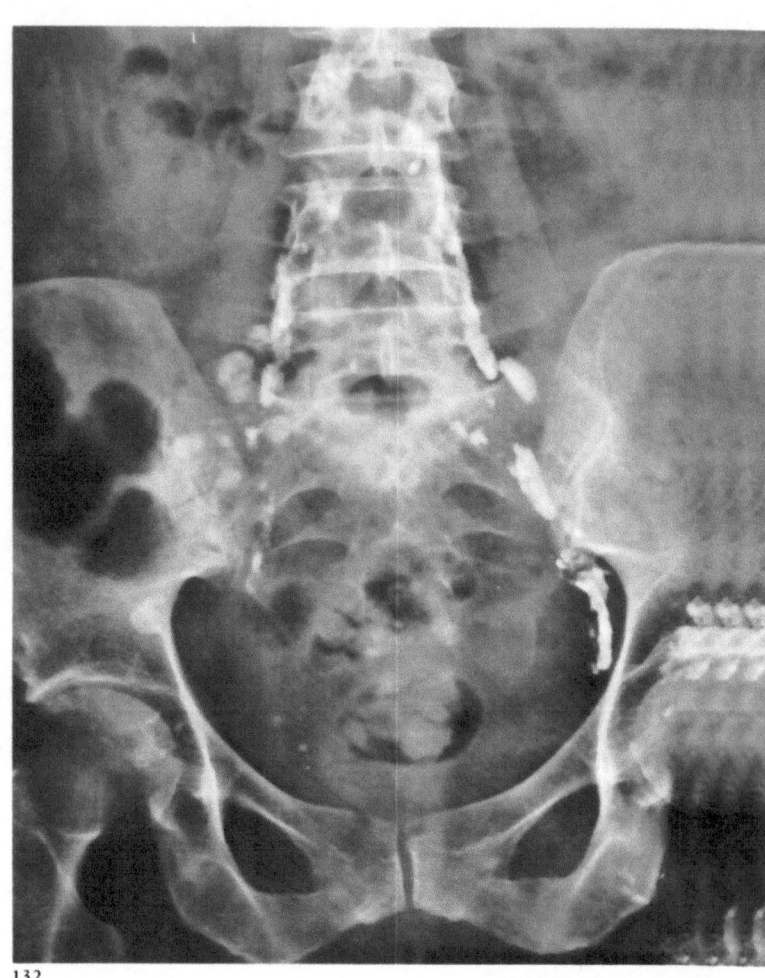

132

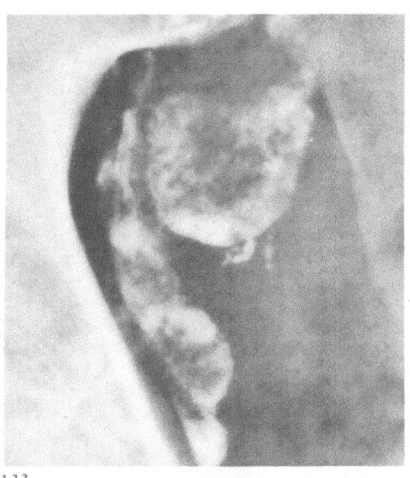

133

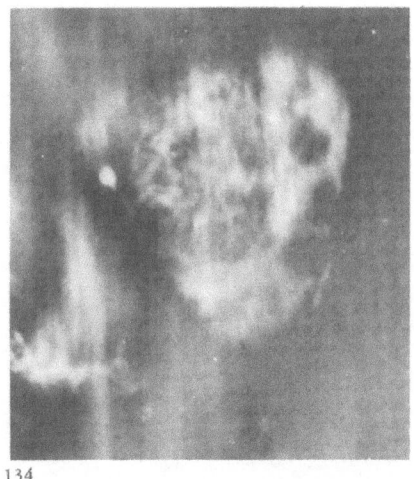

134

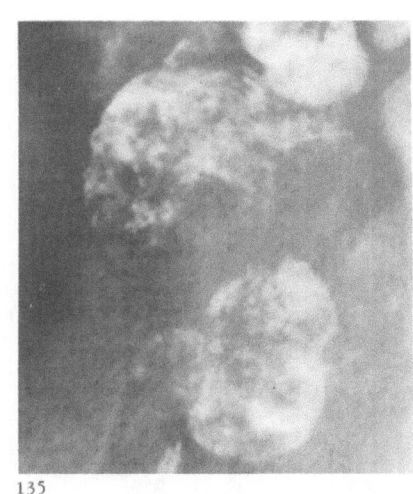

135

figs. 133-141 Lymphadenograms: the lymph nodes in figs. 133-135 are involved by carcinoma but resemble in appearance Hodgkin's disease. The lymph node in fig. 136 is involved by reticulum cell sarcoma which resembles carcinoma. In fig. 137, the lymph nodes are affected by reticulum cell sarcoma which appears to be Hodgkin's disease. The lymph node in fig. 138 is affected by inflammation but suggests Hodgkin's disease. In fig. 139, a lymph node is seen involved by Brill-Symmers' disease which also appears to be Hodgkin's disease. The lymph nodes in fig. 140 are involved by chronic lymphatic leukaemia but they resemble Hodgkin's disease. The lymph node in fig. 141 is affected by lymphosarcoma but resembles involvement by chronic lymphatic leukaemia. *Comment:* Generally the basic types of lymph node described in figs. 110-132 are correct; in practice however the architecture of the pathological lymph nodes sometimes overlaps so that differentiation becomes difficult – especially in lymphoreticular malignancies.

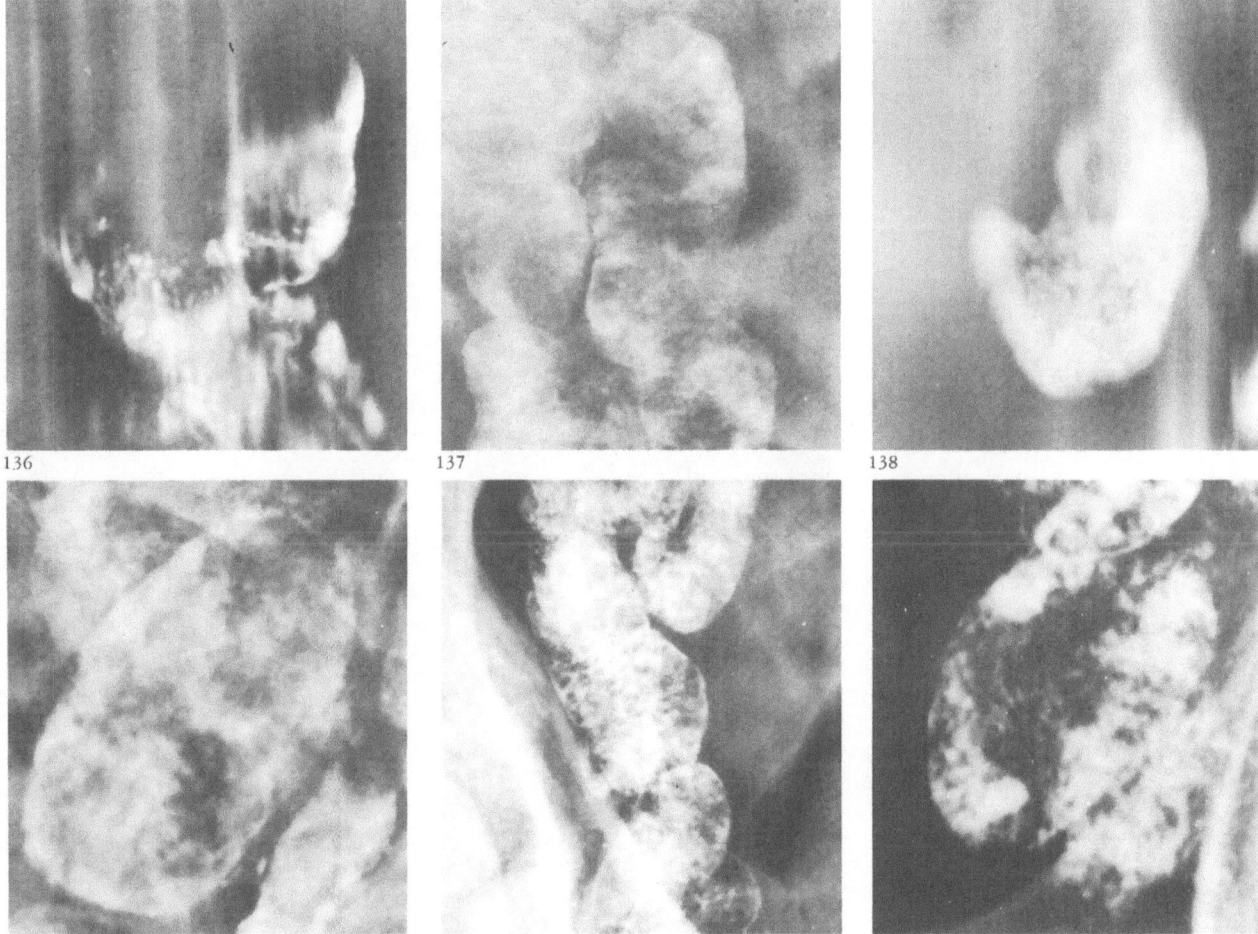

136

137

138

139

140

141

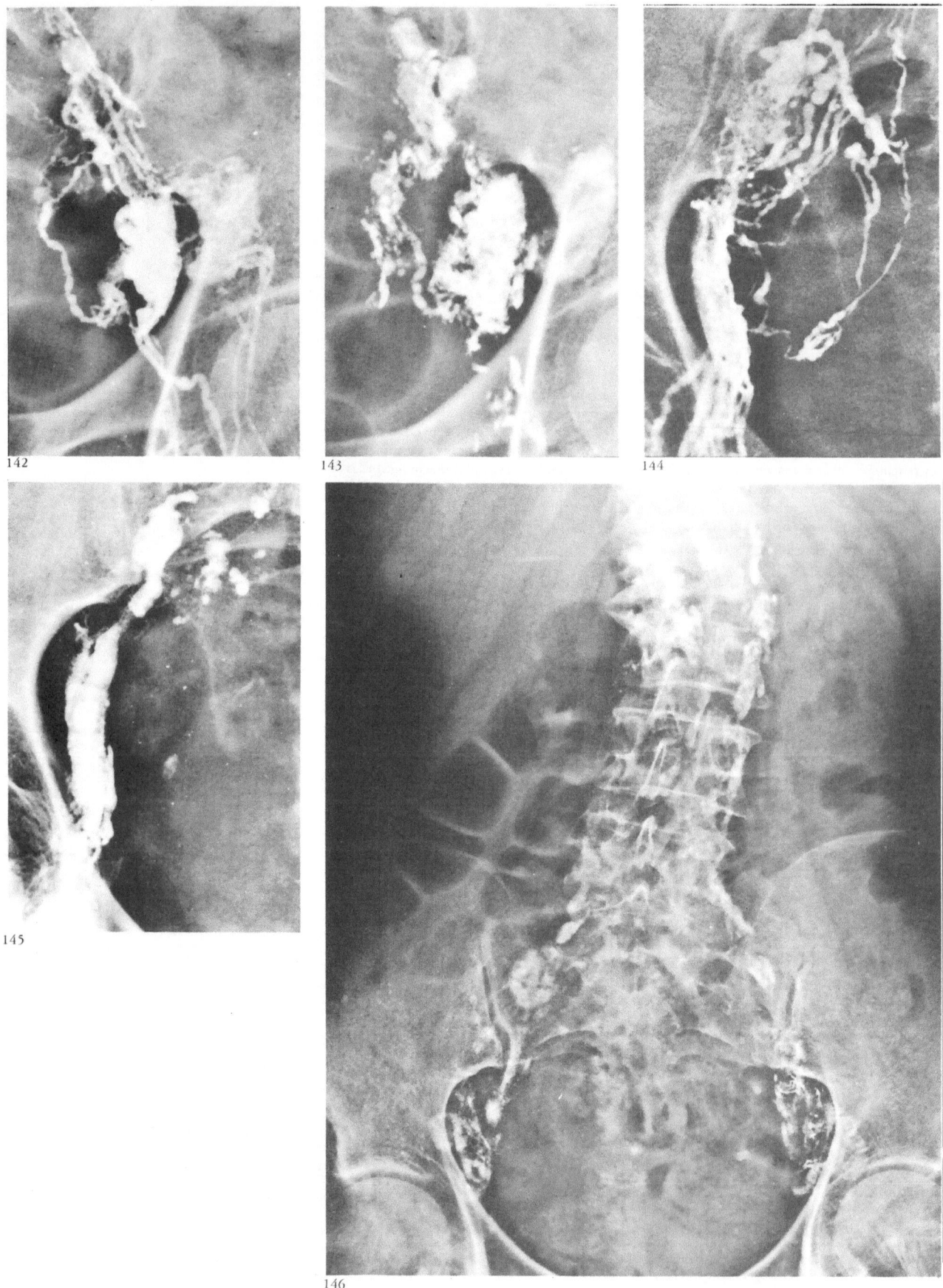

142

143

144

145

146

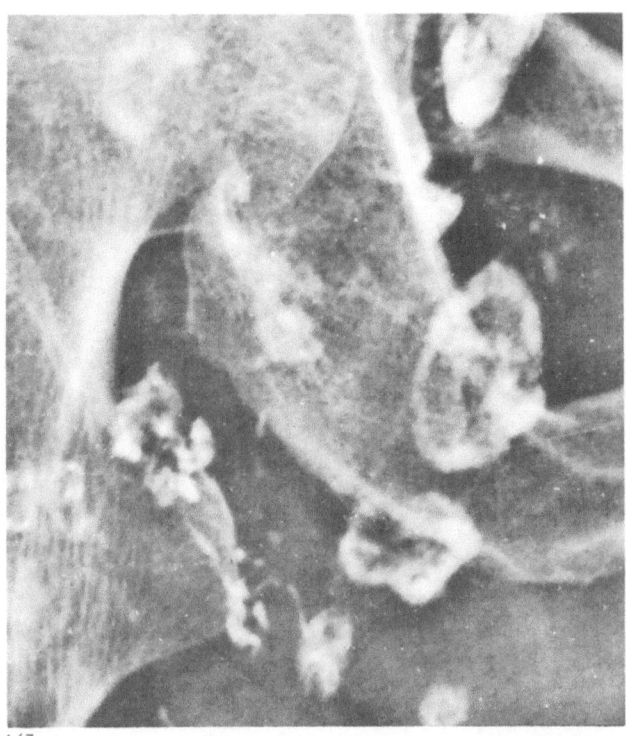

147

figs. 142-145 Non-pathological variations.
Although the presence of collateral lymphatic
channels on the lymphogram (as in figs. 142,
144) usually indicates a pathological disease,
this is not necessarily true if the lymph nodes
on the lymphadenogram (figs. 143, 145) appear
normal and there is no lymphatic obstruction.

fig. 146 Non-pathological variations. The lymphadenogram of old patients can show many
misleading patterns as a result of degeneration
and the development of fat and fibrosis.

fig. 147 Fat and fibrosis in lymph nodes, frequently occurring in the aged, especially in the
inguinal region; it can be confused with involvement by a malignant disease. Follow-up
studies can prove useful (figs. 148-151).

figs. 148-151 Fat and fibrosis in lymph nodes.
Reticulum cell sarcoma. On the lymphadenogram (fig. 148), several lymph nodes (−) seem
to be affected by fat and fibrosis. The general
appearance of the lymph nodes is quiescent.
On the follow-up radiograms taken 3 (fig. 149),
6 (fig. 150) and 8 (fig. 151) weeks later, the
lymph nodes in question show a gradual but
pronounced enlargement and begin to resemble
lymph nodes involved by reticulum cell sarcoma.

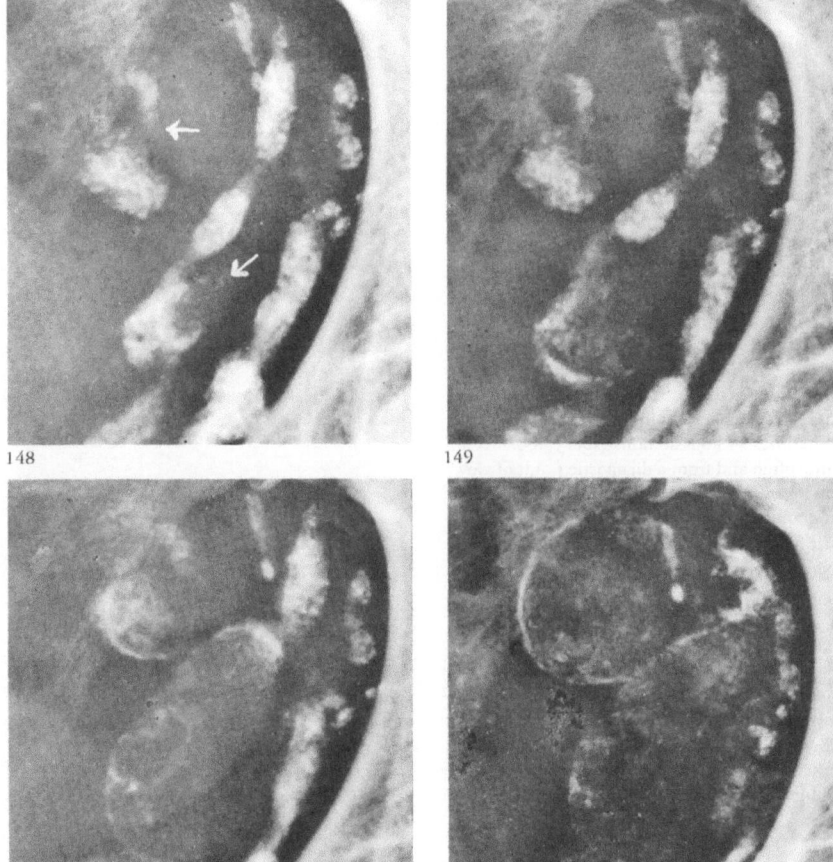

148

149

150

151

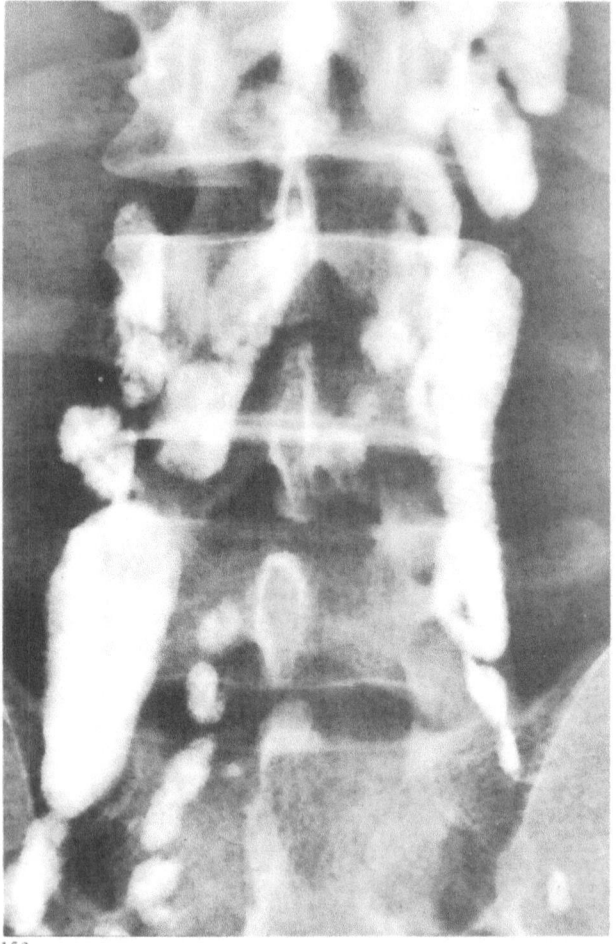

152

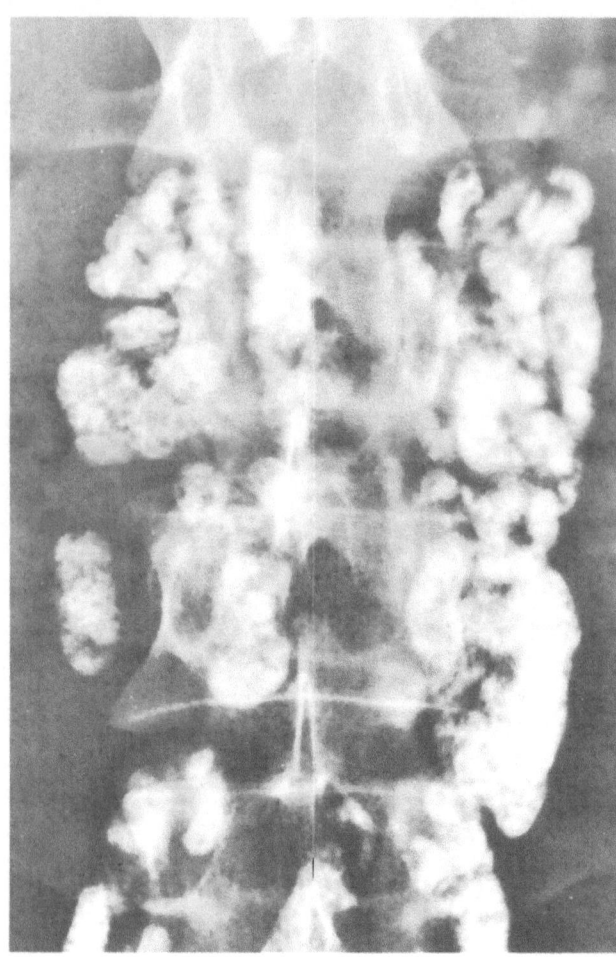

153

figs. 152 and 153 Irritated lymph nodes; lymphadenograms: inflammatory-like changes characterized by enlargement (fig. 152) and a disorderly and irregular appearance of the lymph nodes (fig. 153).

Comment: This type of lymph node shows no indications of involvement by a malignant disease. Found near tumours and infections, and sometimes without demonstrable cause. Occurs quite often and from a diagnostic point of view can be considered normal in the first instance. In doubtful cases, follow-up radiograms can be helpful since this irritated condition may lead to a malignant disease in incidental patients (figs. 154, 155).

figs. 154 and 155 Irritated lymph nodes. Ovarian carcinoma. Lymphadenogram: enlargement of the lymph nodes, no indication of involvement by a malignant disease (fig. 154). Roentgenological follow-up 3 months later: the irritated lymph nodes are now involved by a malignant disease (fig. 155). One of the rare cases.

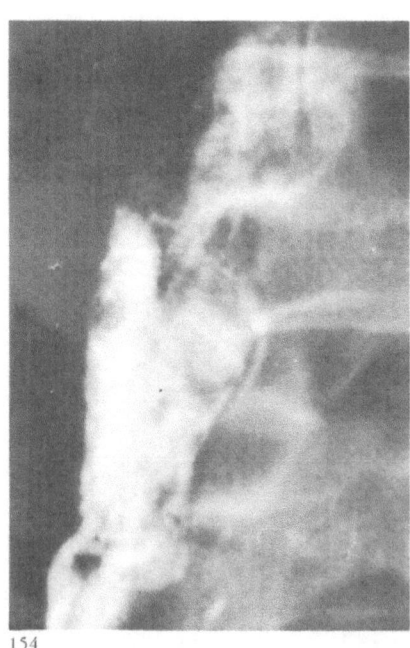

154

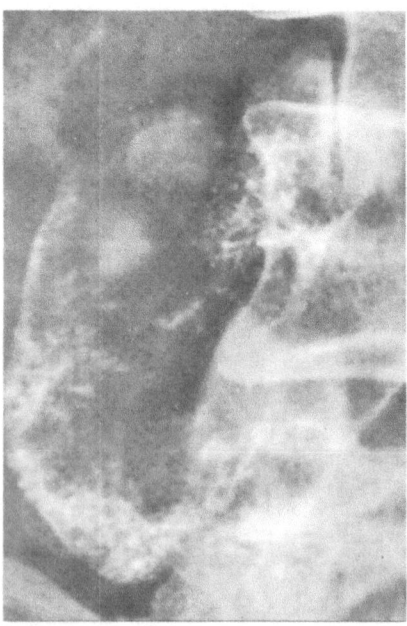

155

fig. 156 Acute inflammation. Catscratch disease. Lymphadenogram.

figs. 157-159 Calcified lymph nodes with old specific inflammations. Before lymphographic examination (fig. 157), after lymphography (fig. 158) and the subtraction technique (fig. 159). *Comment:* Subtraction films are only possible in incidental cases and cannot be used as supplementary routine examination since it is not feasible to make two exactly identical exposures before and after lymphography.

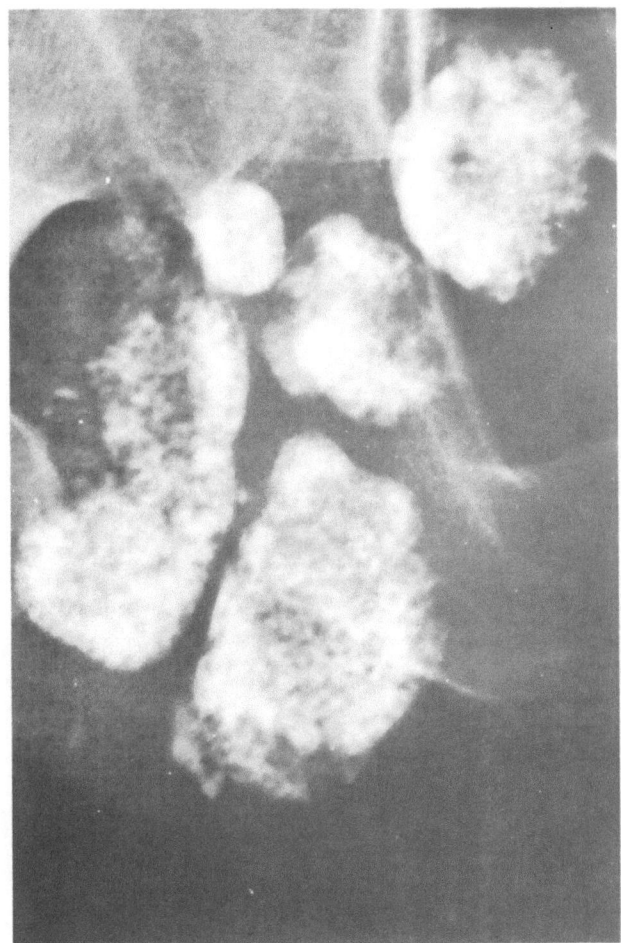

156

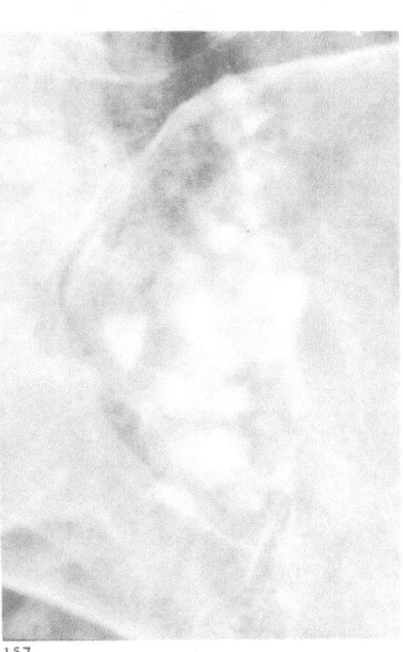

157

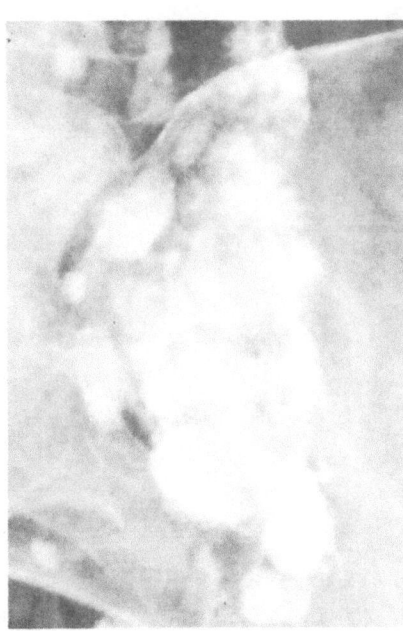

158

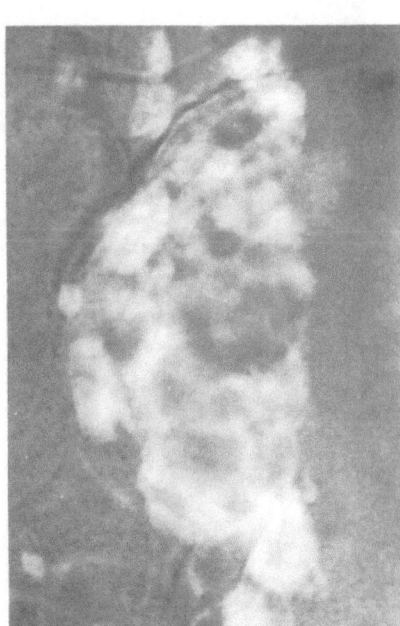

159

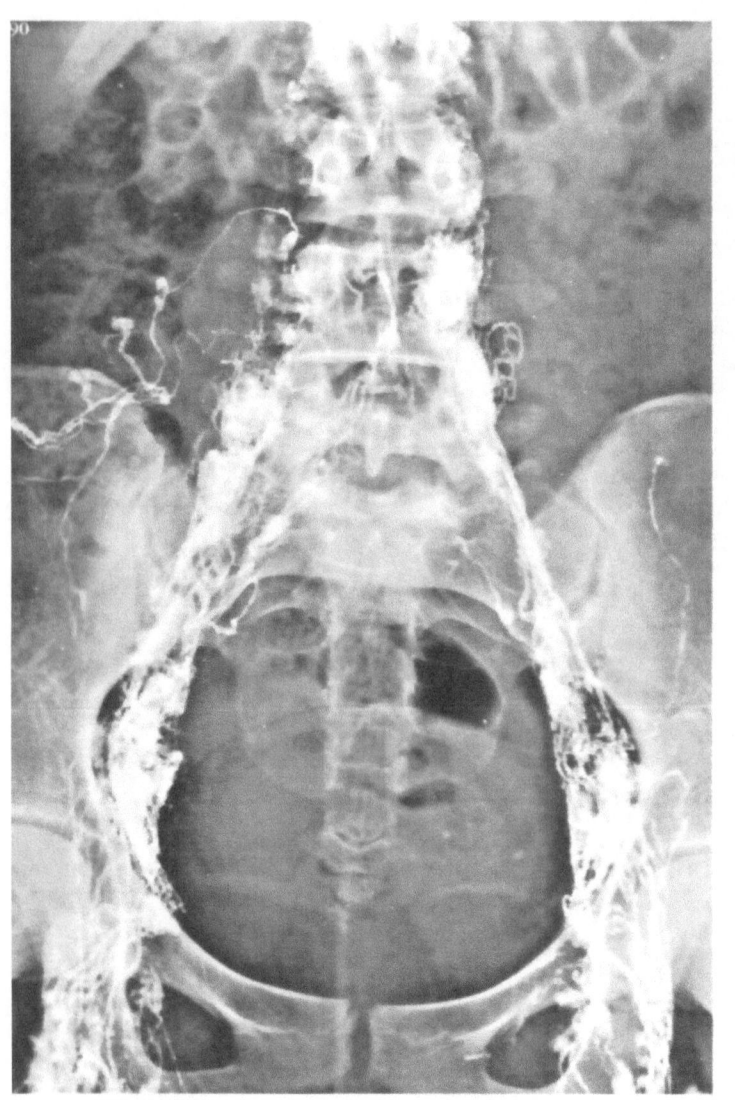

160

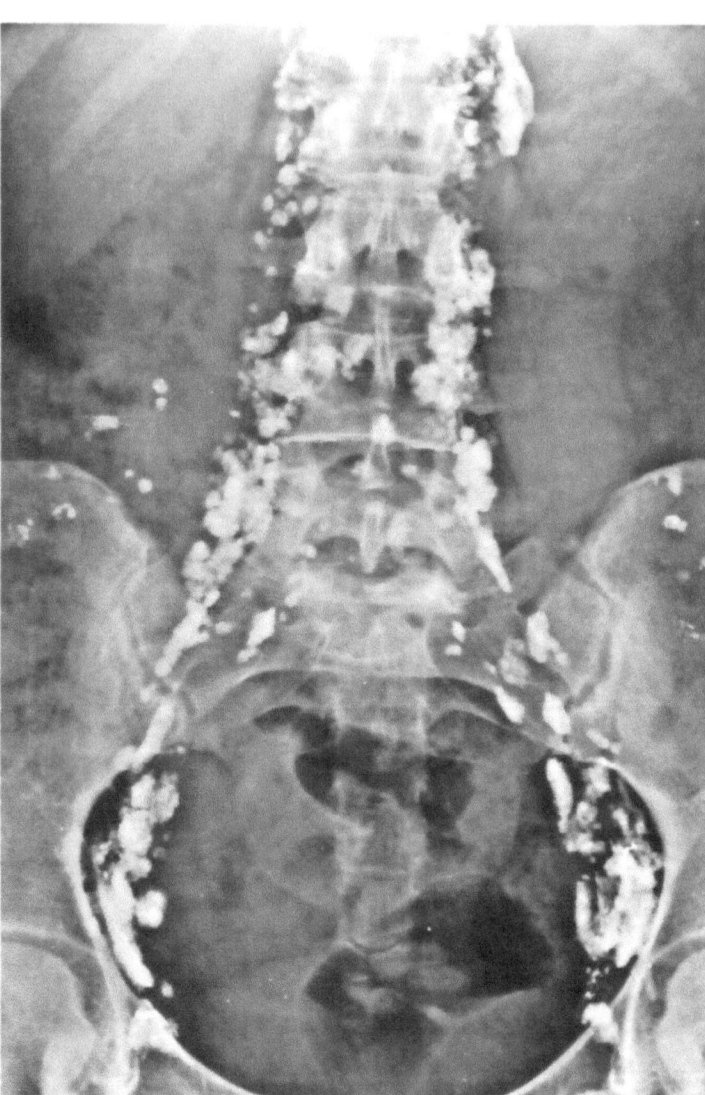

161

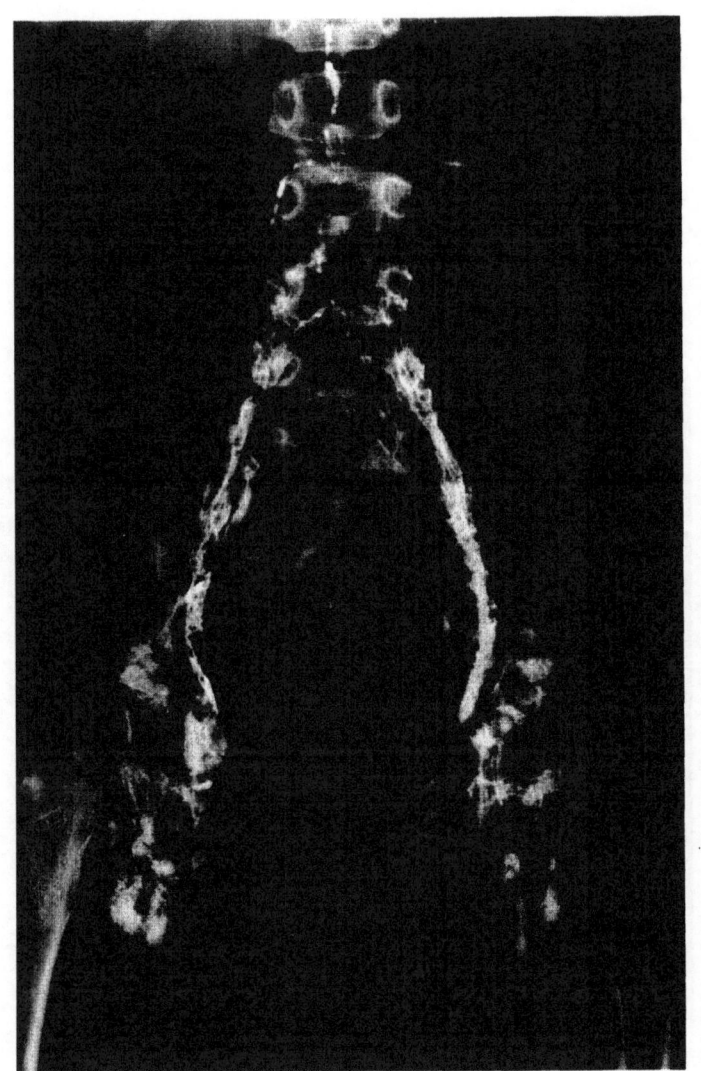

162

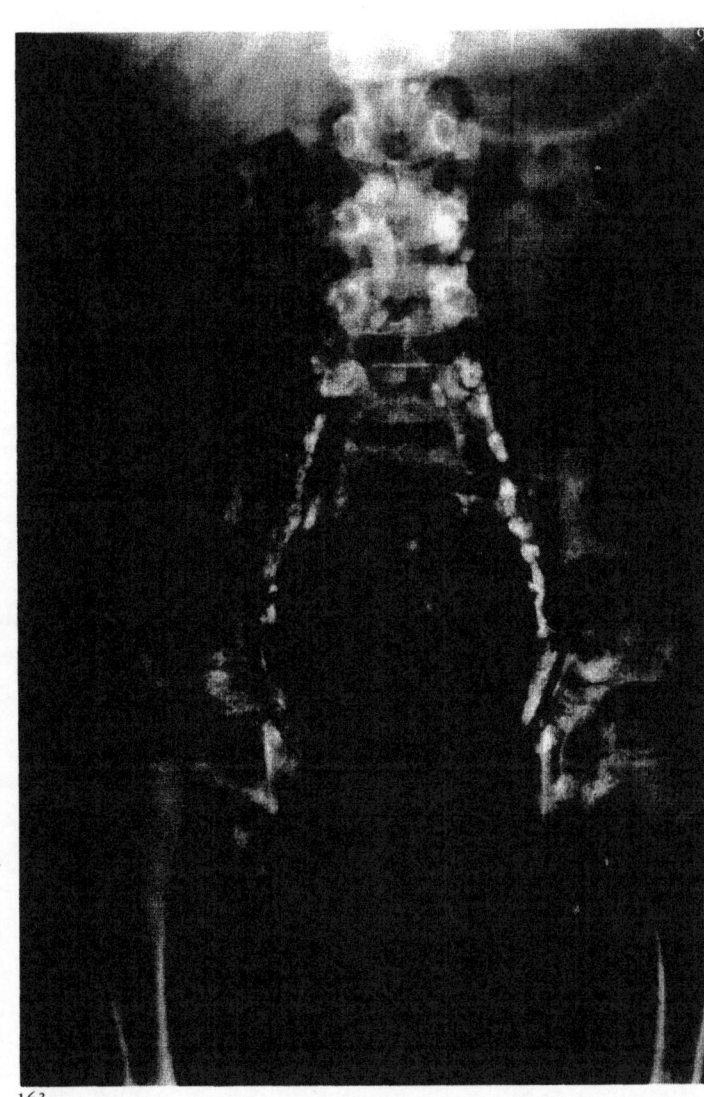

163

figs. 160-167 Hodgkin's disease; lymphograms (figs. 160, 162, 164, 166) and lymphadenograms (figs. 161, 163, 165, 167). Diverse types of involvement of lymph nodes ranging from first patient (figs. 160, 161) – not distinguishable from irritated lymph nodes – to last patient (figs. 166, 167) – extensive involvement.

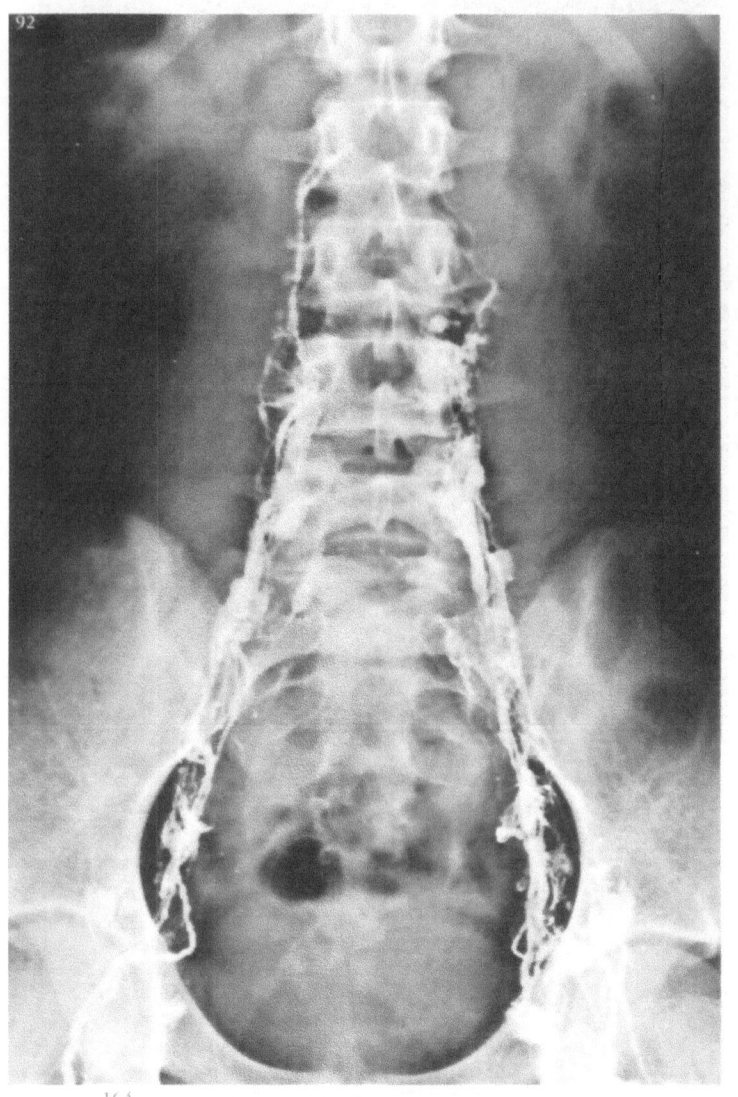

164

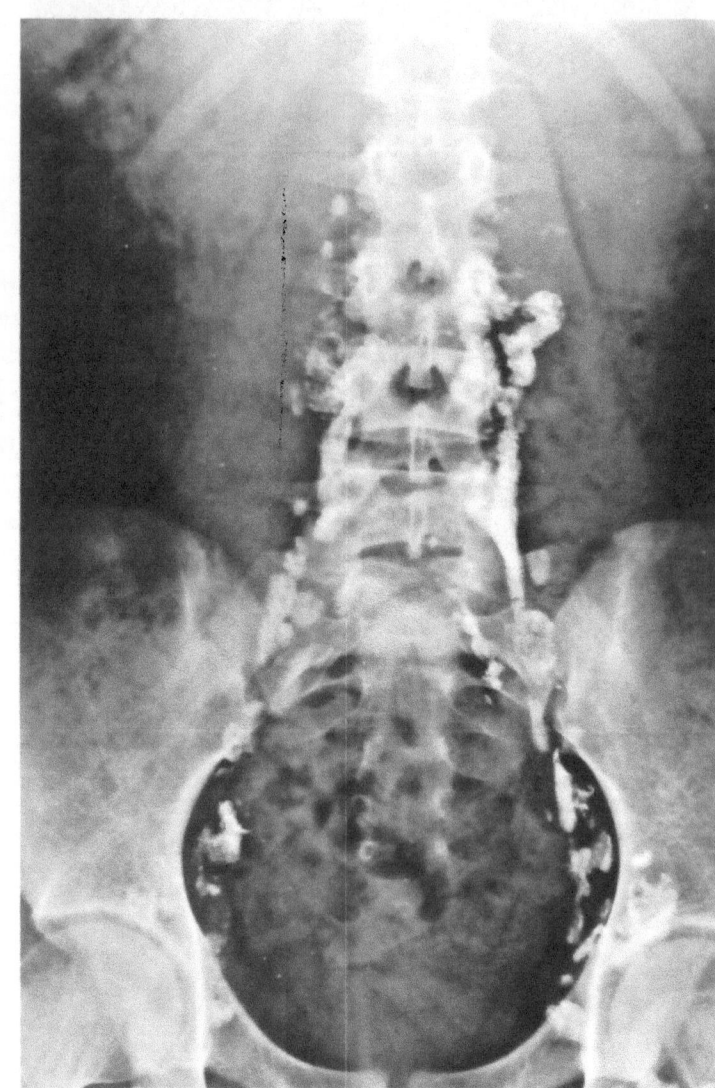

165

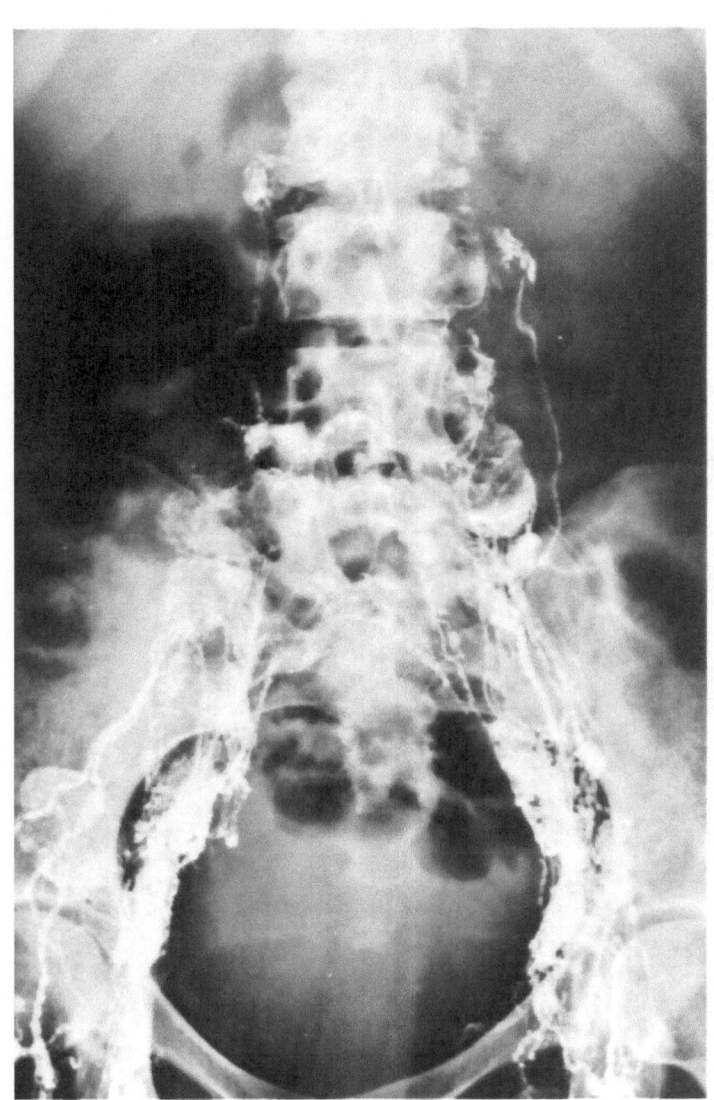

166

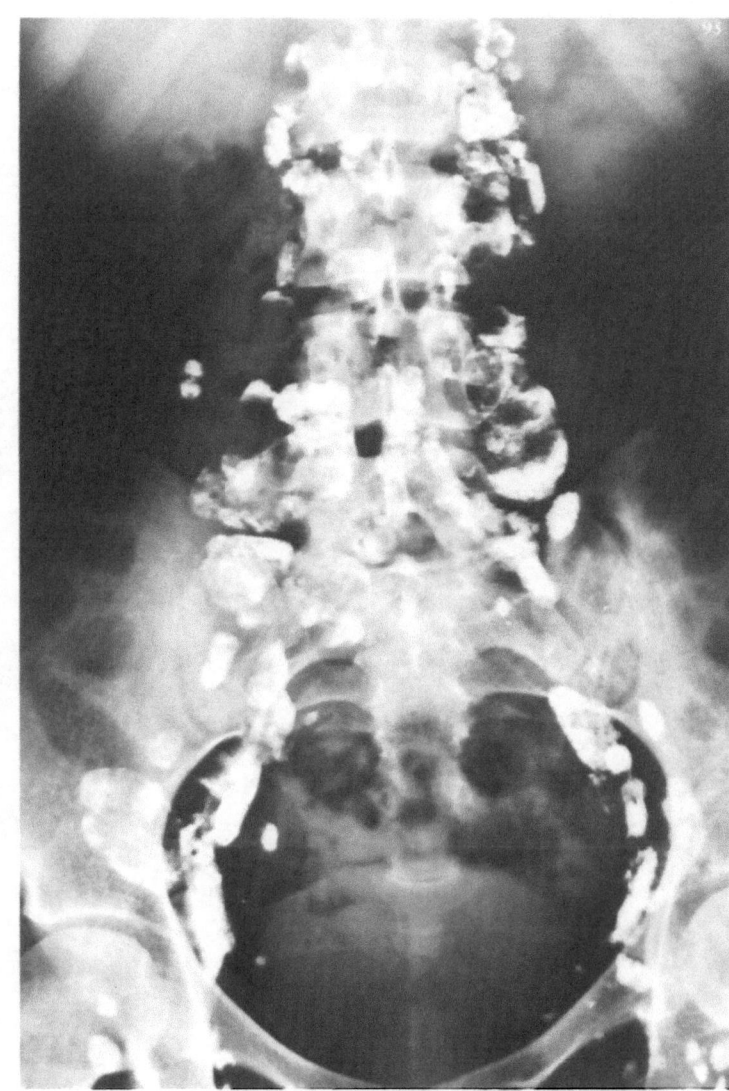

167

on pages 94 and 95

figs. 168 and 169 Hodgkin's disease; lymphogram and lymphadenogram: extensive involvement of paralumbar and para-aortic lymph
nodes.

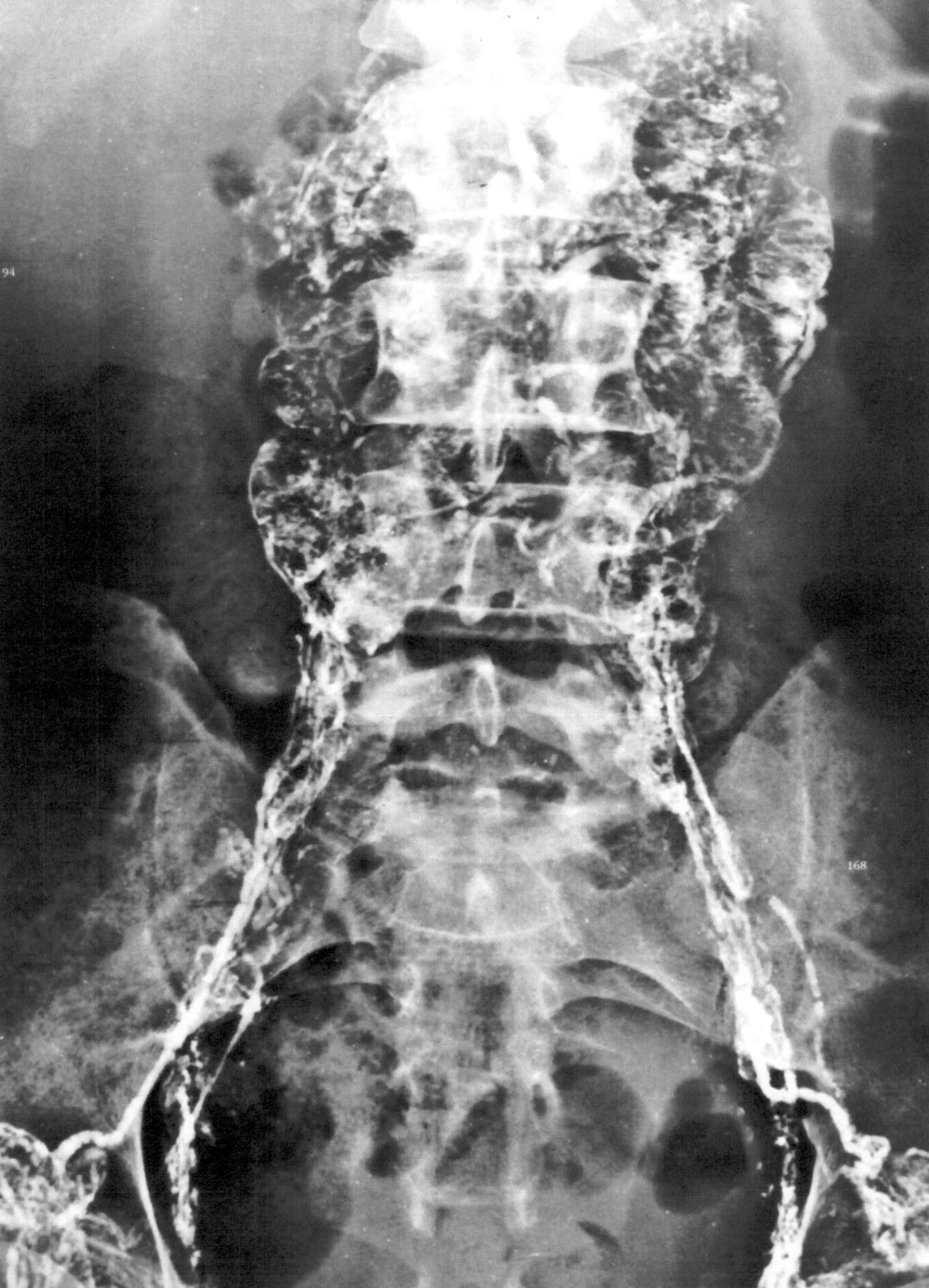

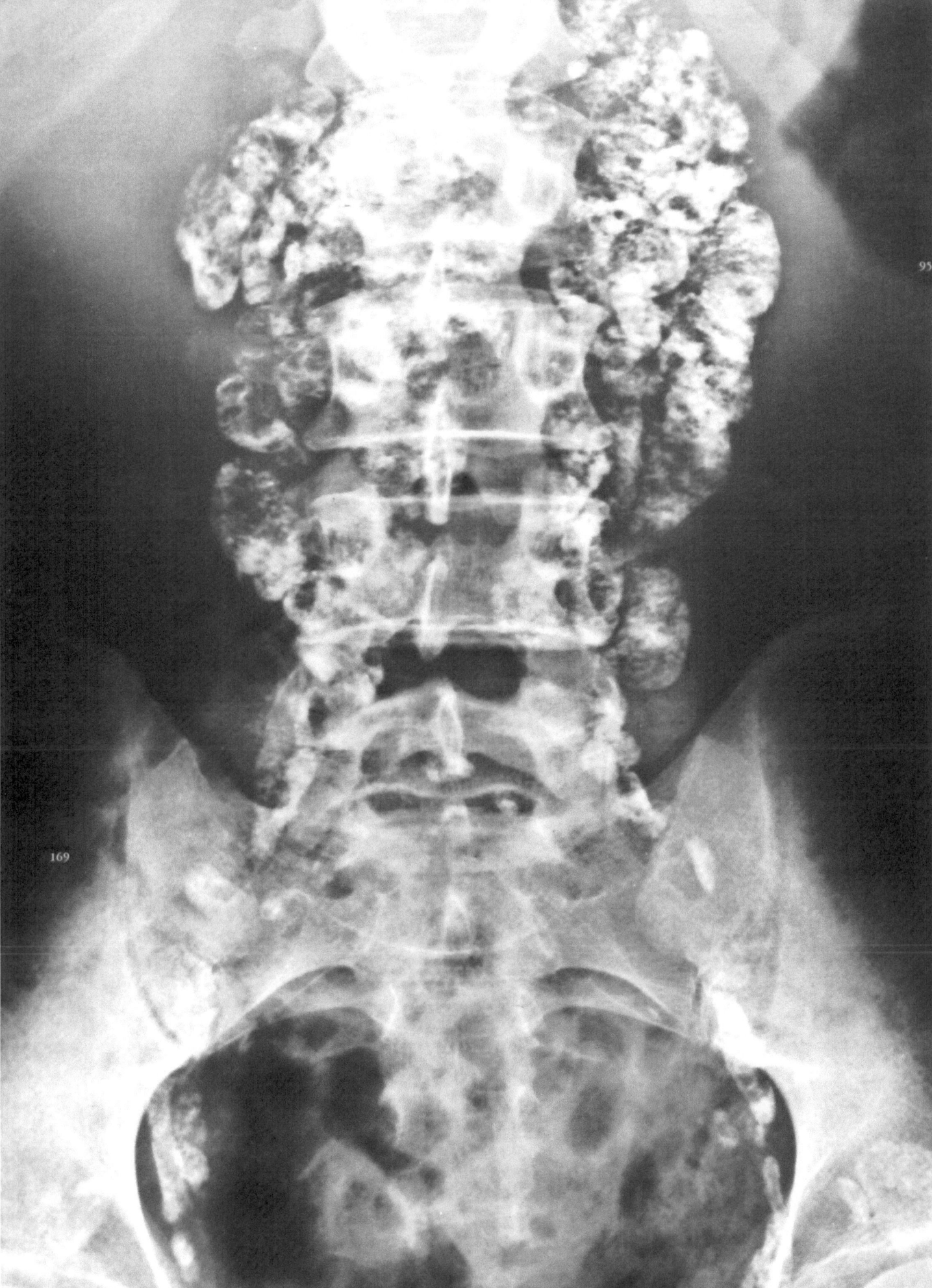

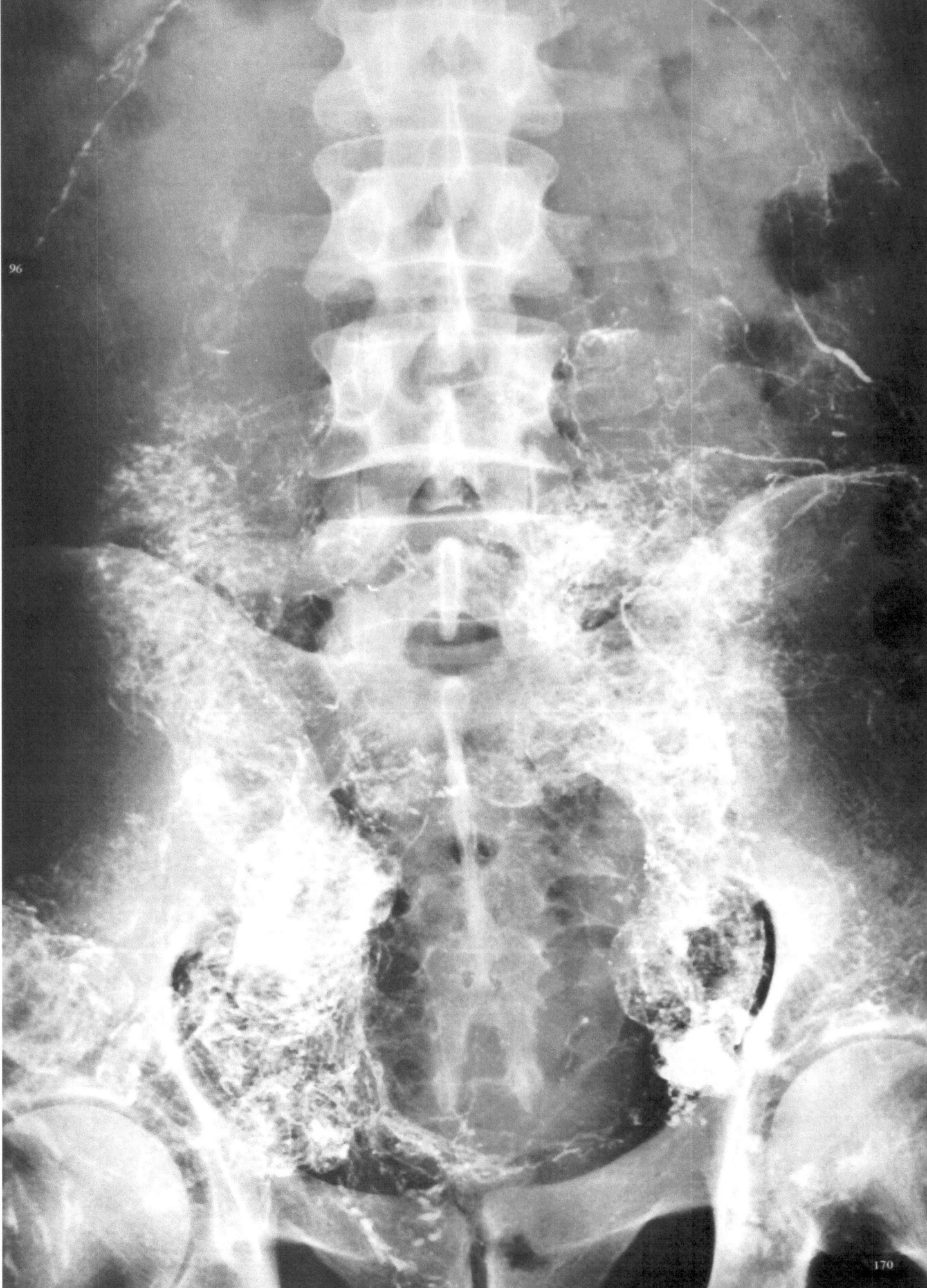

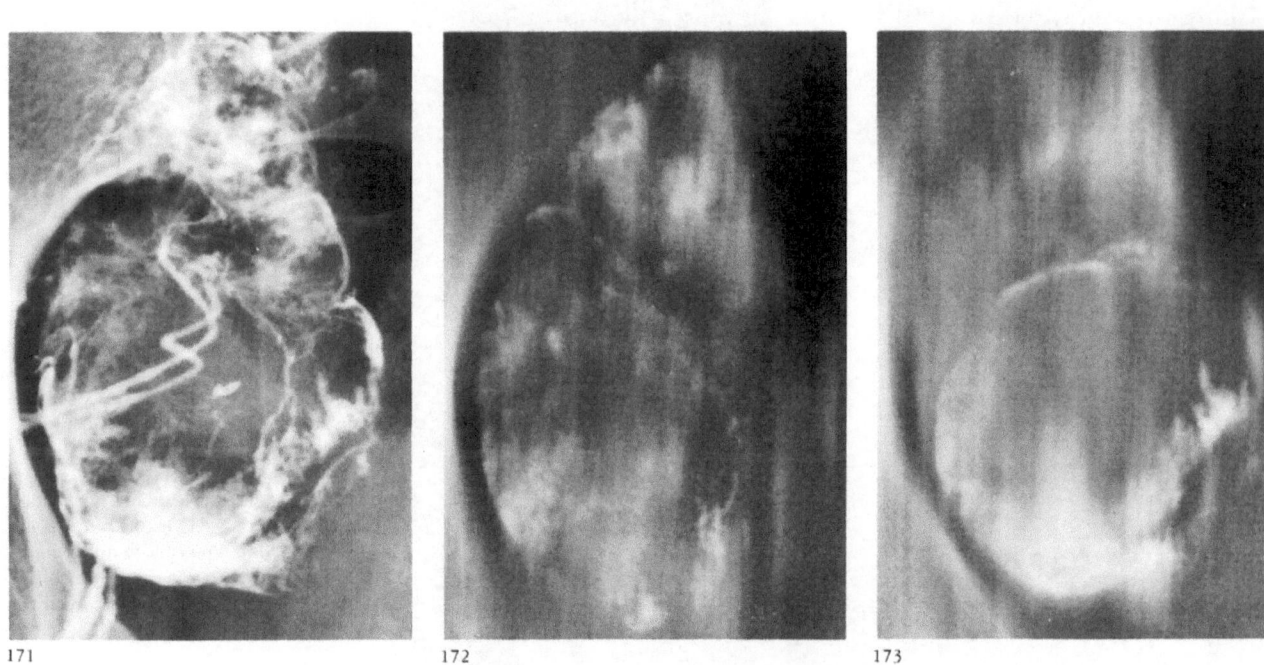

171

172

173

fig. 170 Hodgkin's disease; lymphadenogram:
extensive lymph node abnormalities with drainage obstruction at L3.

fig. 171-173 Hodgkin's disease. Matted lymph
nodes. Lymphadenogram (fig. 171): one greatly
enlarged pathological lymph node; tomograms
(figs. 172, 173): the lymph node is shown to
consist of at least three pathological lymph
nodes matted together.

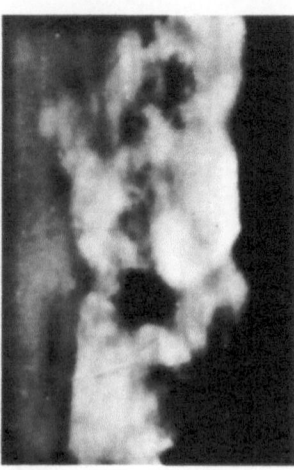

175

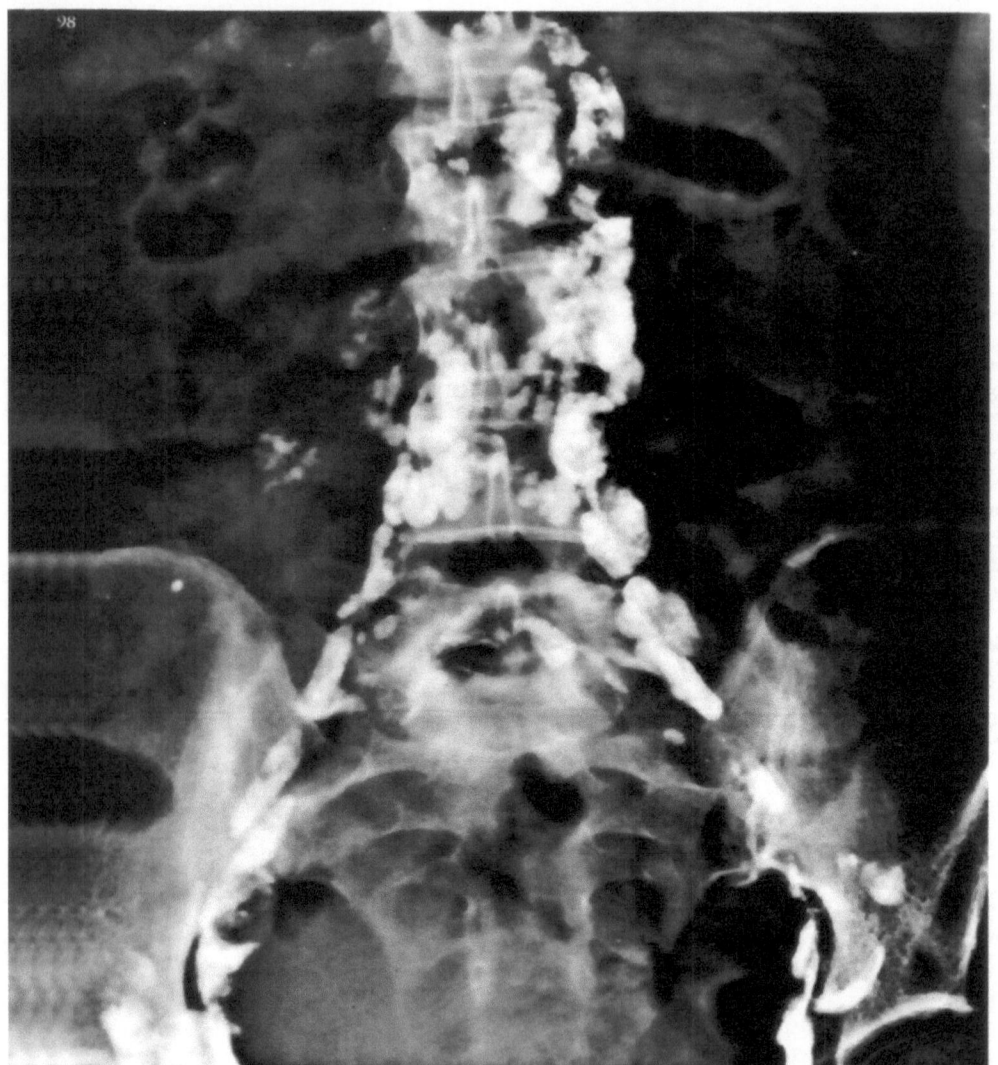

98

174

figs. 174-176 Patient with ascites and gastric tumour. Cytological examination of ascitic fluid: malignant disease, differentiation not possible. Clinical diagnosis: peritoneal carcinosis. Lymphography: pathological lymph nodes on the lymphadenogram (fig. 174), left paralumbar nodes (tomogram, fig. 175) and right iliac nodes (tomogram, fig. 176). Roentgenological diagnosis: Hodgkin's disease. Pathological-anatomical diagnosis at autopsy: Hodgkin's sarcoma.
Comment: It is not possible to differentiate on the lymphogram between paragranuloma, Hodgkin's disease and Hodgkin's sarcoma.

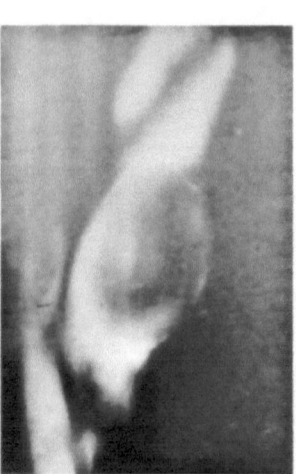

176

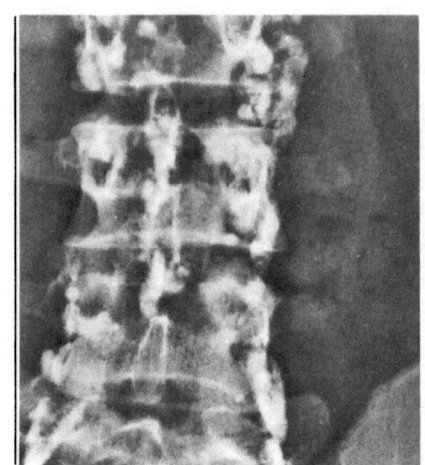

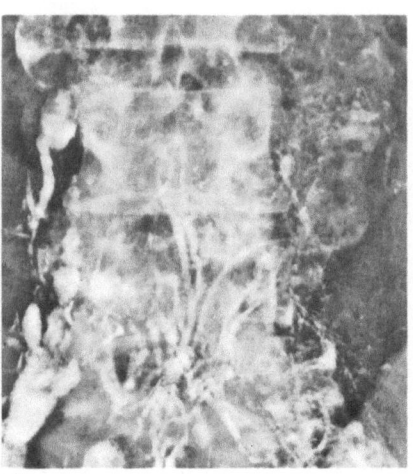

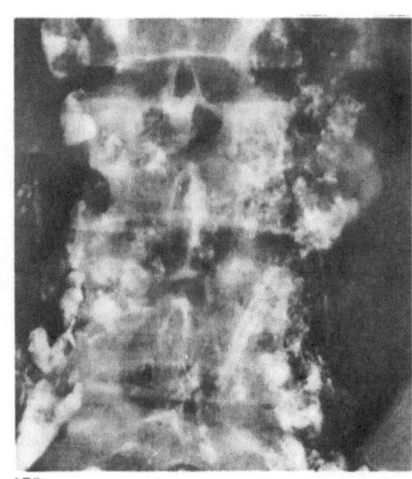

177

178

179

figs. 177-179 Hodgkin's disease; lymphadenogram (fig. 177): normal. Repeat lymphography 6
months later: pathological lymphadenogram
(fig. 178). Follow-up radiogram (fig. 179) after radiation therapy (tumour dose 3000 r.): significant
reduction in size of pathological lymph nodes.

figs. 180 and 181 Hodgkin's disease; lymphadenogram: greatly enlarged pathological lymph
nodes (fig. 180). Reduction after radiation therapy (tumour dose 3000 r) (fig. 181).

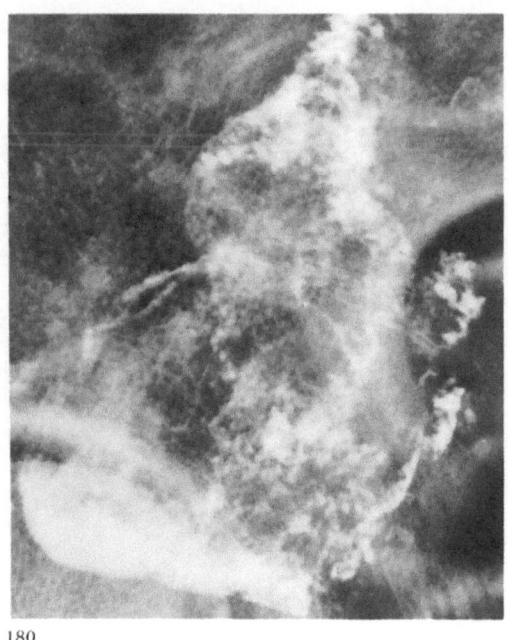

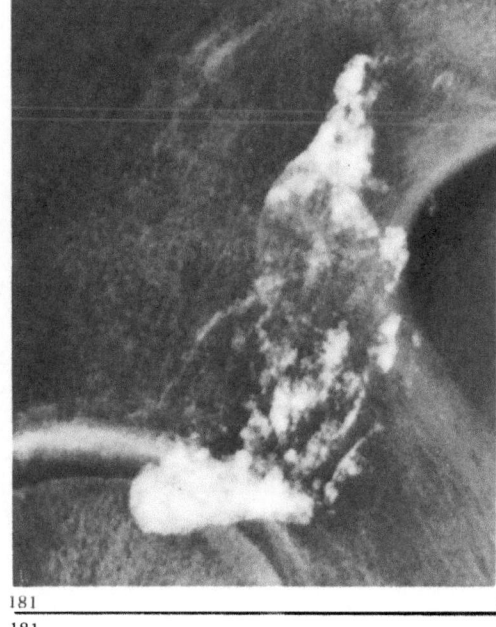

180

181

180

181

100   figs. 182-184 Brill-Symmers' disease; lymphogram (fig. 182), lymphadenogram (fig. 183) and follow-up radiogram after radiation therapy (tumour dose 3000 r.) (fig. 184): these pathological lymph nodes cannot be differentiated from Hodgkin's disease.

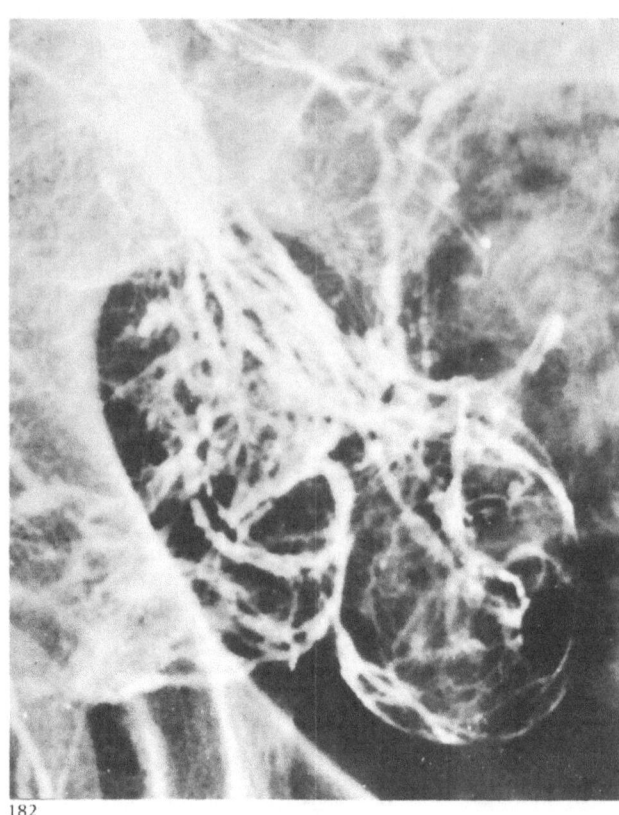

182

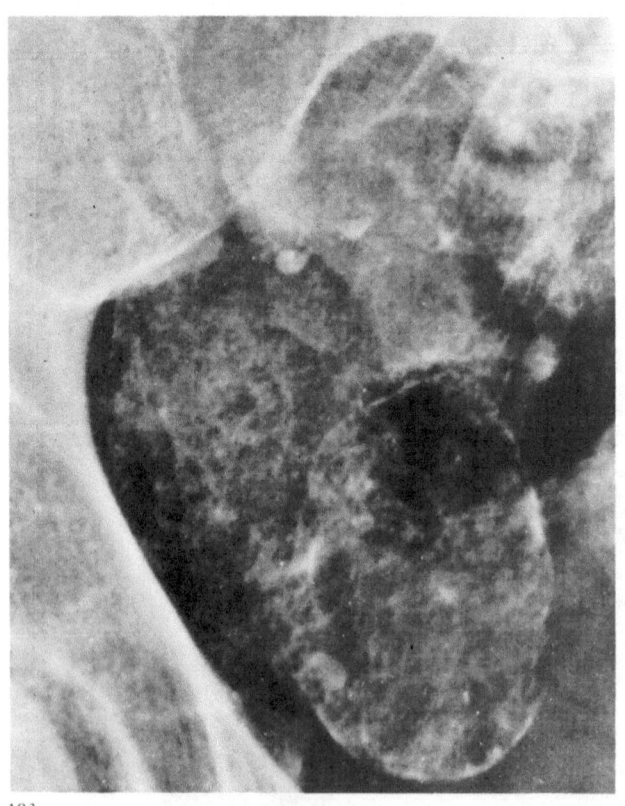

183

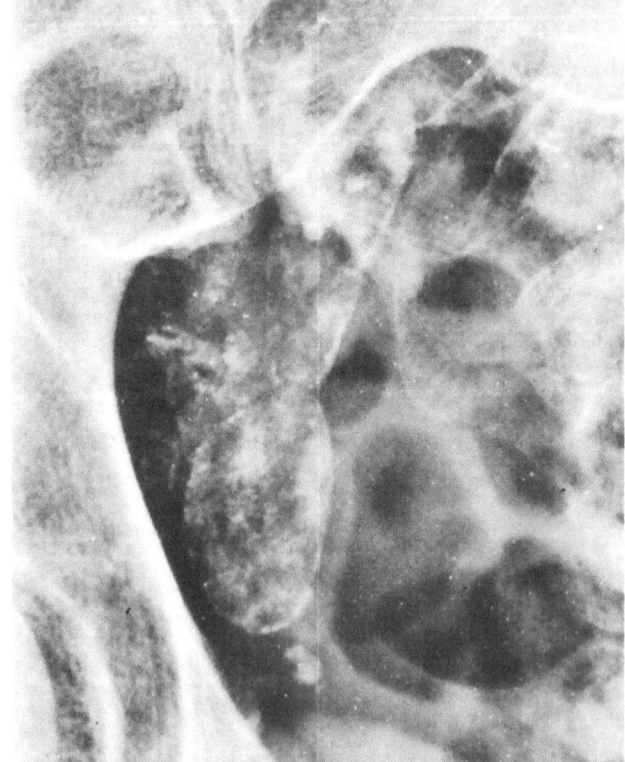

184

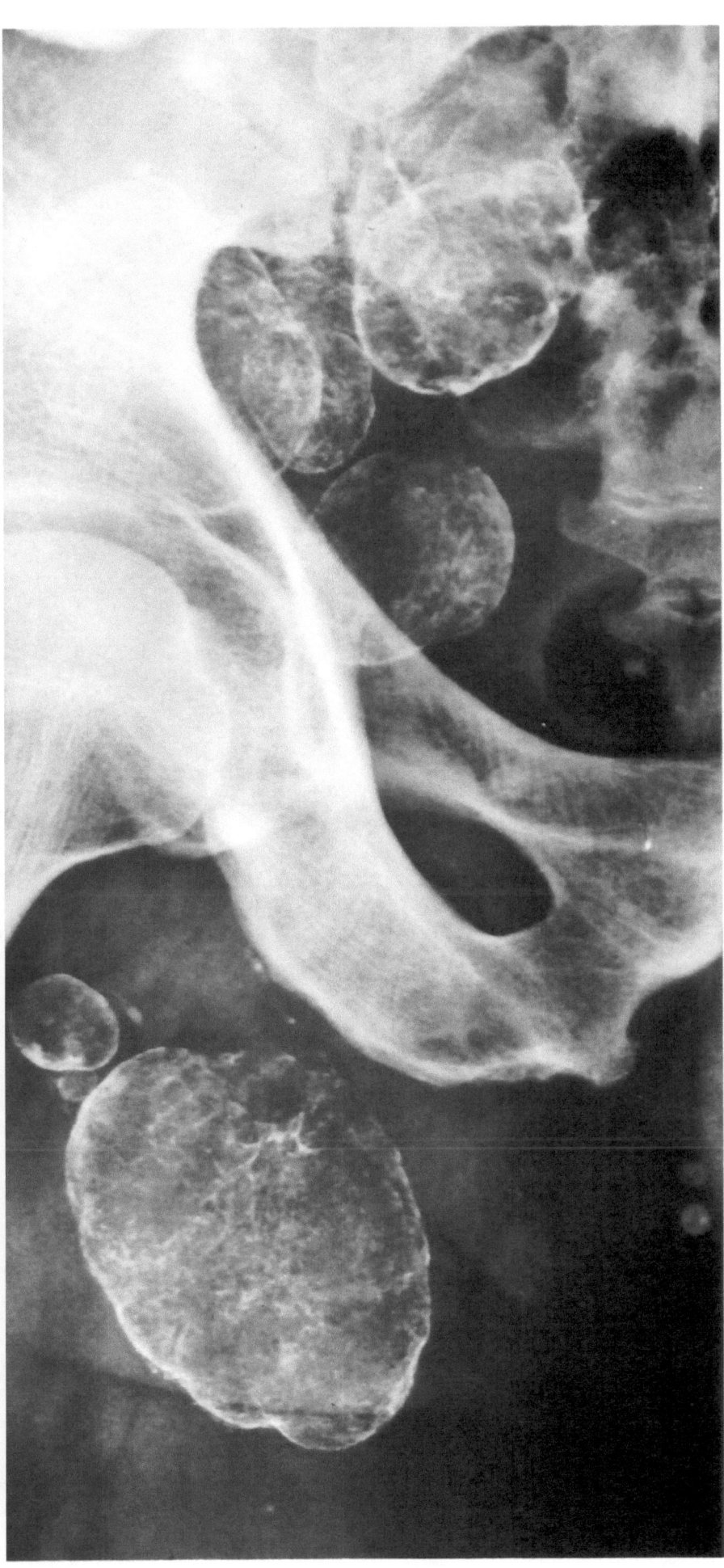

fig. 185 Whipple's disease; lymphadenogram.

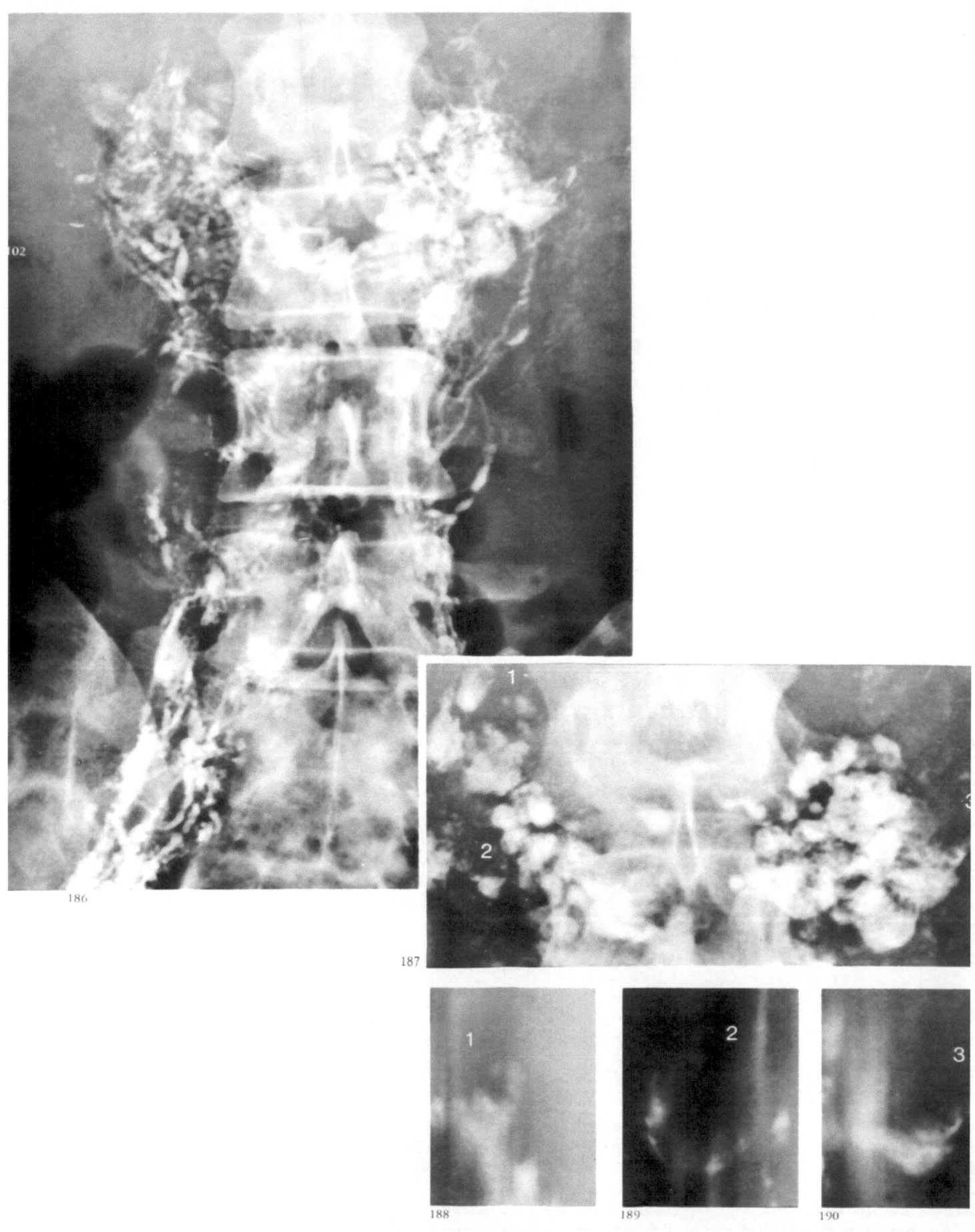

102

186

187

1

2

3

188 1

189 2

190 3

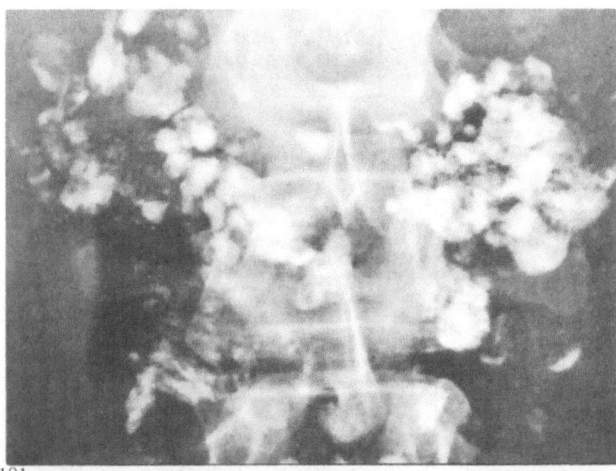

191

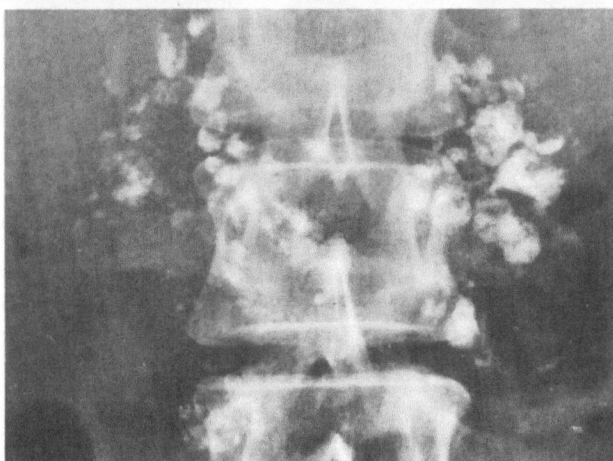

192

figs. 186-190 Reticulum cell sarcoma. Pathological paralumbar lymph nodes on lymphogram (fig. 186) and lymphadenogram (fig. 187). Lymph nodes could not be evaluated due to superposition: (1), (2) and (3). The tomograms (figs. 188, 189, 190) clarify the situation and the roentgenological diagnosis reticulum cell sarcoma could be established.

figs. 191 and 192 Reticulum cell sarcoma; lymphadenograms before and after radiation therapy.

figs. 193-197 Reticulum cell sarcoma. Pathological lymph nodes on lymphadenogram (fig. 193), (a), (b), (c) and (d) among others, appeared on the tomograms (figs. 194, 195, 196 and 197) to be lymph nodes with the typical structural changes characteristic of reticulum cell sarcoma.

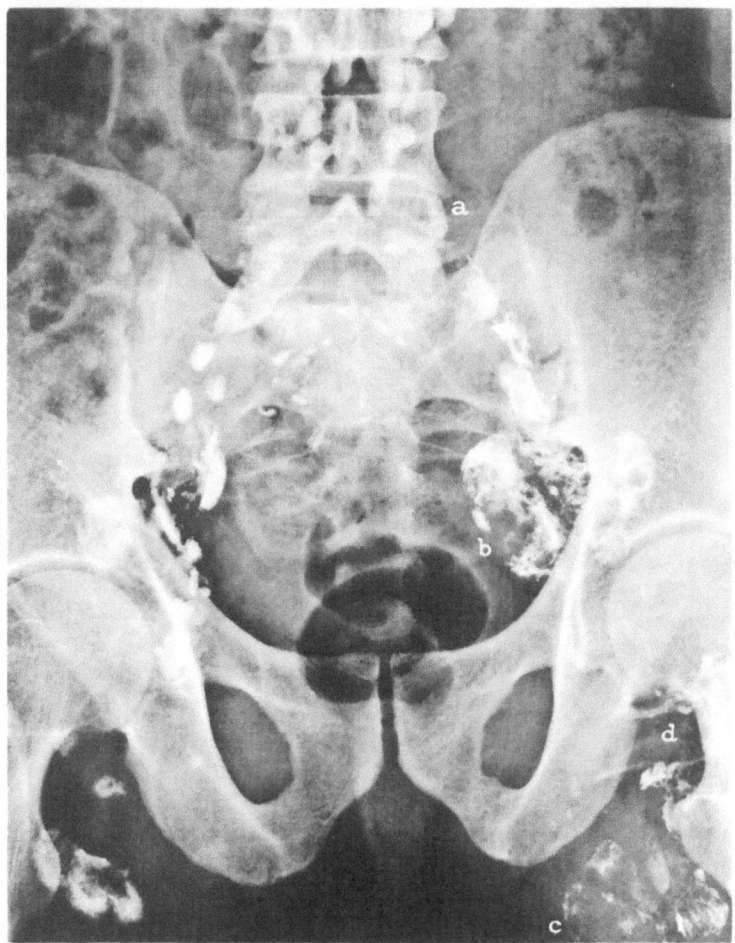

193

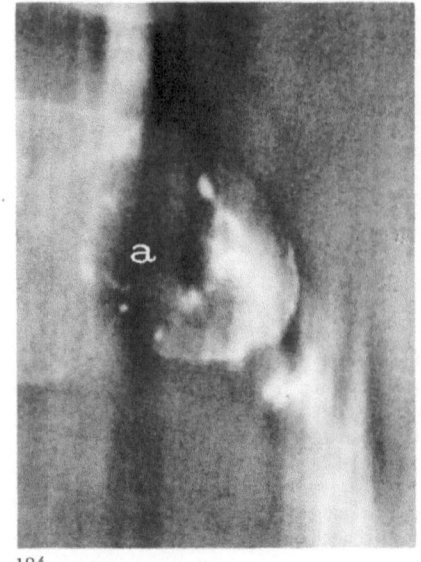

194

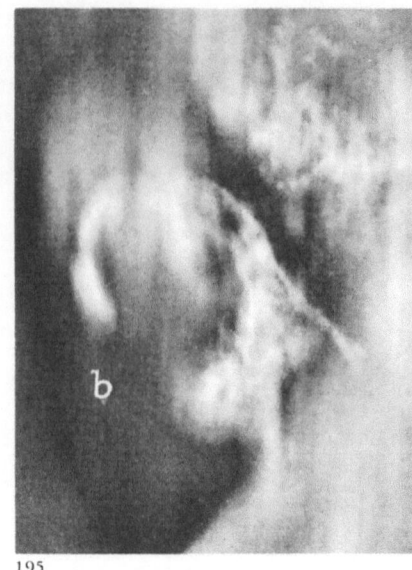

195

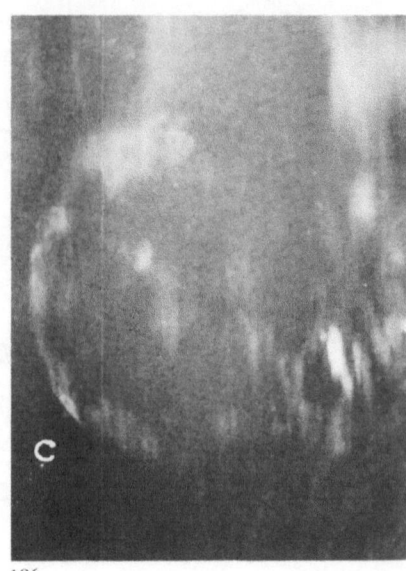

196

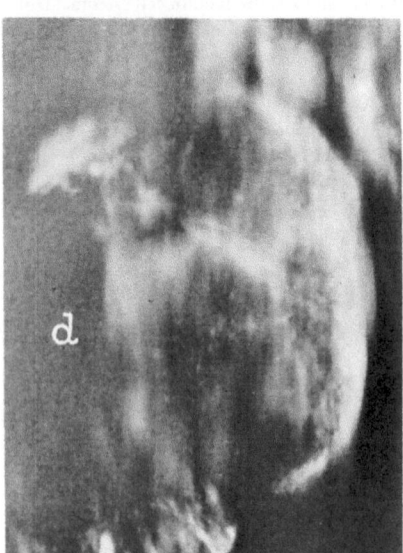

197

fig. 198-203 Reticulum cell sarcoma. On the lymphogram (fig. 198) and lymphadenogram (fig. 199) a configuration is visible in the right paralumbar region which must result from a greatly enlarged involved pathological lymph node or a peculiar arrangement of normal nodes. Tomograms (figs. 200, 201) provide no clarification. The normal cavogram (anteroposterior and lateral: figs. 202, 203) rules out a large pathological lymph node. Roentgenological diagnosis: normal lymphogram. Confirmed at autopsy.

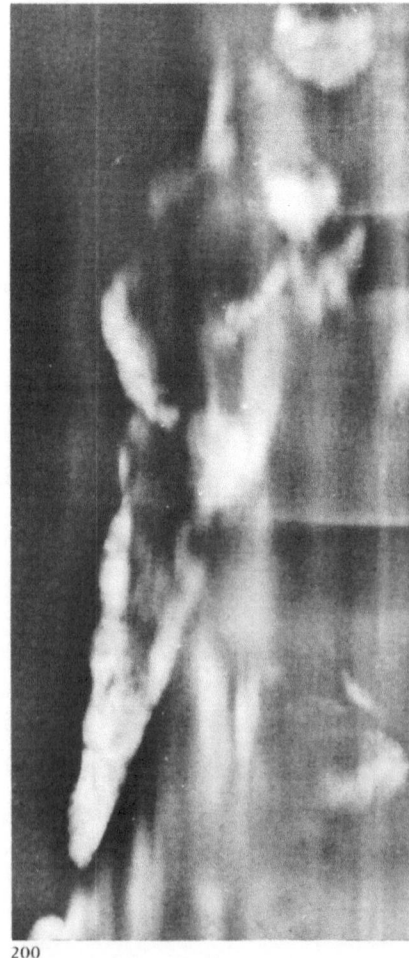

200

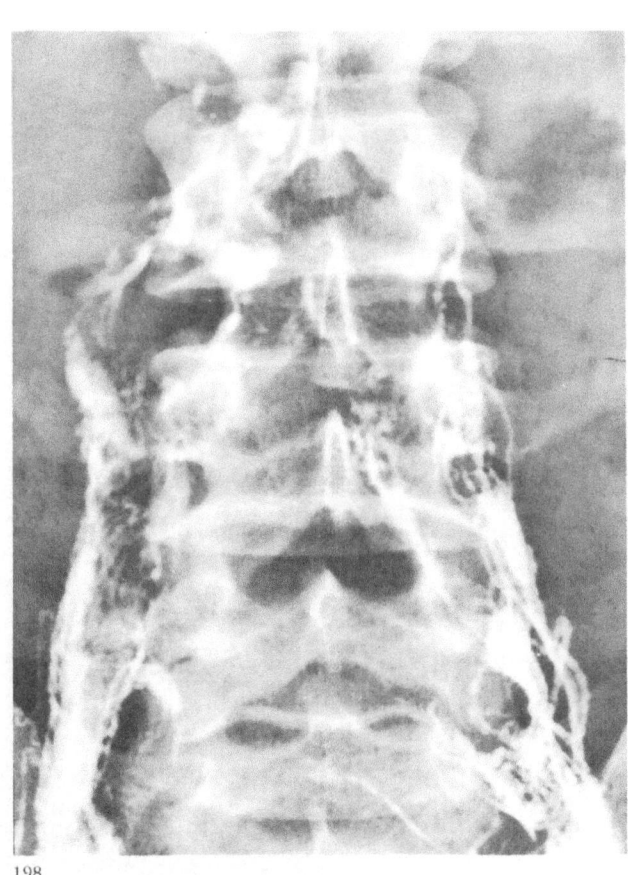

198

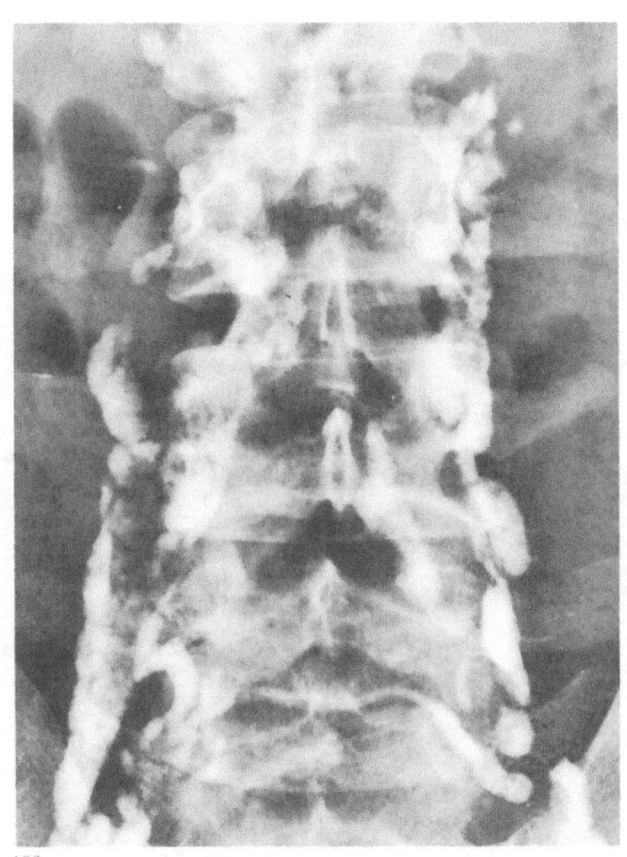

199

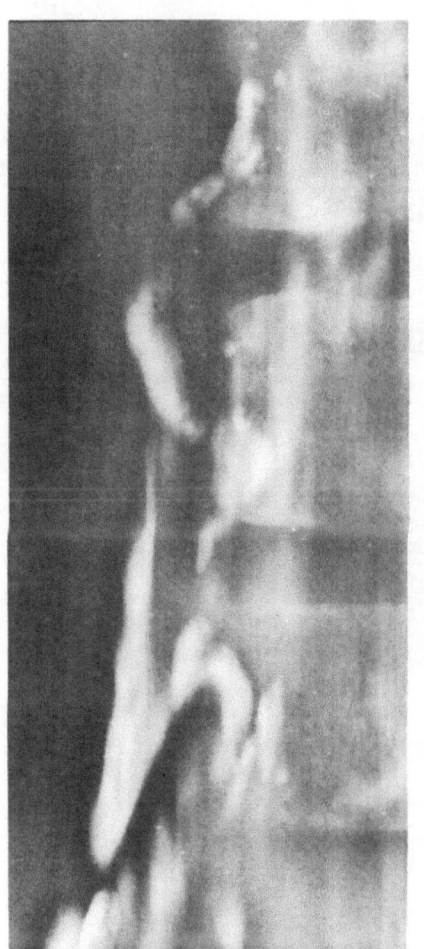

201

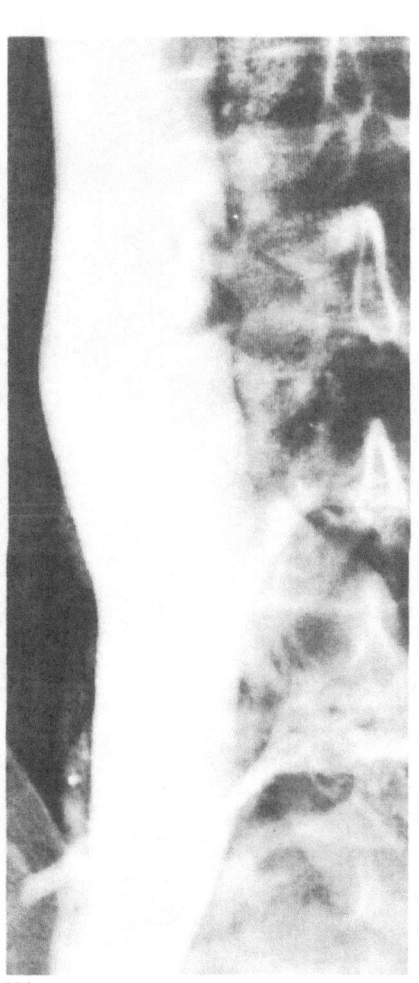

202

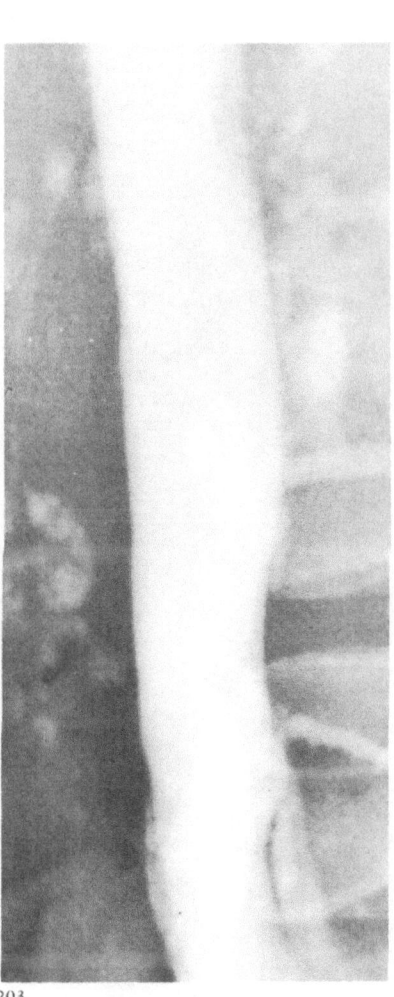

203

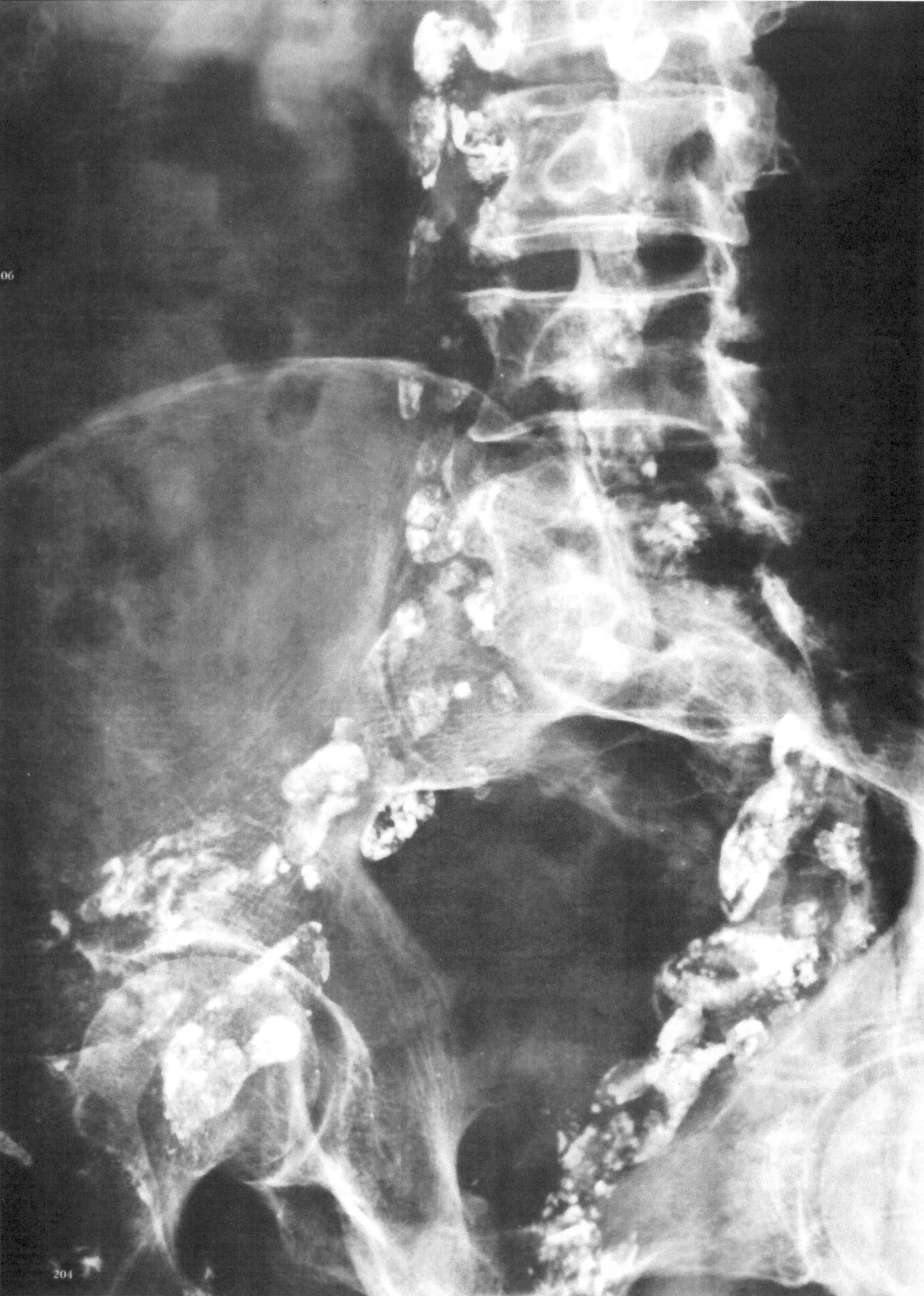

fig. 204 Chronic lymphatic leukaemia; oblique lymphadenogram: typical pathologically affected lymph nodes.

fig. 205 Chronic lymphatic leukaemia; oblique lymphadenogram: typical greatly enlarged pathological lymph nodes.

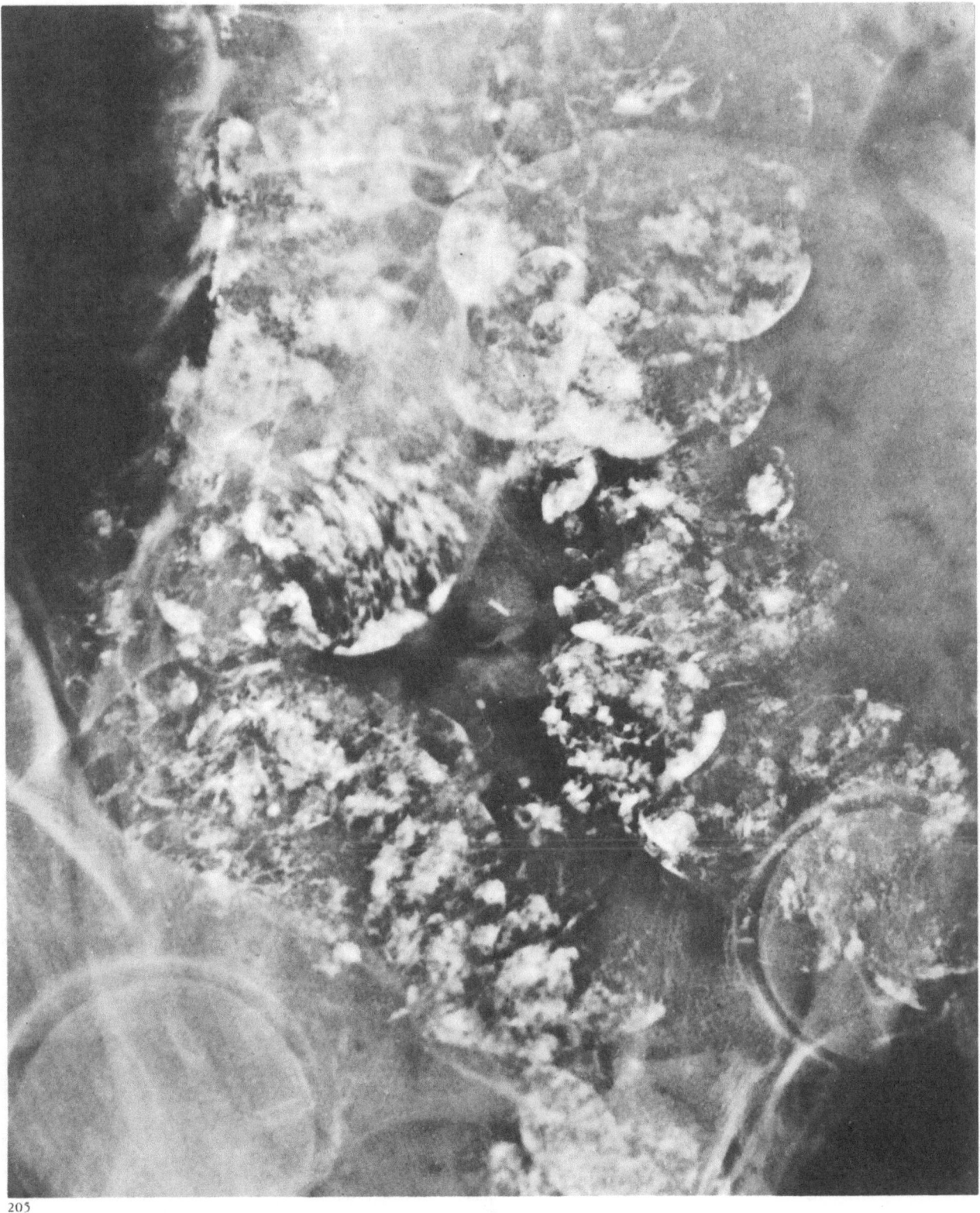

205

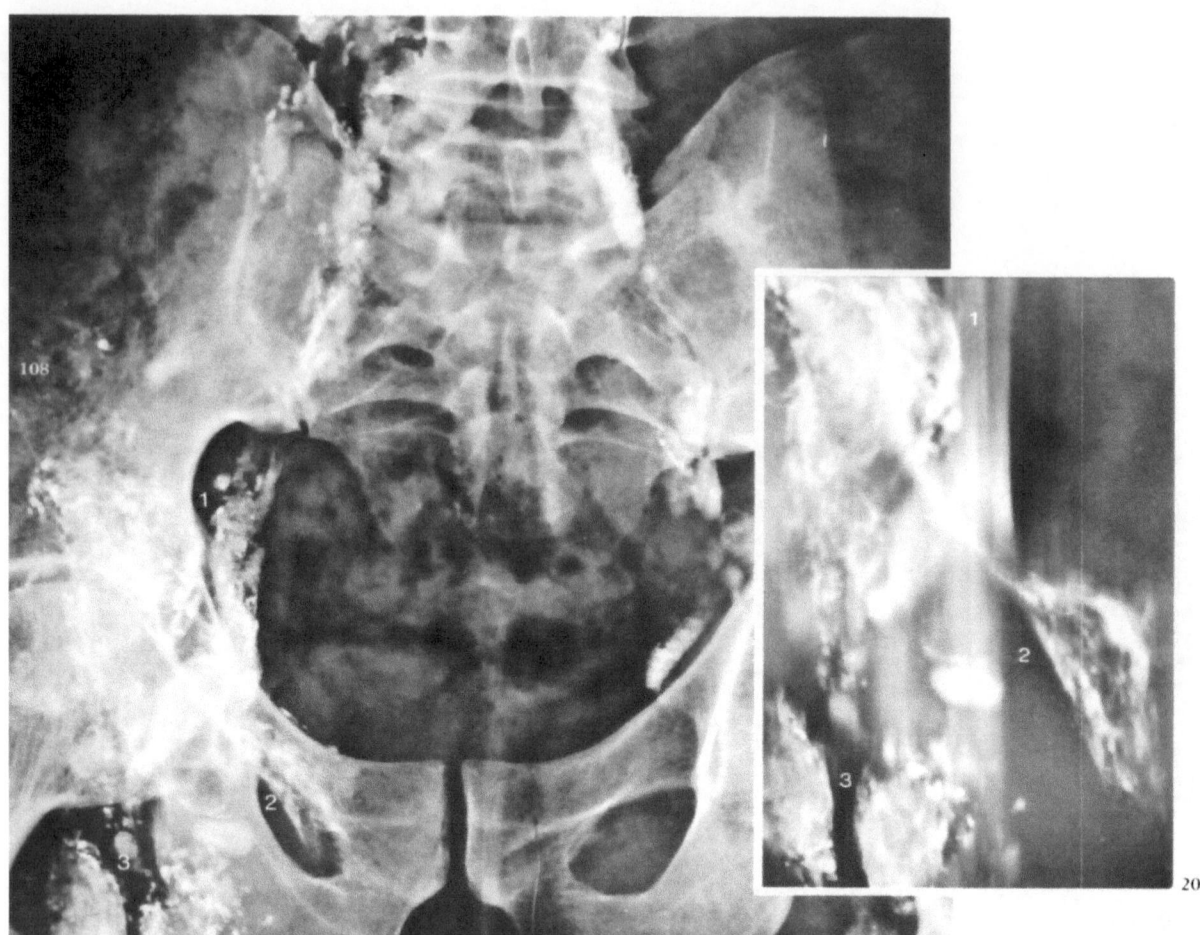

206

207

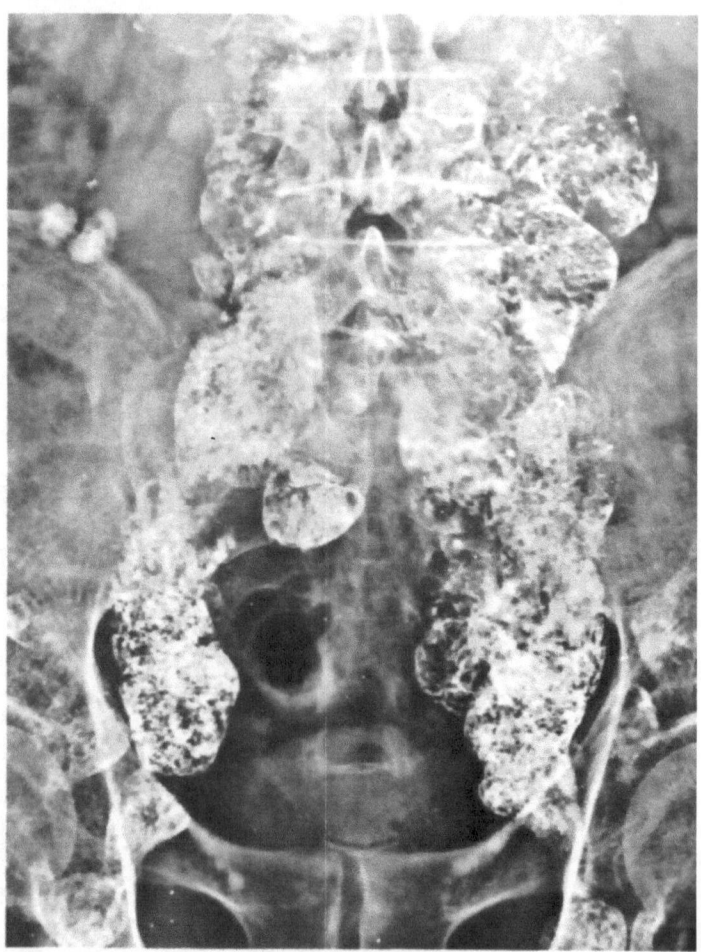

208

figs. 206 and 207 Chronic lymphatic leukaemia. Interpretation of pathological lymph nodes
on lymphadenogram (fig. 206) not possible due
to superposition over parts of the skeleton, (1), (2)
and (3) among others. Clearly visible on tomogram (fig. 207).

figs. 208-210 Chronic lymphatic leukaemia;
lymphadenograms before radiation therapy (fig.
208), during radiation therapy (tumour dose 1500
r) (fig. 209) and after radiation therapy (tumour
dose 3000 r.) (fig. 210).

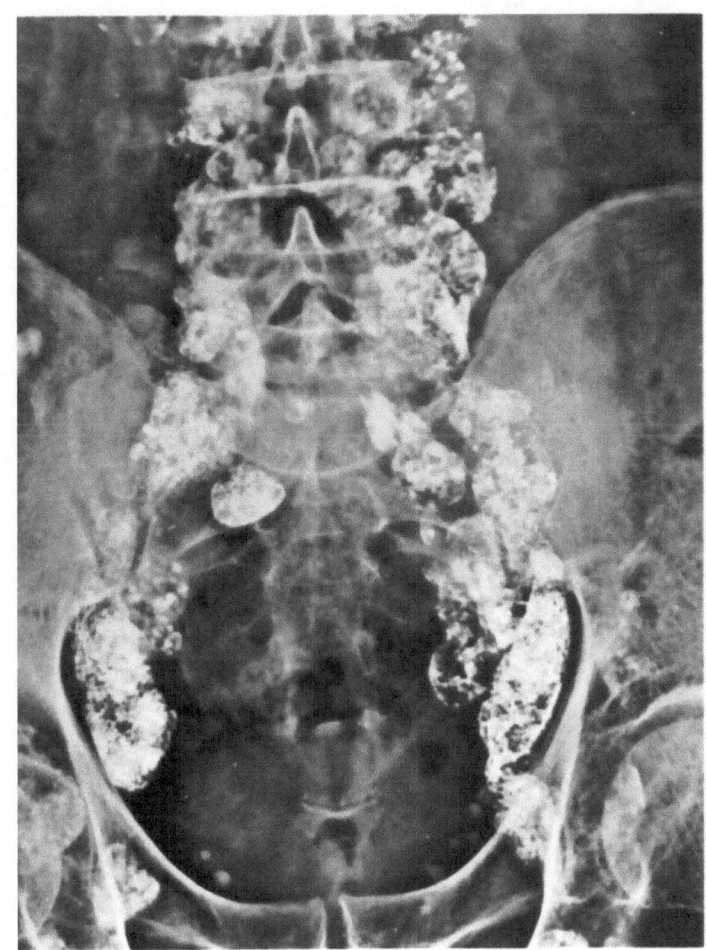

209

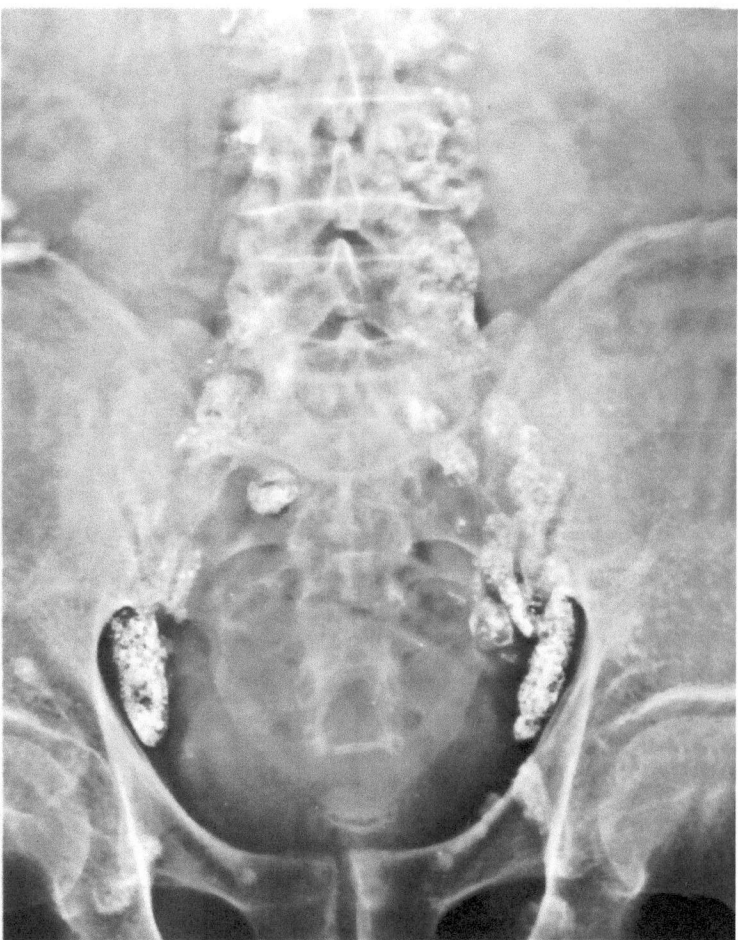

210

fig. 211 Lymphosarcoma; lymphadenogram: all lymph nodes in pelvis and abdomen involved; lymph nodes moderately enlarged.

fig. 212 Lymphosarcoma; lymphadenogram: greater enlargement of lymph nodes than in fig. 211.

fig. 213 and 214 Lymphosarcoma; lymphogram and lymphadenogram: localizations in left pelvis minor.

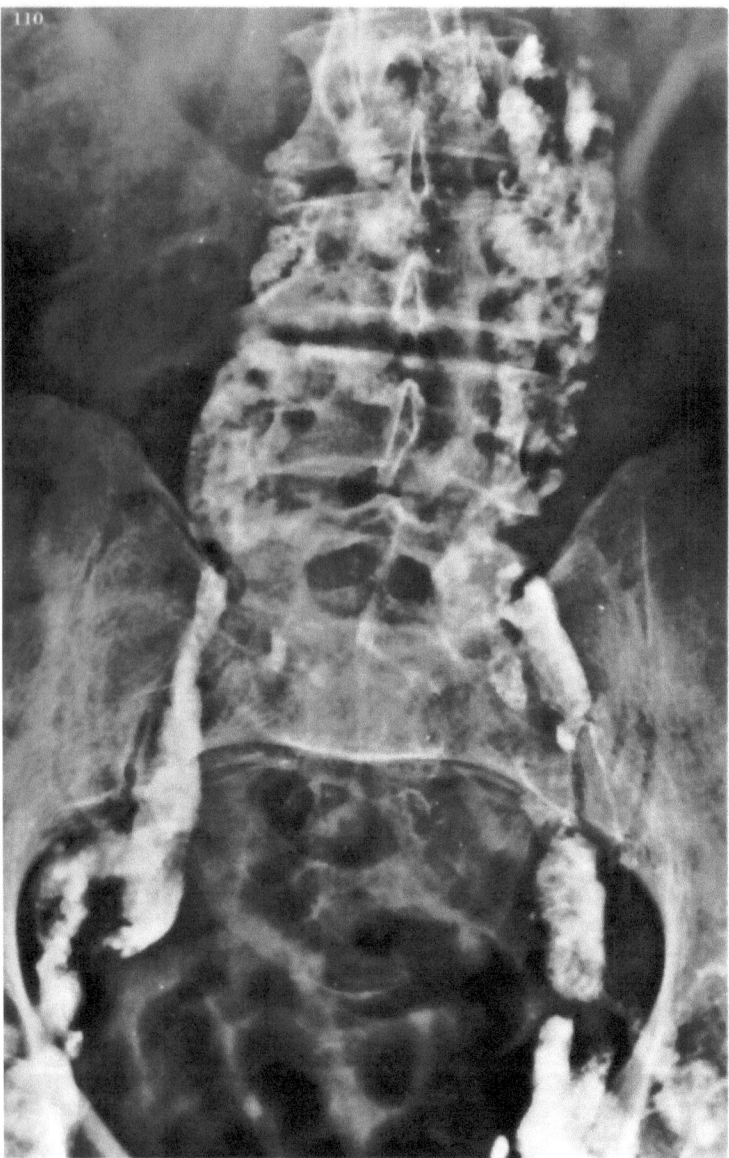

211

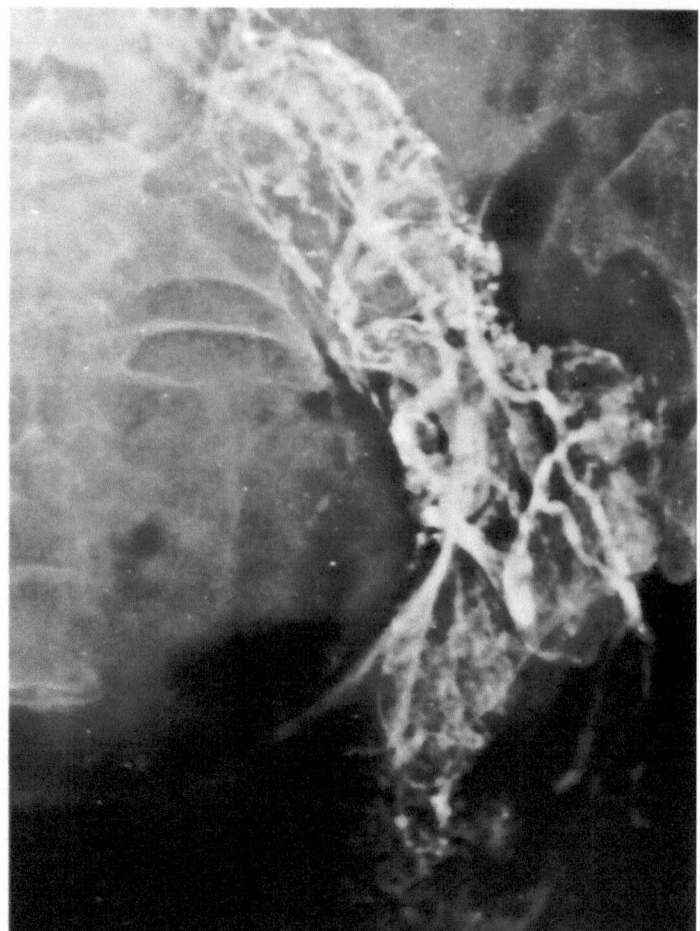

213

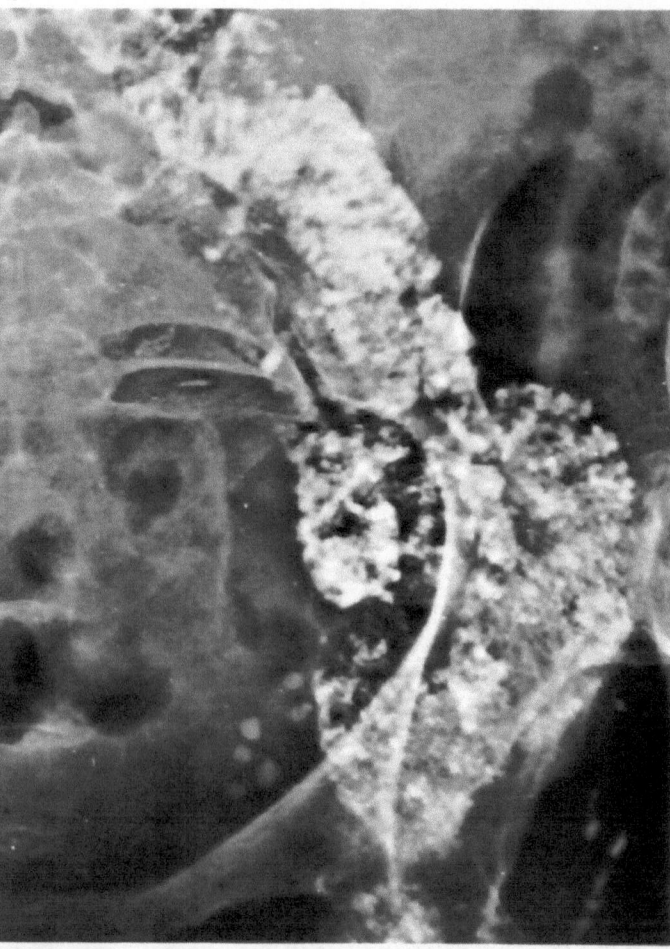

214

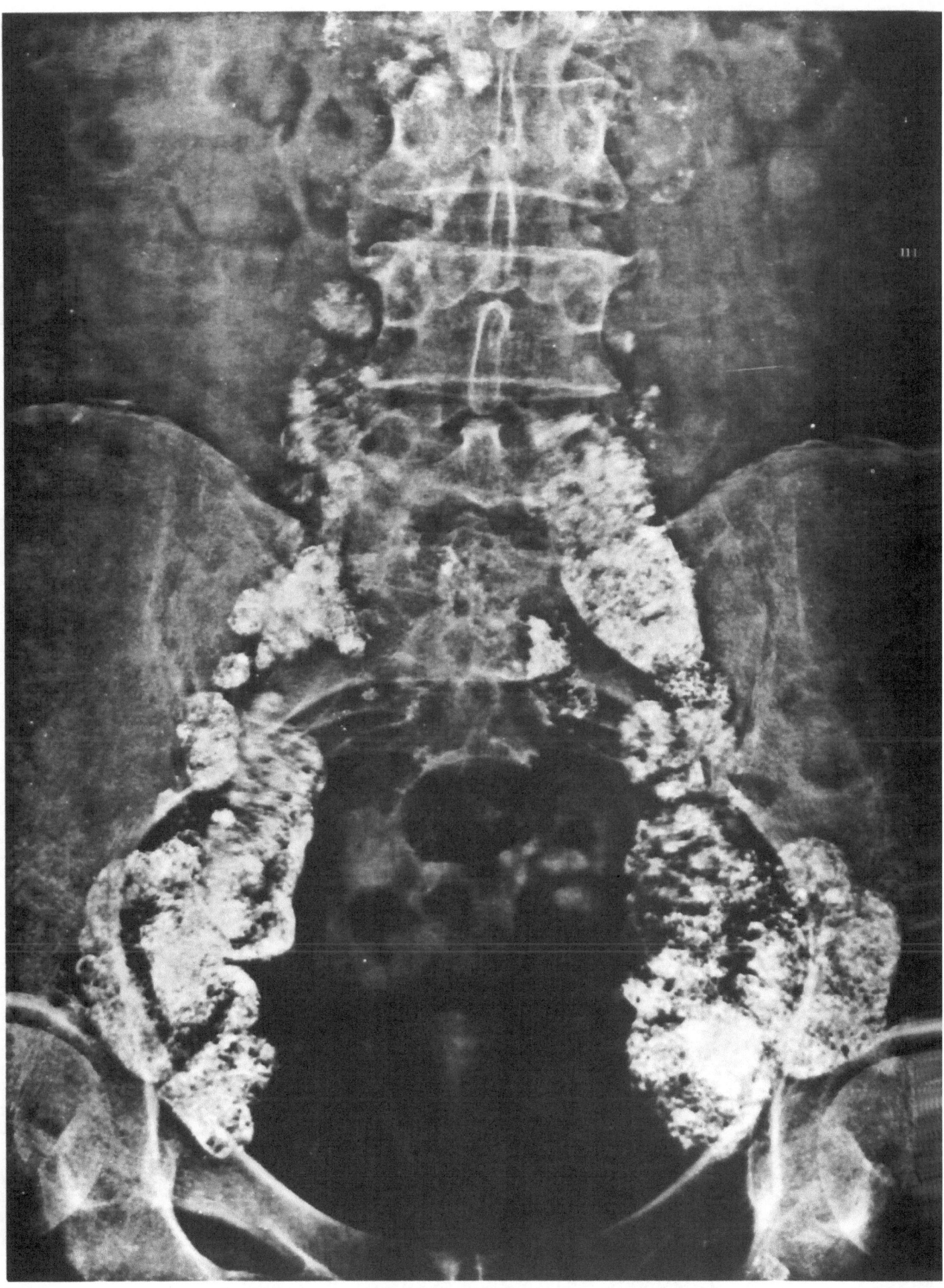

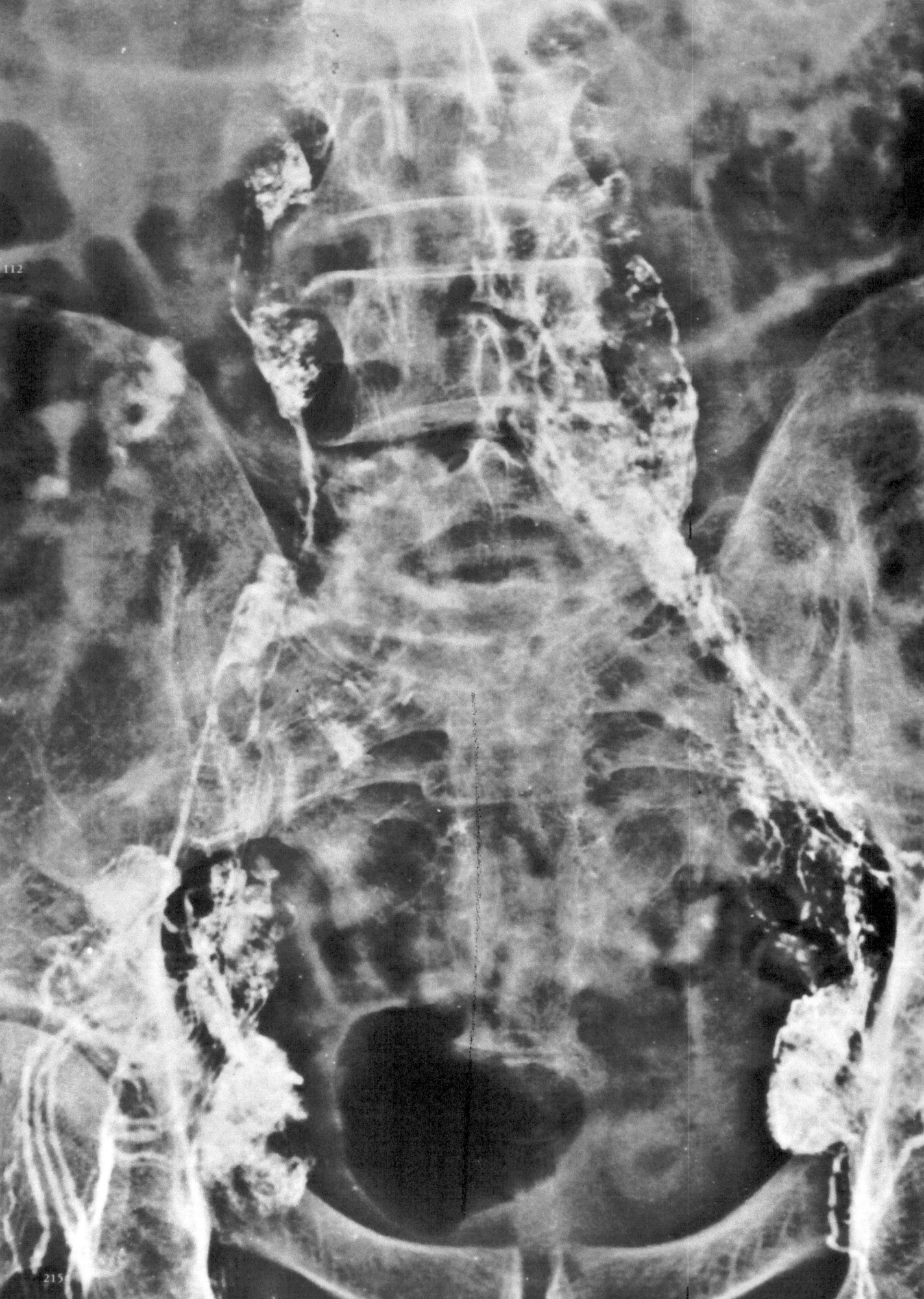

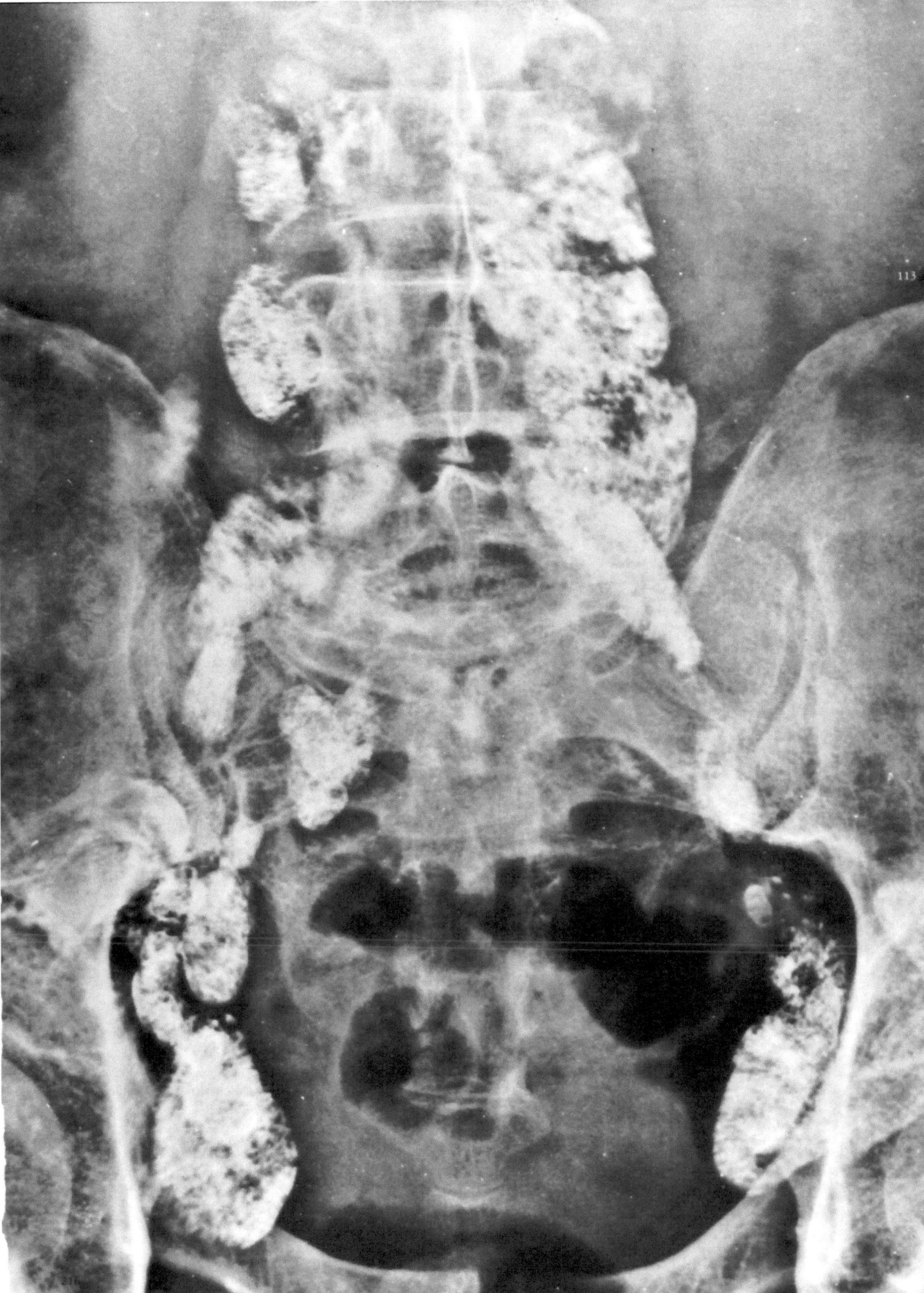

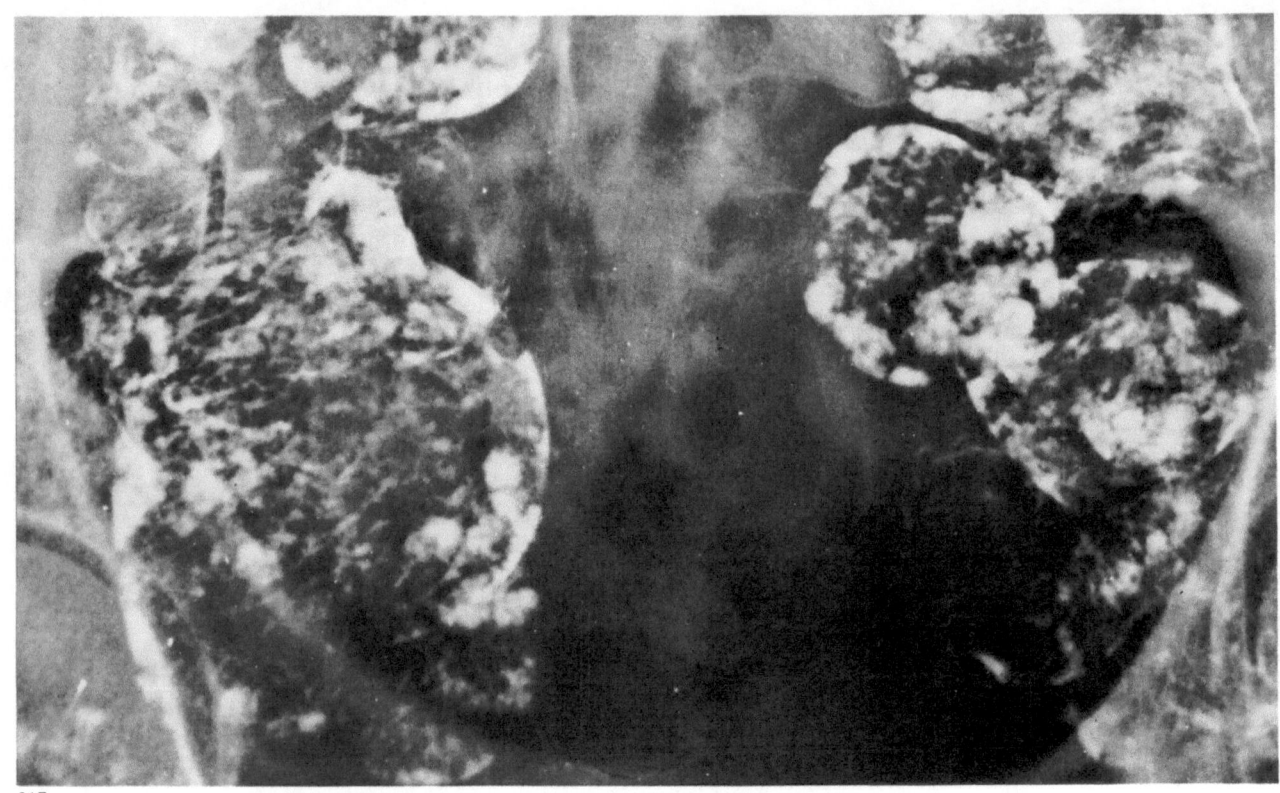

217

fig. 217 Lymphosarcoma; lymphadenogram:
greatly enlarged lymph nodes with partially interrupted marginal sinus.

fig. 218 Lymphosarcoma; lymphadenogram:
extensive localizations. Somewhat similar to fig.
205 (chronic lymphatic leukaemia), the lymph
node structure is however grosser.

on preceding pages 112 and 113
figs. 215 and 216 Lymphosarcoma; lymphogram and lymphadenogram.

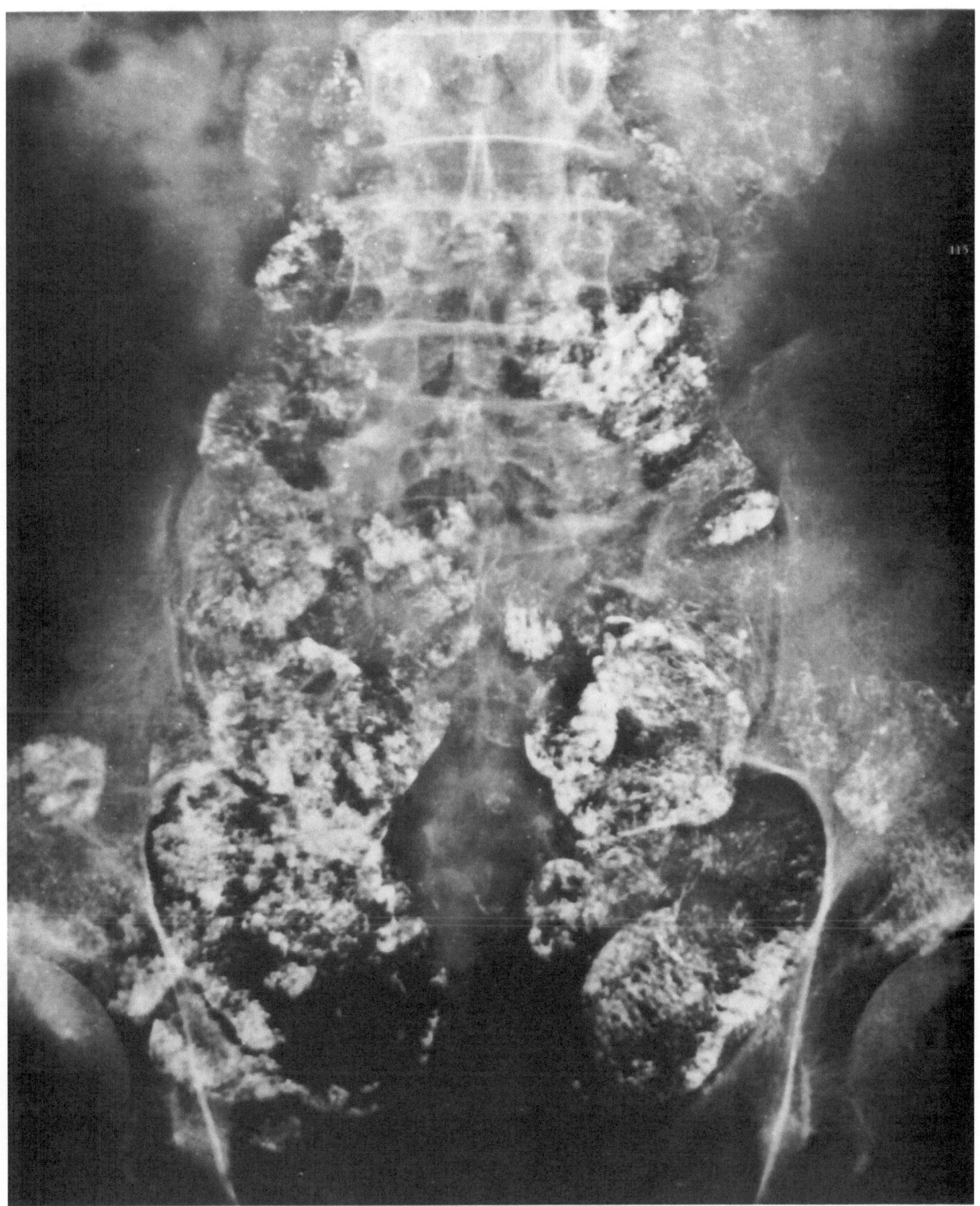

116

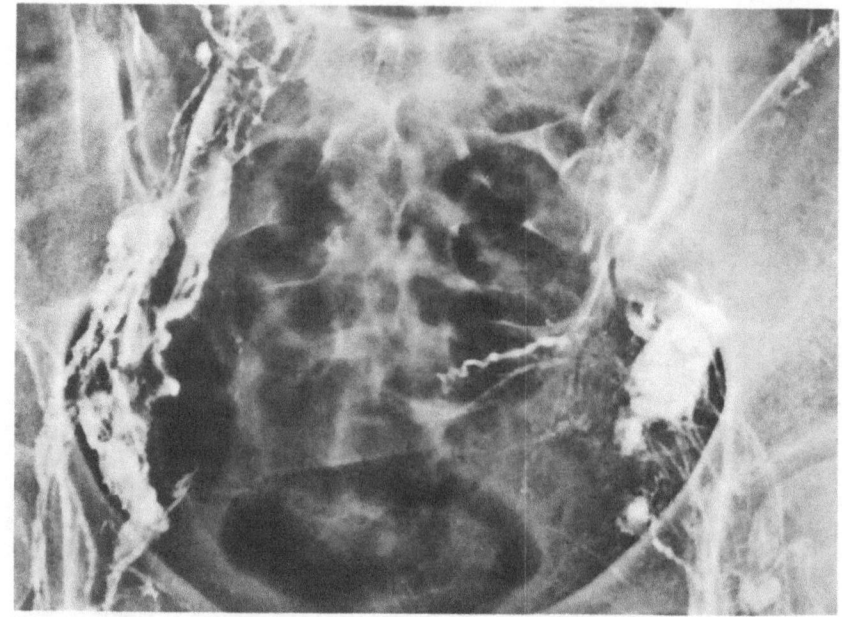

219

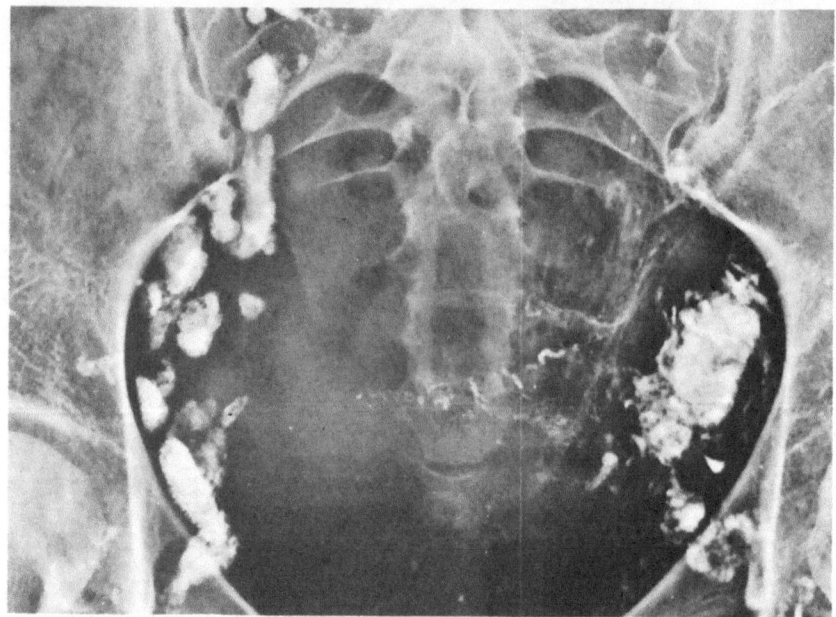

220

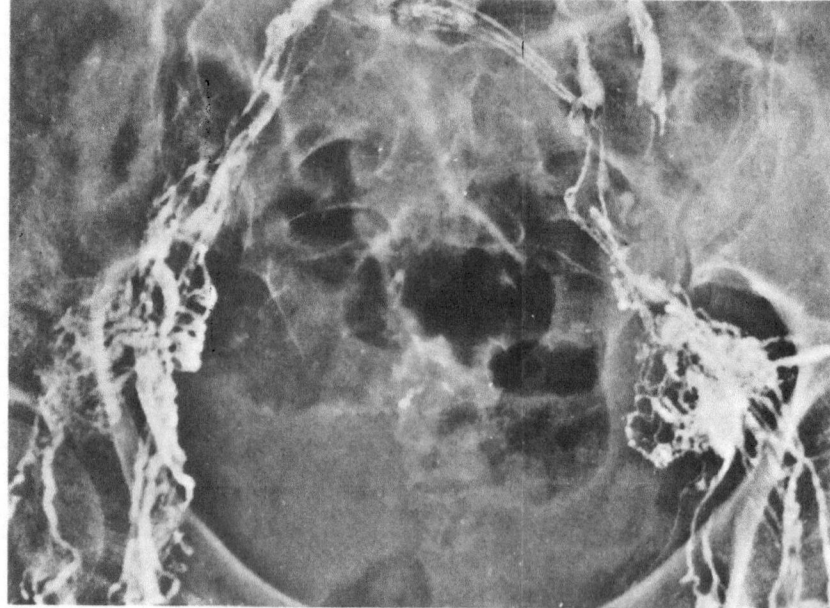

221

fig. 219-224 Carcinoma of the cervix uteri; lymphograms and lymphadenograms: 3 patients with extensive metastases in the left para-iliac region, drainage obstruction on the lymphadenograms and collateral lymphatics on the lymphograms. For patients 1 (figs. 219, 220) and 3 (figs. 223, 224), the lymphographic results agreed with the clinical. For patient 2 (figs. 221, 222), metastases were not suspected clinically.

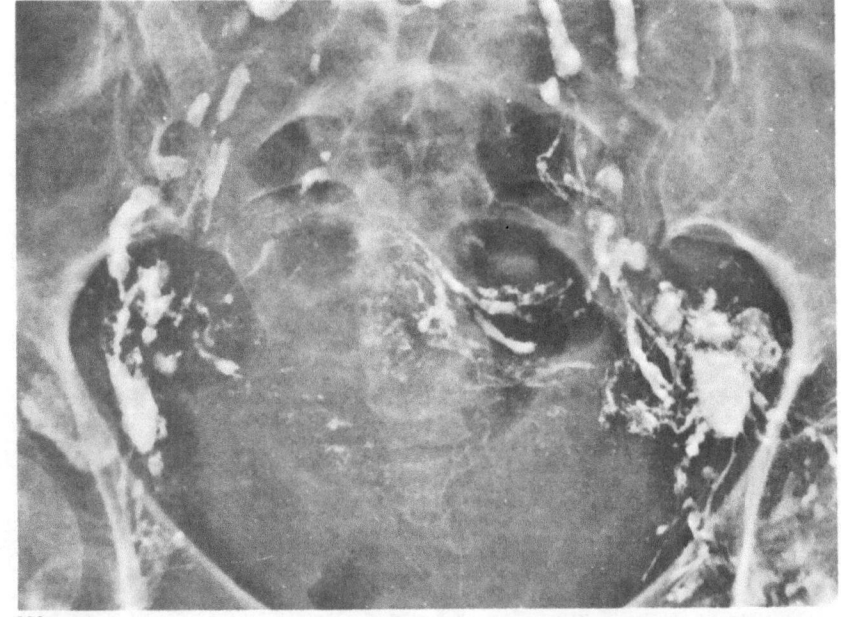

222

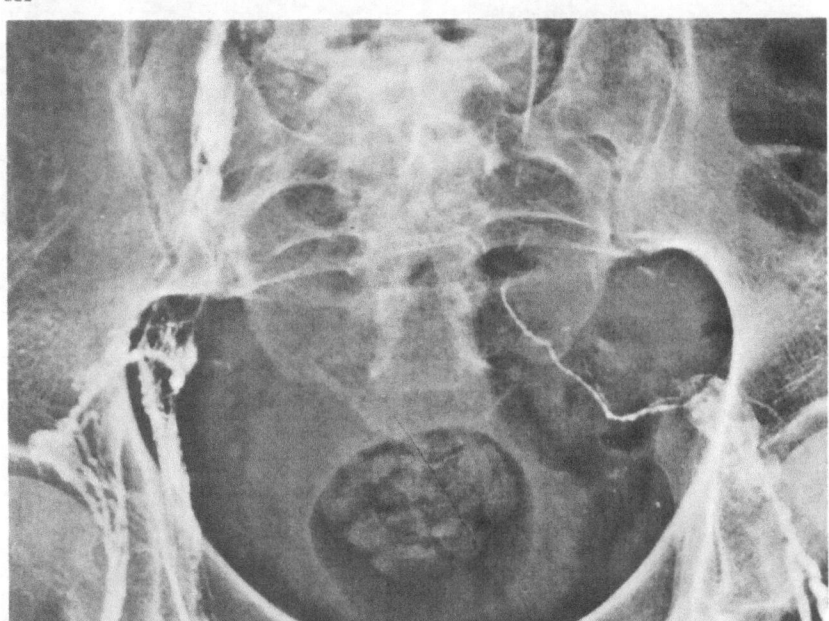

223

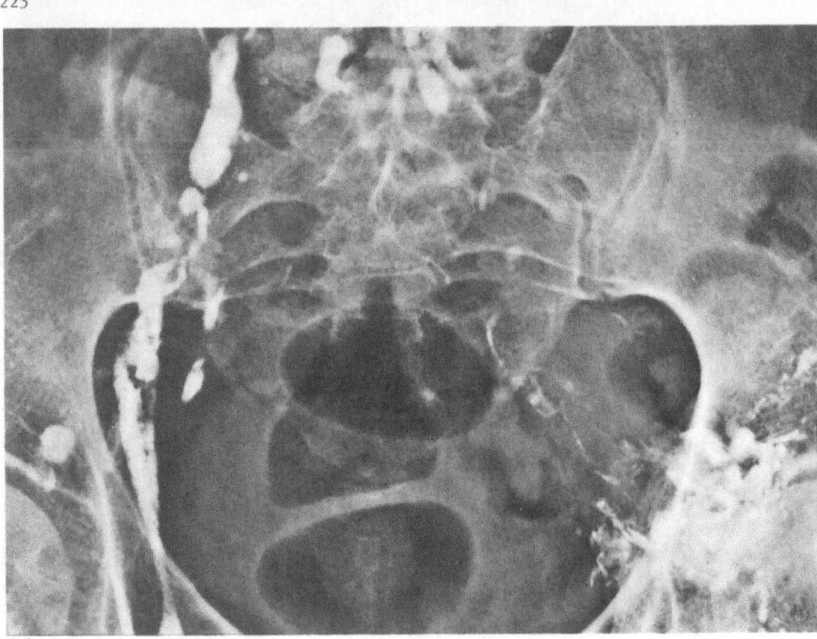

224

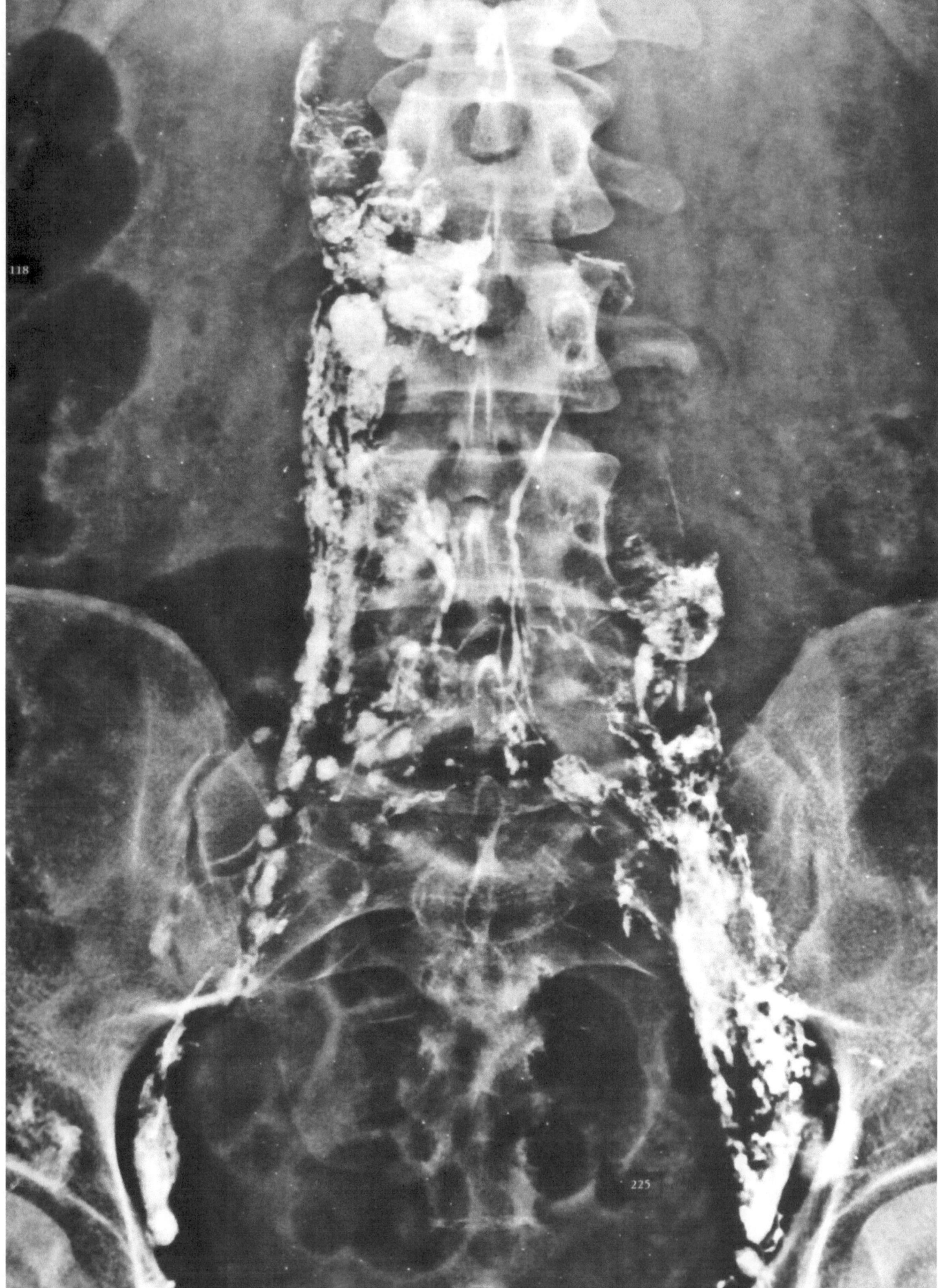

figs. 226-229 Carcinoma of the cervix uteri; lymphadenogram (fig. 226) and tomogram (fig. 227) show an interruption of the lymph node chain in the right paralumbar region. All visible lymph nodes are normal. Supplementary anteroposterior cavogram (fig. 228) also reveals no abnormalities; the lateral exposure of the vena cava reveals an indentation on the ventral side due to a pathological lymph node mass at the location of the interruption in the lymphatic chain. (fig. 229). Confirmed after surgery and pathological-anatomical examination.

fig. 225 Carcinoma of the cervix uteri; lymphadenogram: extensive metastases, especially in the right and left paralumbar regions.

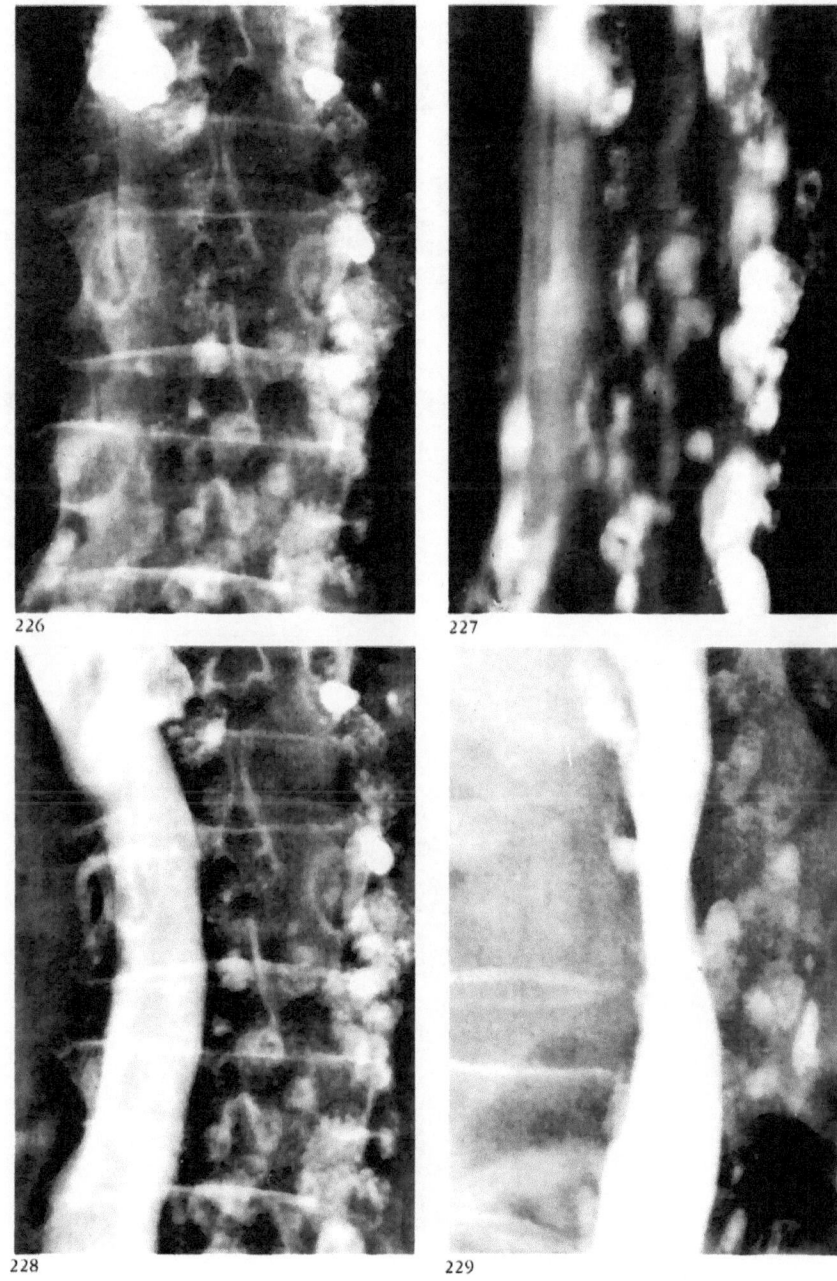

226

227

228

229

figs. 230 and 231 Carcinoma of the cervix uteri; An empty area above obstruction of the lymphatic system. Total block in the lower right iliac region on the lymphadenogram (fig. 230). The vena iliaca externa (fig. 231) narrows just above the last filled lymph nodes and arches out in a medial direction because of pathological lymph node masses.

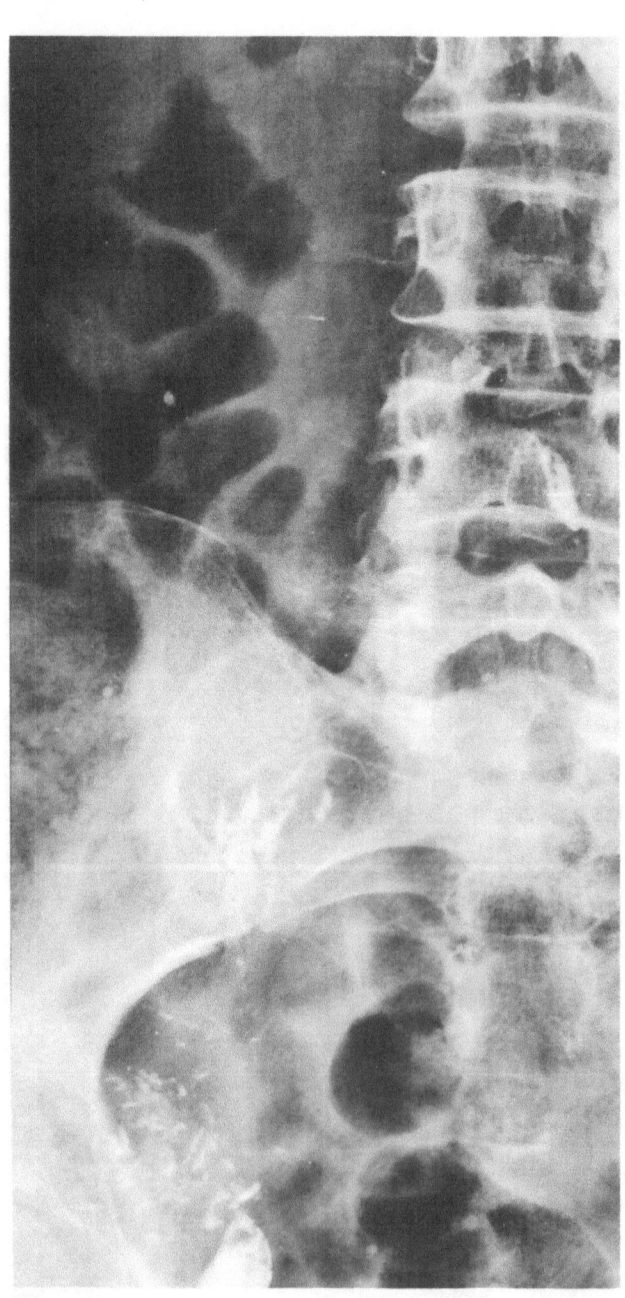

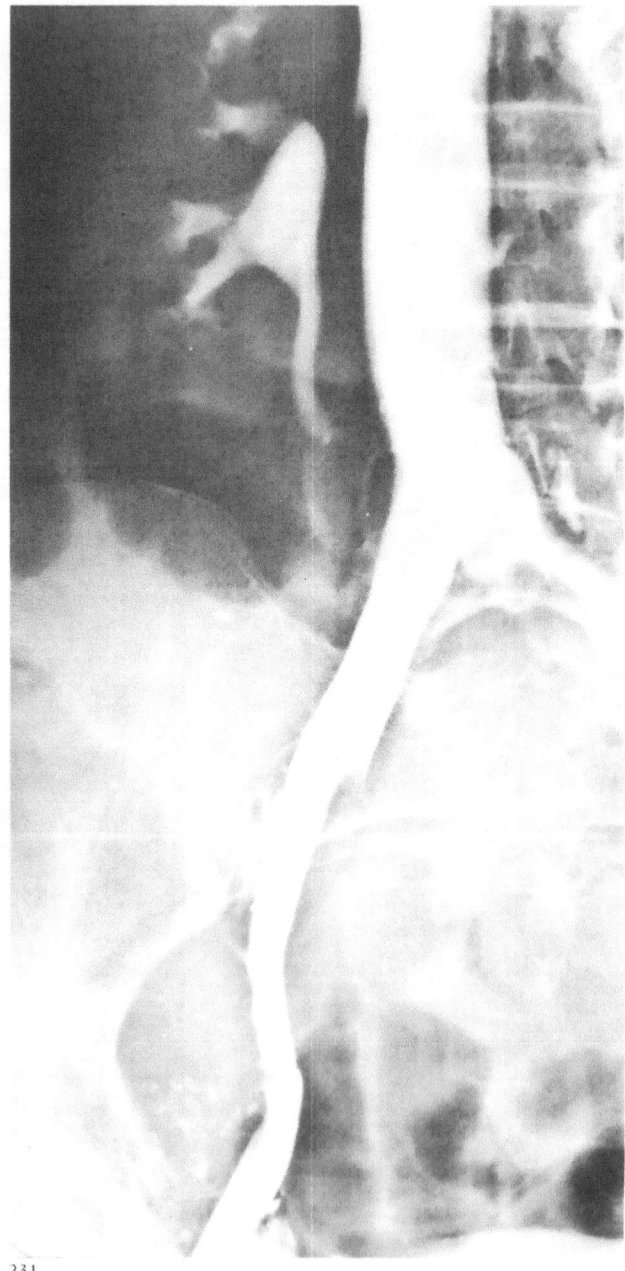

230   231

fig. 232 Carcinoma of the cervix uteri; Lymph nodes outside the drainage area. Aortography: above the obstruction seen on the lymphogram, displacement and narrowing of the arteria iliaca interna (as well as the arteria iliaca externa et communis) due to pathological lymph node masses are visible.

figs. 223-239 Carcinoma of the cervix uteri; Anteroposterior (fig. 233), oblique (fig. 234) and lateral (fig. 235) lymphadenograms of an apparently enlarged lymph node involved by metastases in the paralumbar region. Tomograms (figs. 236, 237, 238, 239) of this lymph node (sections at 10, 10½, 11, 11½ cm., respectively): first an elongated lymph node (1), then two oval round lymph nodes (2) and (3), and finally several small spots of contrast medium. Roentgenologically there is no question of involvement by metastases but instead a misleading superposition of normal lymph nodes.

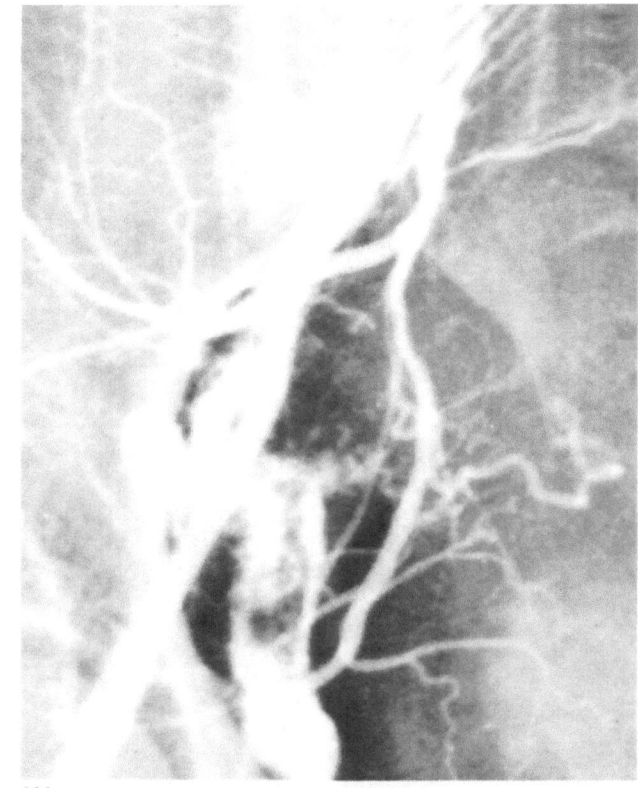

232

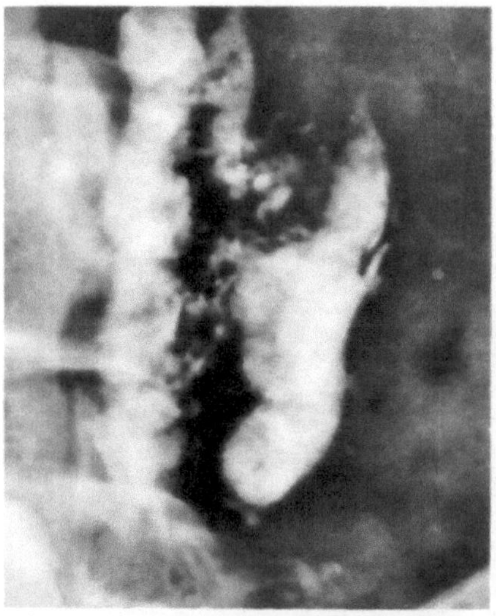

121

233

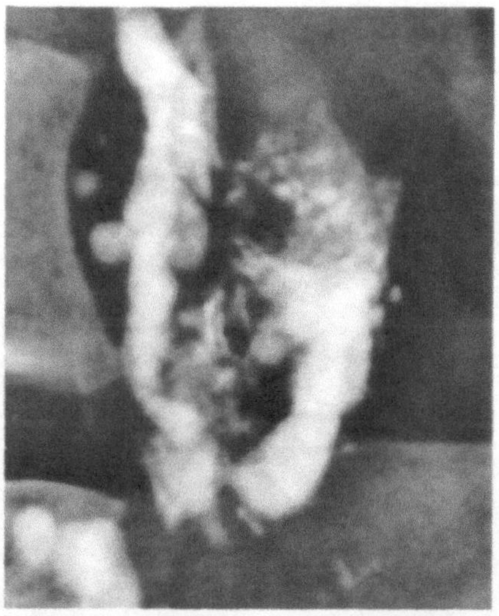

234

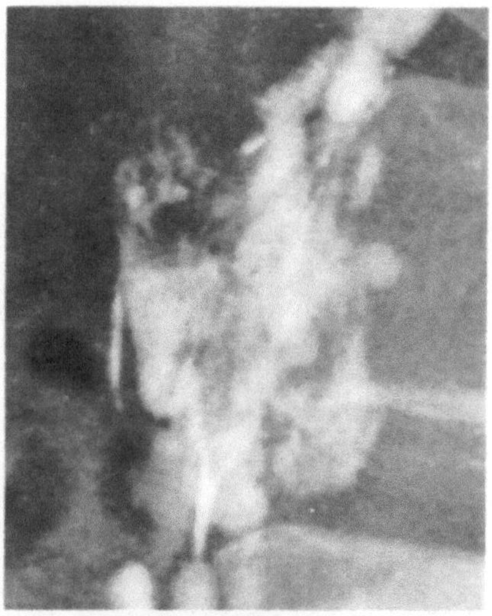

235

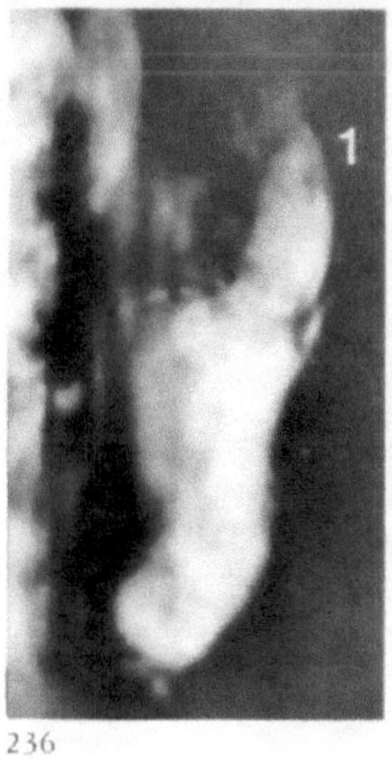

236

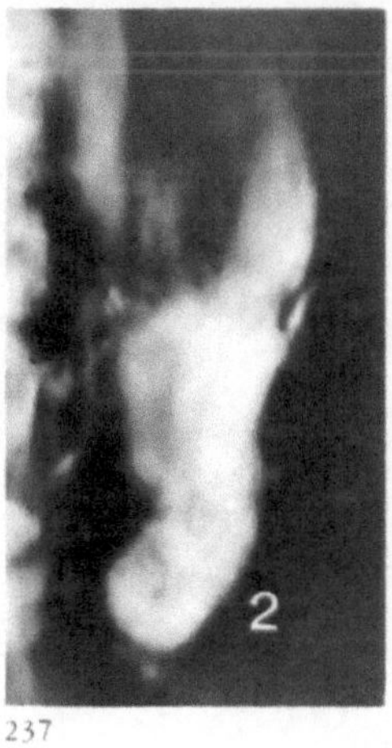

237

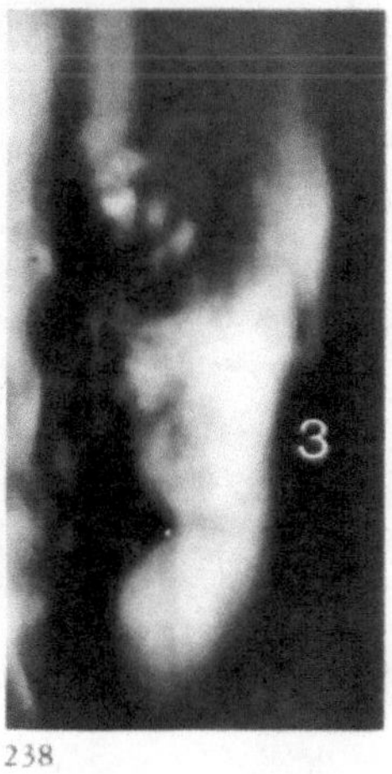

238

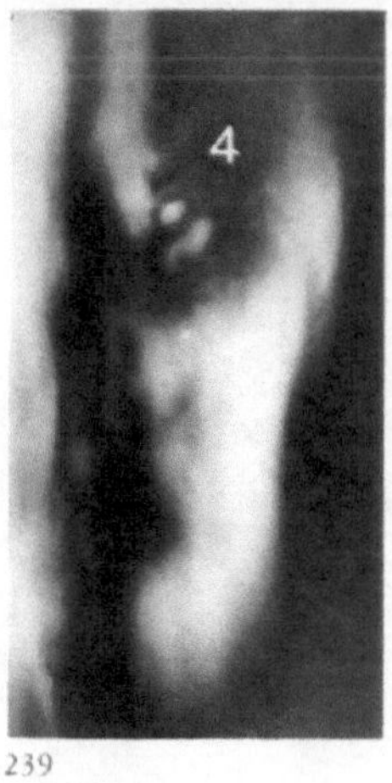

239

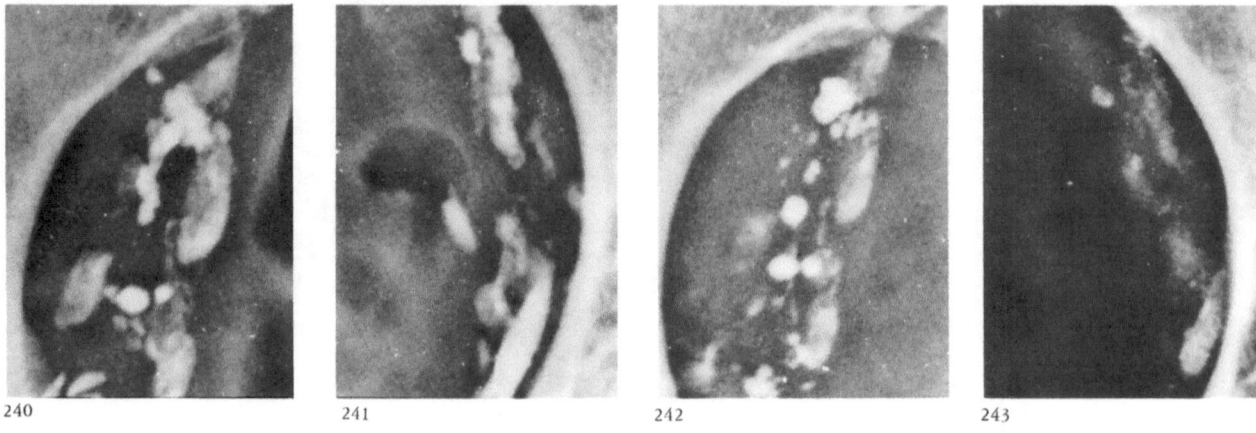

240   241   242   243

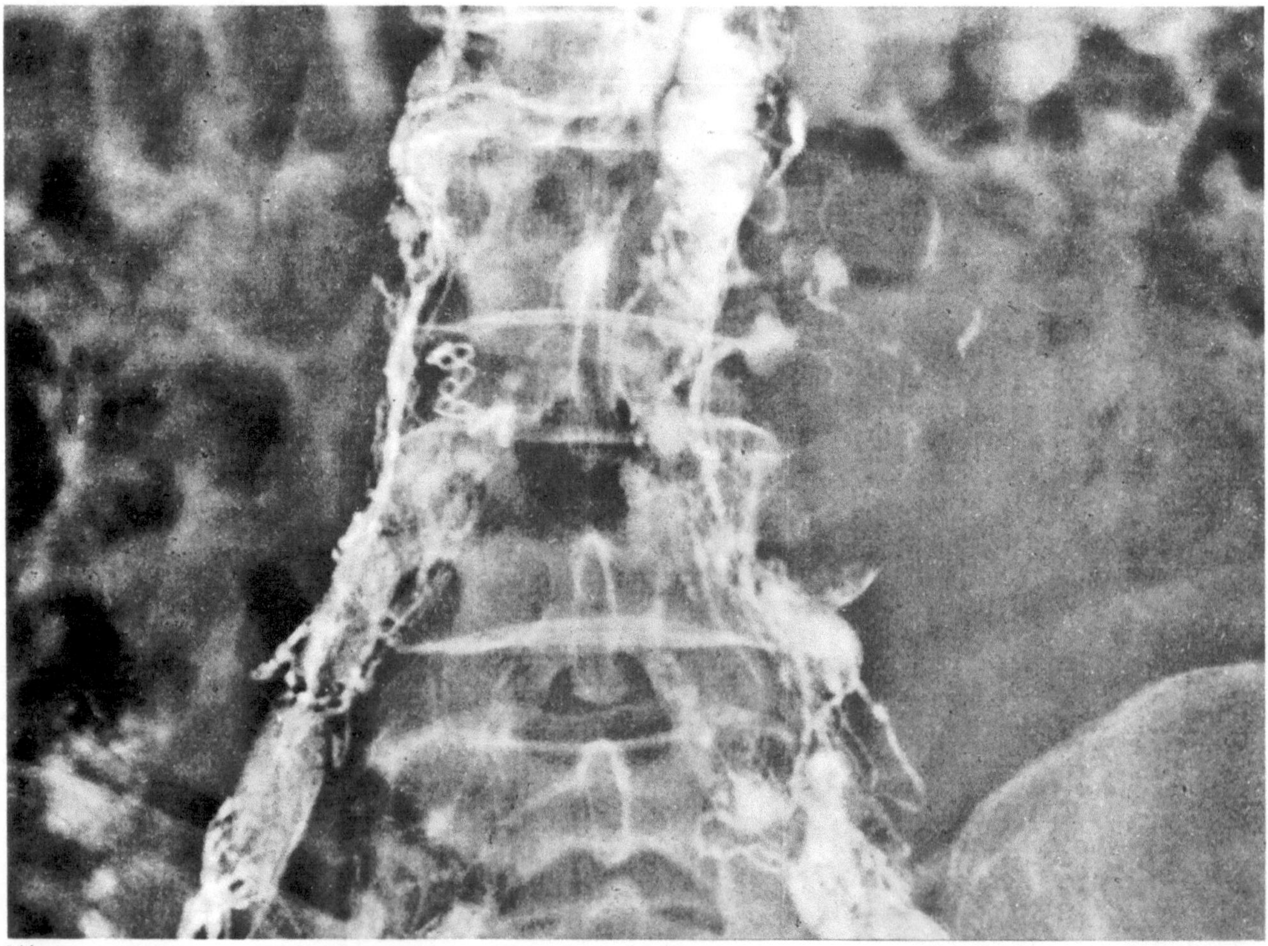

244

figs. 240-243 Carcinoma of the cervix uteri;
Normal lymph nodes in the left and right para-
iliac regions on the lymphadenograms (figs. 240,
241). Films taken of the same area at the end of
the operation (figs. 242, 243) whereby total
lymph node excision was carried out.
Comment: It is obvious therefore that in practice an adequate total lymph node excision is
difficult without previous lymphographic examination and control films during the operation.

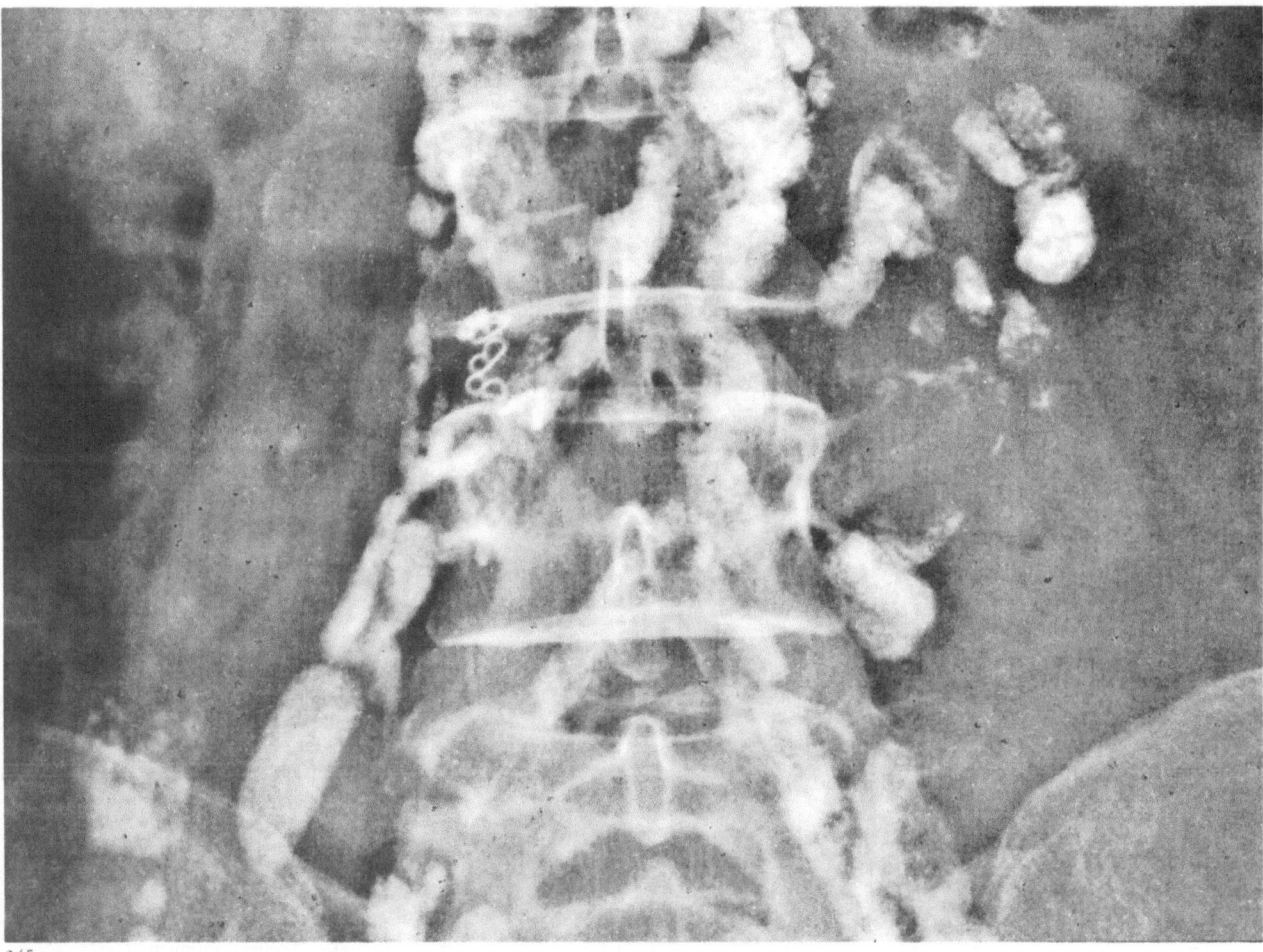

245

figs. 244 and 245 Carcinoma of the corpus uteri;
lymphogram and lymphadenogram: extensive
metastasizing in the left paralumbar region.

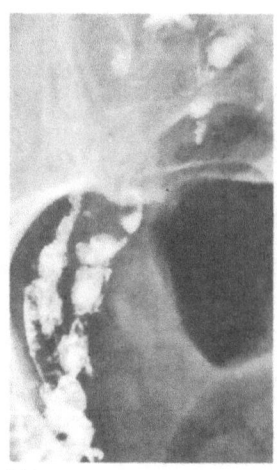
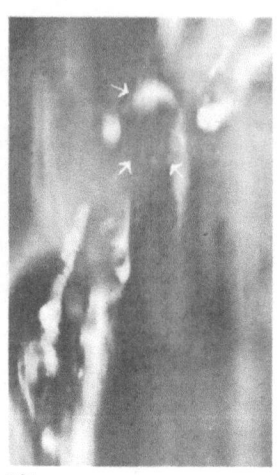

246   247

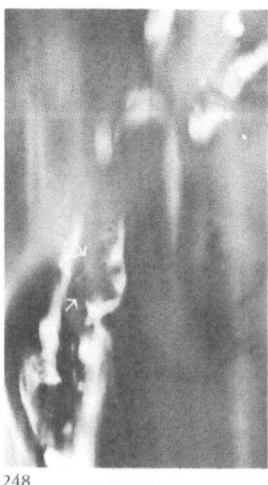
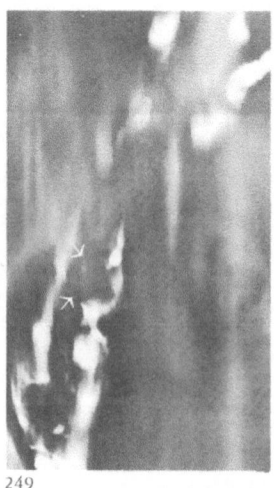

248   249

figs. 246-249 Carcinoma of the corpus uteri.
The lymphadenogram (fig. 246) shows an empty
area at the level of the arteria iliaca communis
bordered above and below by small lymph nodes.
It is not clear whether this region contains small
normal lymph nodes or partly involved large
lymph nodes. The tomograms (figs. 247, 248,
249) reveal not only small normal lymph nodes
but also several lymph nodes involved by metastases; the marginal sinus of the latter is mostly
broken (→). Confirmed after surgery and pathological-anatomical examination.

fig. 250 Ovarian carcinoma; lymphadenogram:
extensive metastasizing in the right and left paralumbar regions.

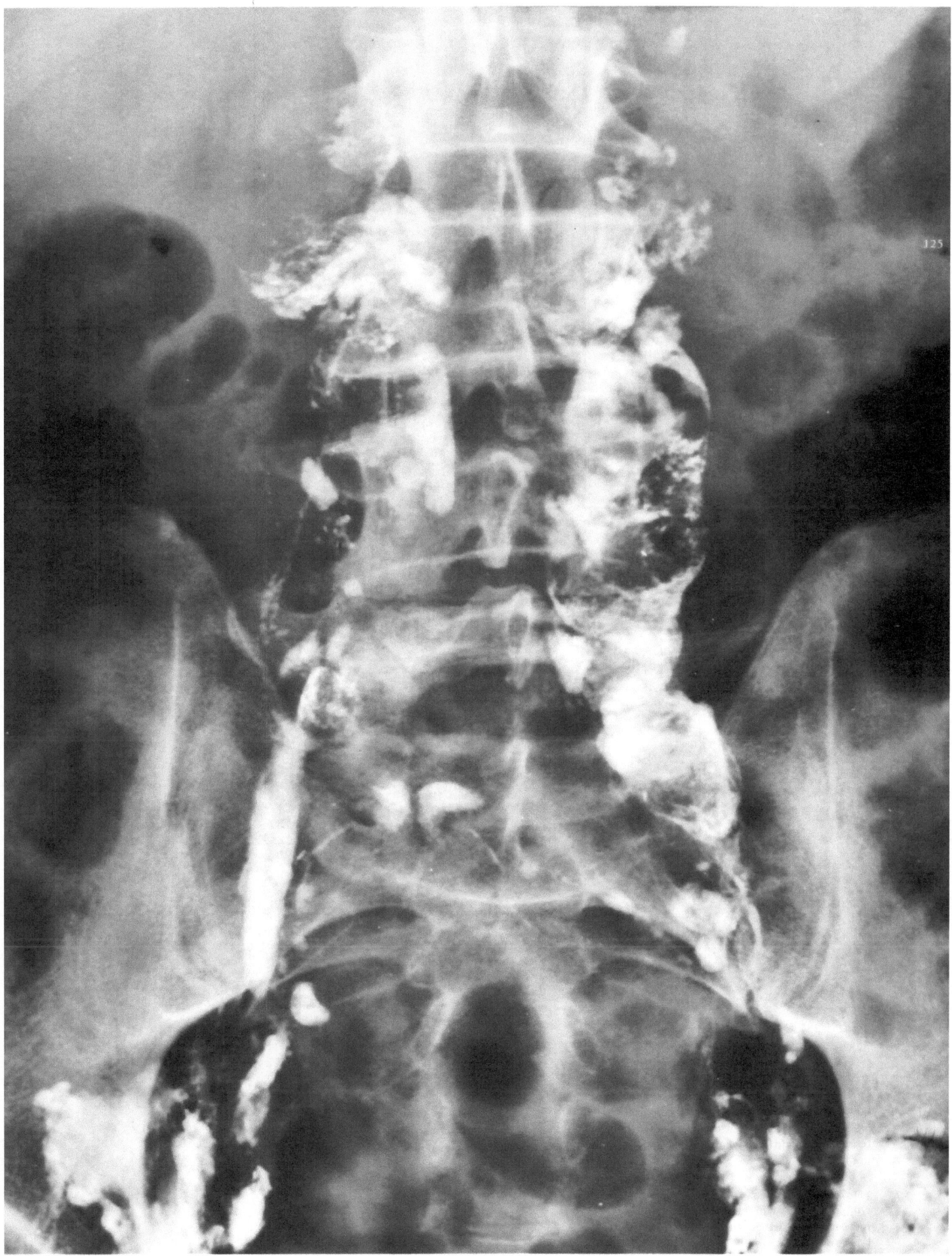

126

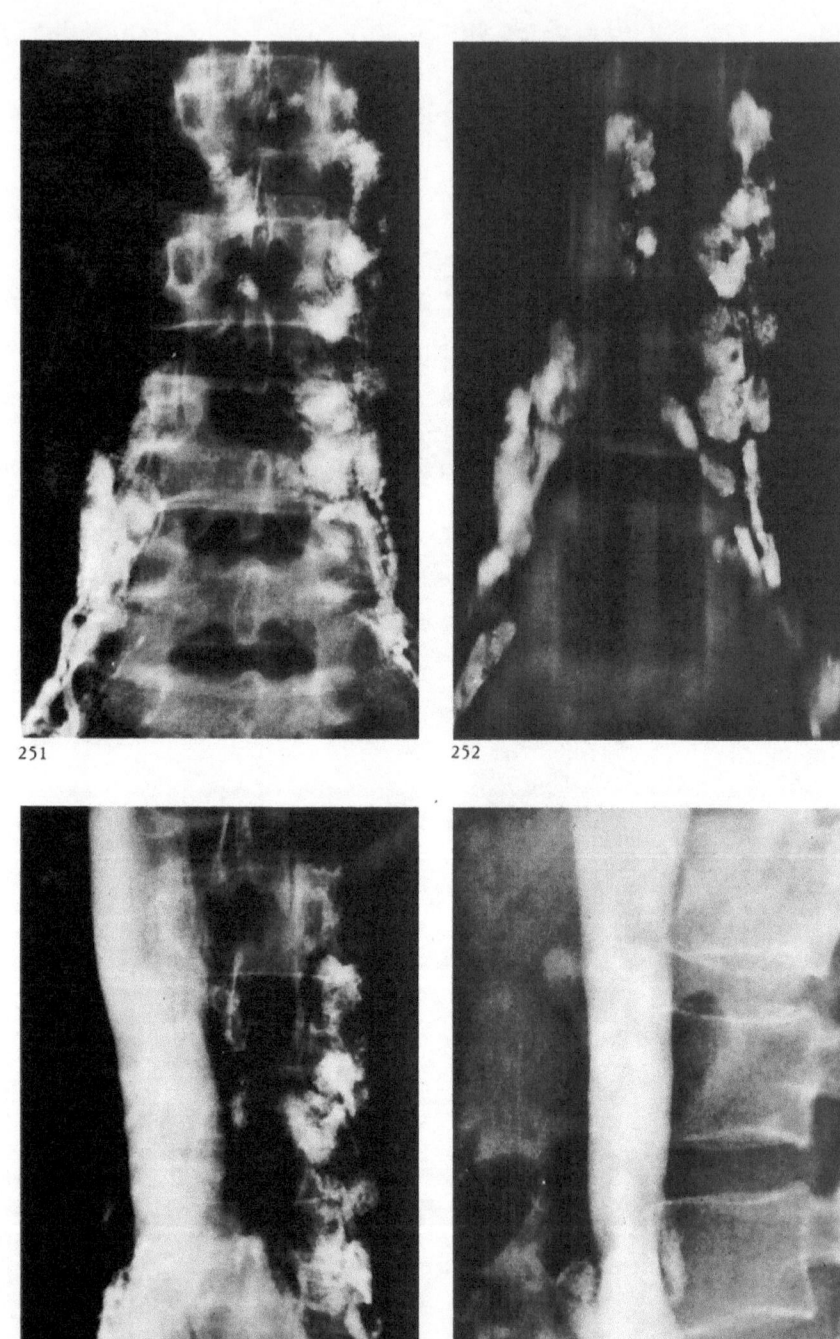

251

252

253

254

figs. 251-254 Ovarian carcinoma; on the lymphadenogram (fig. 251) and tomogram (fig. 252), several lymph nodes affected by inflammation are seen in the lower right paralumbar region. An empty area is found above these nodes on the lymphogram; it is not caused by a pathological lymph node mass since the cavogram (anteroposterior: fig. 253 and lateral: fig. 254) is completely normal.

figs. 255 and 256 Carcinoma of the bladder; lymphogram and lymphadenogram: extensive metastasizing in left iliac region (lymph nodes no longer recognizable) with retrograde filling of the lymph nodes of the bladder.

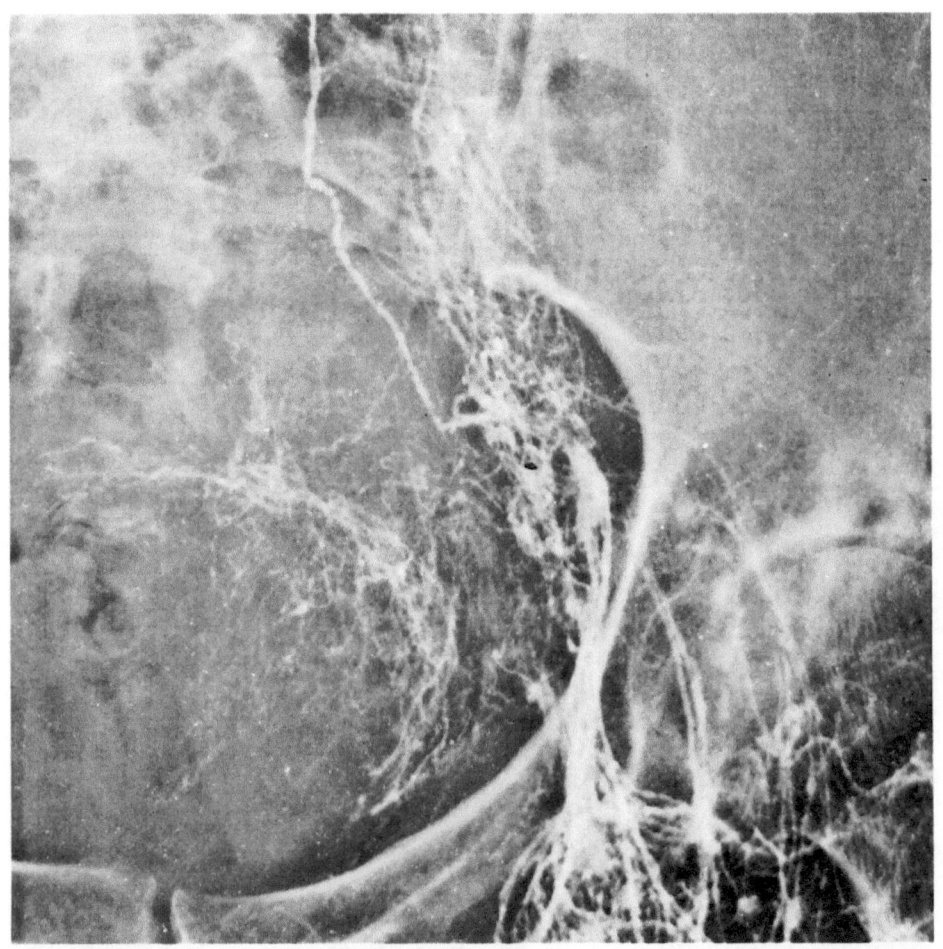

255

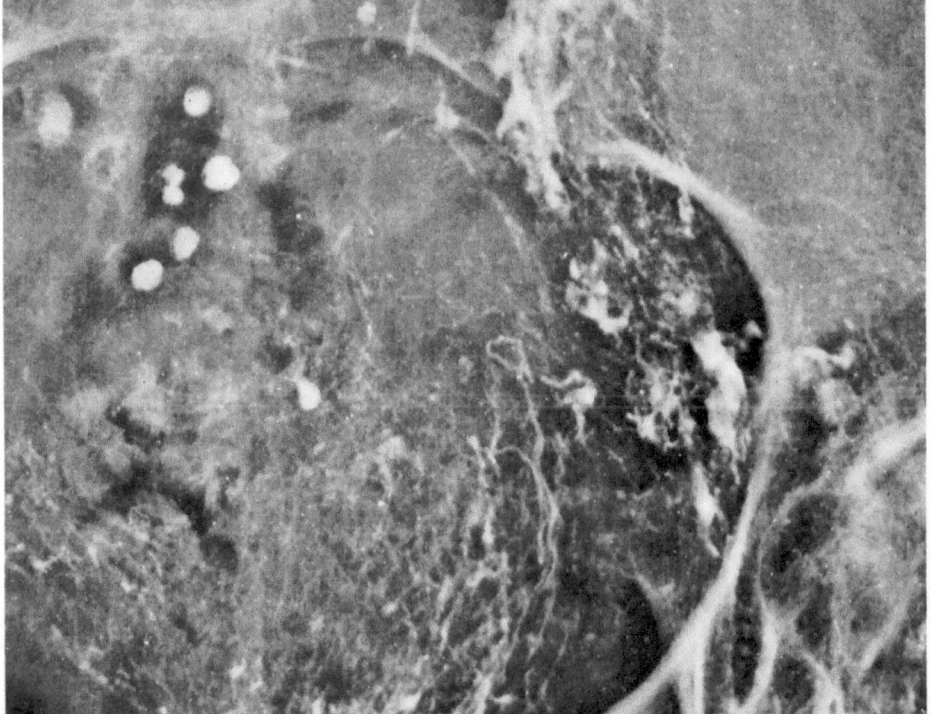

256

figs. 257-260 Carcinoma of the bladder. Metastases in the right pelvis minor suspected clinically. The lymphogram (fig. 257), lymphadenogram (fig. 258) and tomogram (fig. 259) reveal a suspicious area in the right iliac region but involved lymph nodes are not recognized so that the presence of metastases remains questionable. The phlebocavogram (fig. 260) is normal. Roentgenological diagnosis: no metastases. Confirmed after surgery and pathological-anatomical examination.

figs. 261-263 Carcinoma of the bladder. Metastases in the right pelvis minor suspected clinically. On the lymphadenogram (fig. 261) and tomogram (fig. 262) is an empty area in the right iliac lymph node chain. The phlebocavogram (fig. 263) is normal. The tip of the catheter is positioned just before the area to be examined to ensure maximum distension and filling of the vena iliaca in the suspect area. Roentgenological diagnosis: no metastases. Confirmed after surgery and pathological-anatomical examination.

figs. 264 and 265 Renal carcinoma. Clinically palpable swelling in the abdomen to the left of the vertebral column. No definite diagnosis. Intravenous pyelogram (fig. 265): normal excretion, left kidney enlarged and displaced laterally. Lymphadenogram (fig. 264): large pathological lymph node mass to the left next to L3. Roentgenological diagnosis: in view of the typical location of the lymph node mass, metastases of a testicle tumour were suspected; renal carcinoma was second choice since large metastases of renal carcinoma do not occur rapidly. The se-

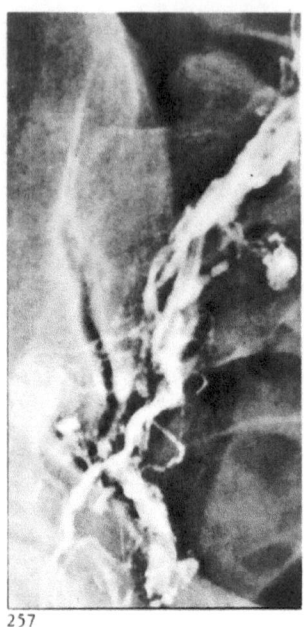

257

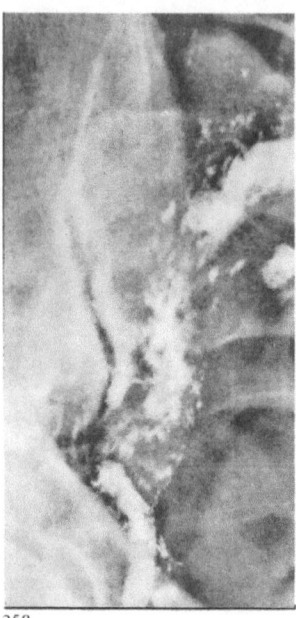

258

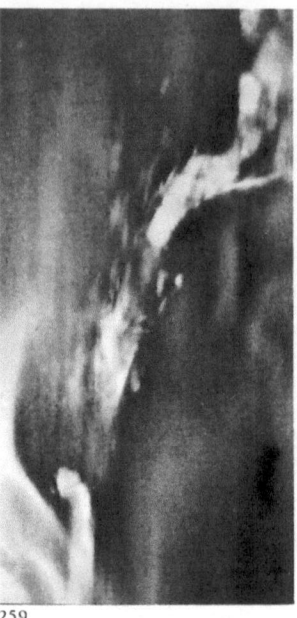

259

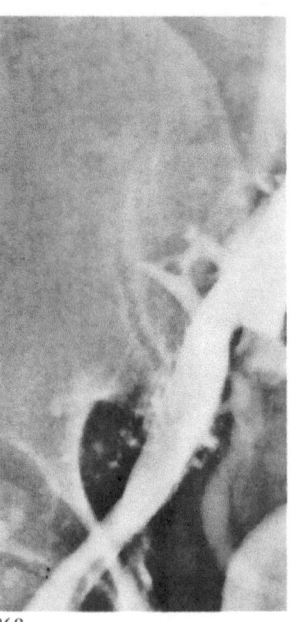

260

lective arteriogram of the left kidney taken 3 weeks later (fig. 264) shows a large renal carcinoma (in contrast to the previous intravenous pyelogram) which occupies the entire upper and middle poles of the kidney.

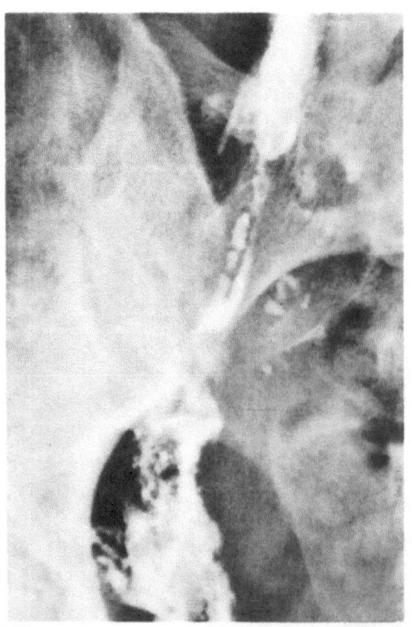

261

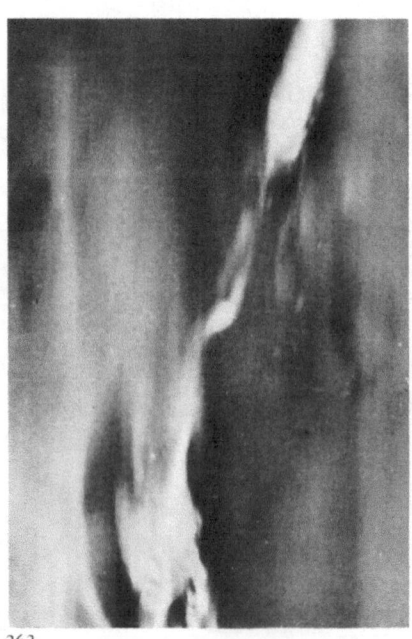

262

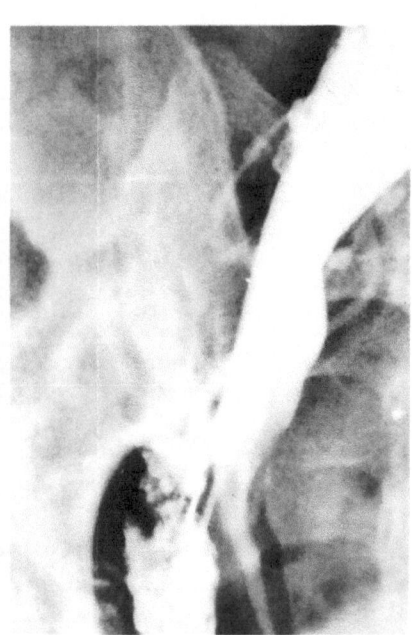

263

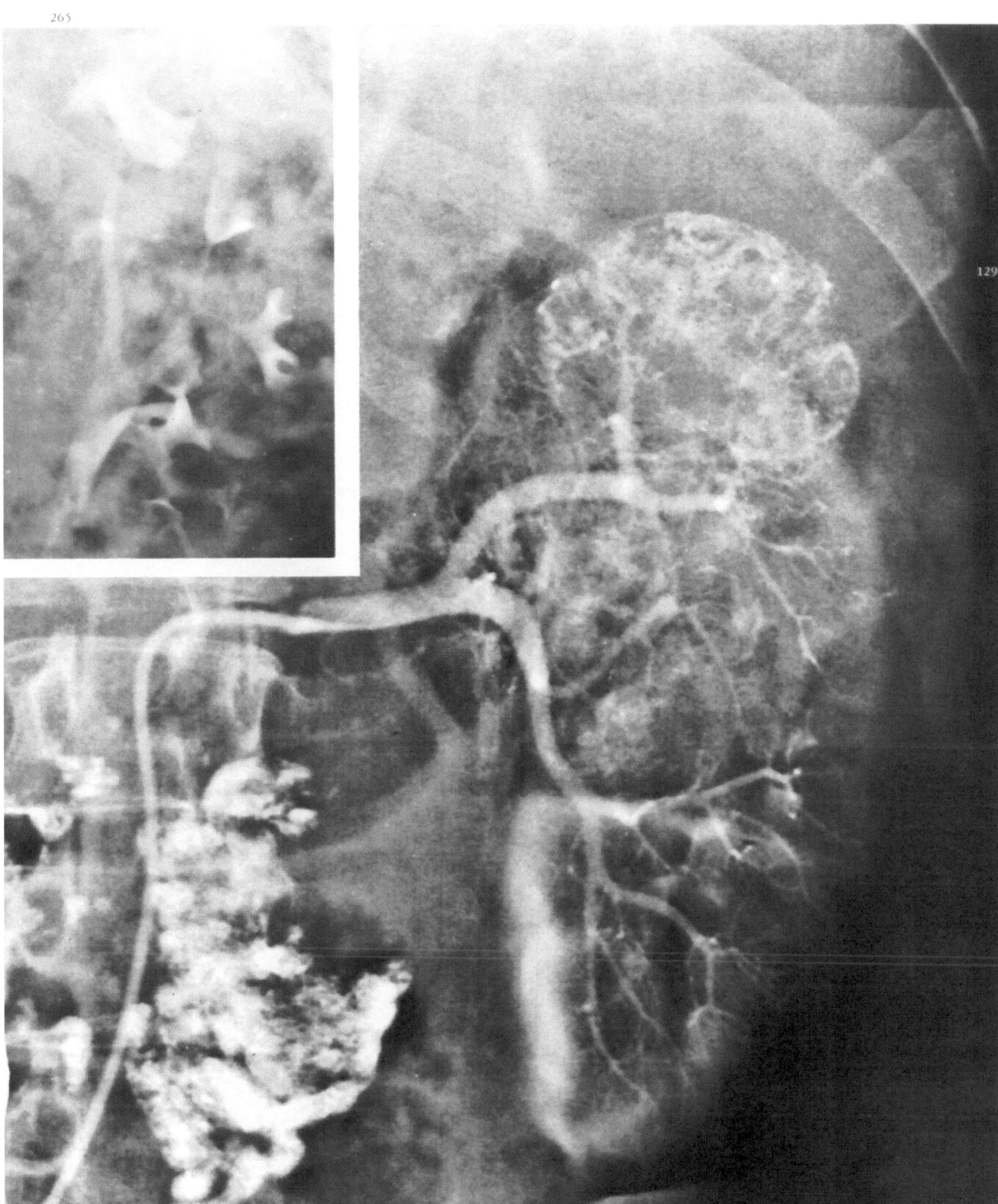

265

130

266

267

figs. 266-269 Renal carcinoma. Renal carcinoma does not metastasize rapidly to the lymphatic system. Large renal carcinoma (selective arteriography of the kidneys: figs. 266, 268) with a few metastases in one patient (fig. 267) and none at all in another (fig. 269).

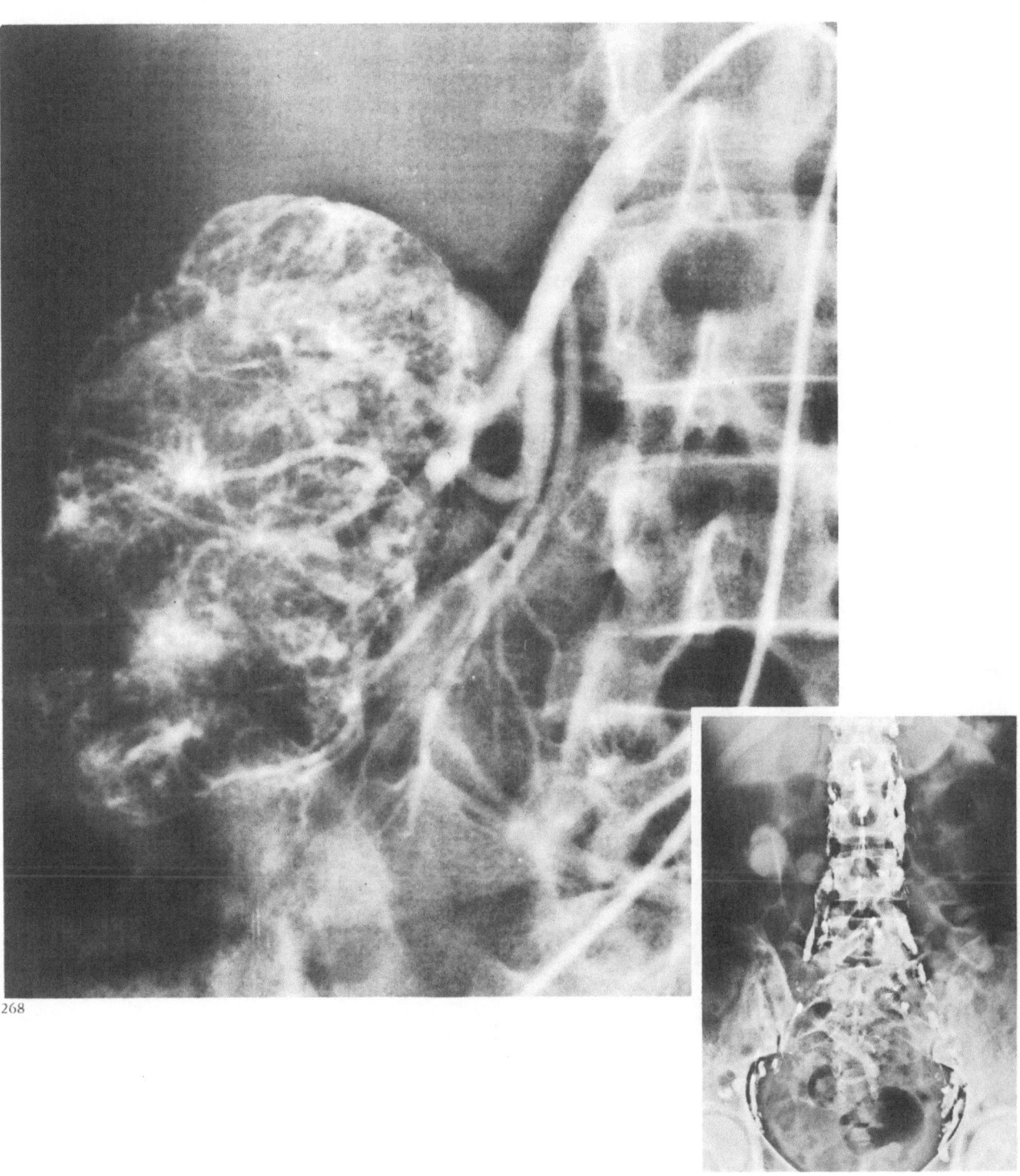

268

269

figs. 270 and 271 Adenocarcinoma of the adrenal gland. Selective arteriography of the right kidney shows (fig. 270) a large carcinoma of the adrenal gland causing an indentation in the kidney. The lymphogram is normal. Above the last filled lymph node (→), which is just visible, the vena cava arches (fig. 271) outwards and is narrowed. Diagnosis, confirmed after surgery and pathological-anatomical examination: no lymph node metastases..

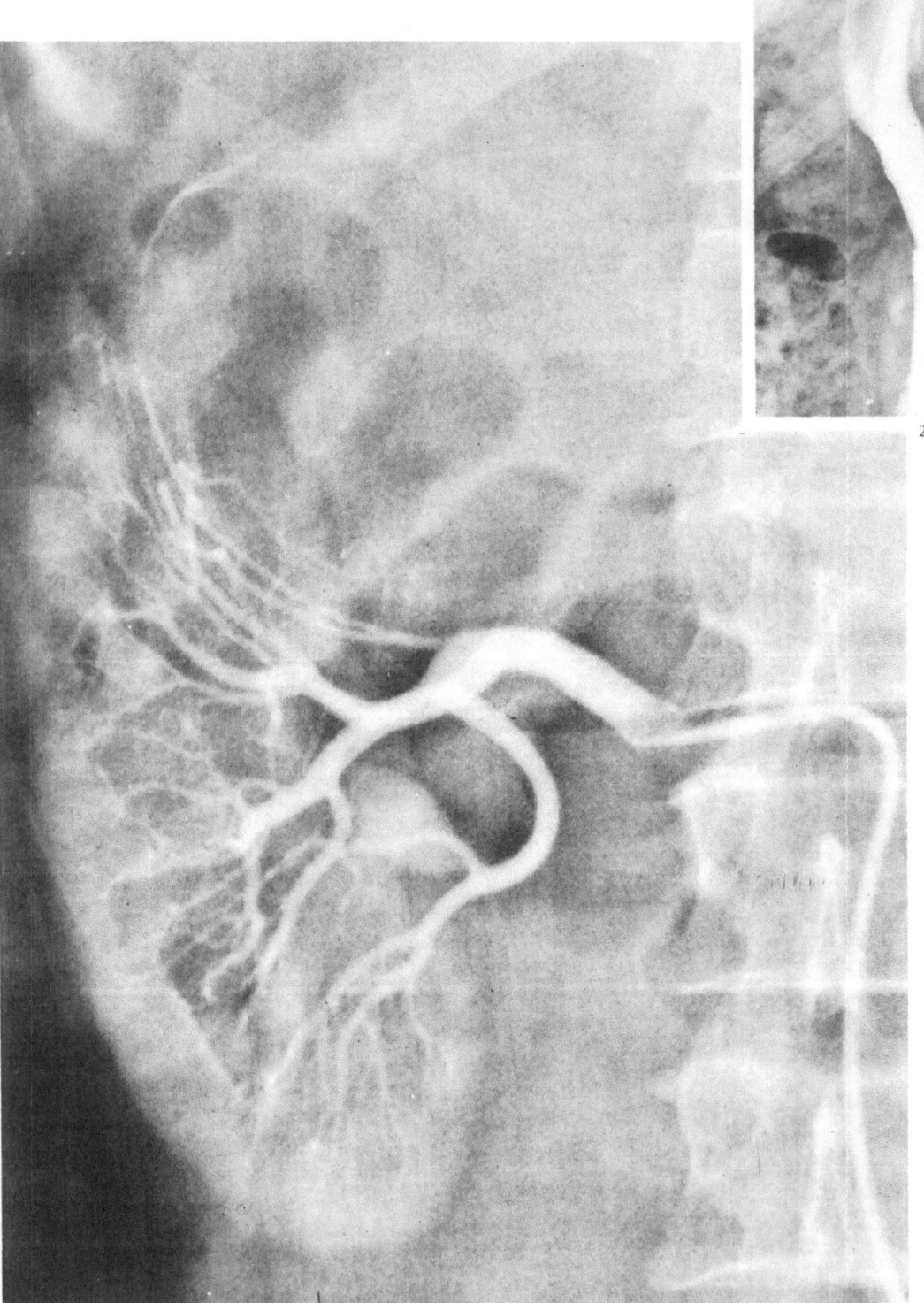

271

270

fig. 272 Carcinoma of the pancreas; lymphadenogram: extensive metastases in the left paralumbar region.

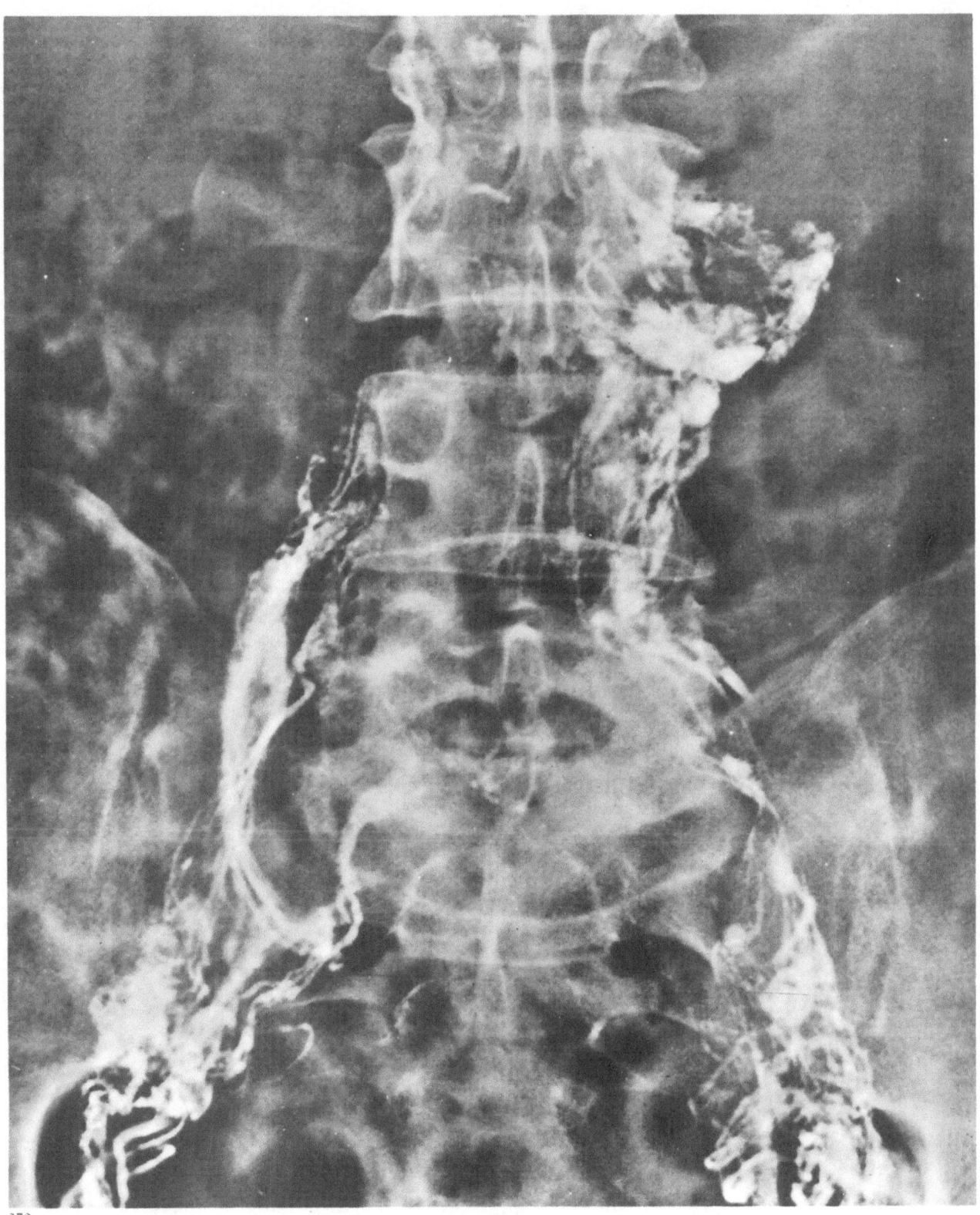

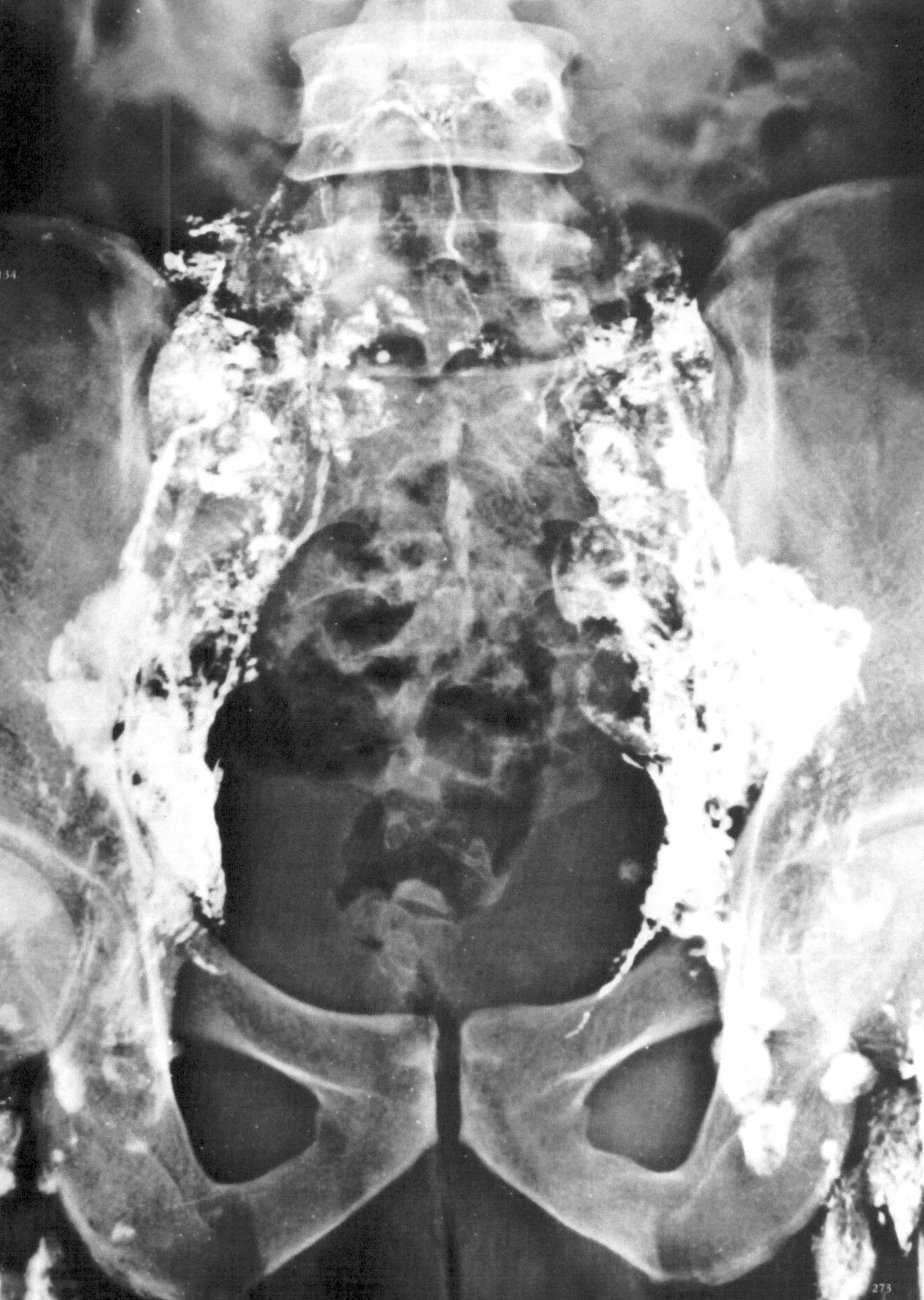

fig. 273 Carcinoma of the large bowel; lymphadenogram: extensive metastases with distension
and lymphatic obstruction.

on pages 136 and 137

figs. 274 and 275 Large gastric carcinoma; lymphogram and lymphadenogram: extensive metastases in paralumbar region with dilatation
and lymphatic obstruction.

on pages 138 and 139

figs. 276 and 277 Tumour of the right testicle
(seminoma); lymphogram and lymphadenogram: extensive formation of metastases in the
right paralumbar L5 region and, because of the
transverse lymphatic channels on the contra-
lateral side of the vertebral column, the left paralumbar L2-L4 region.

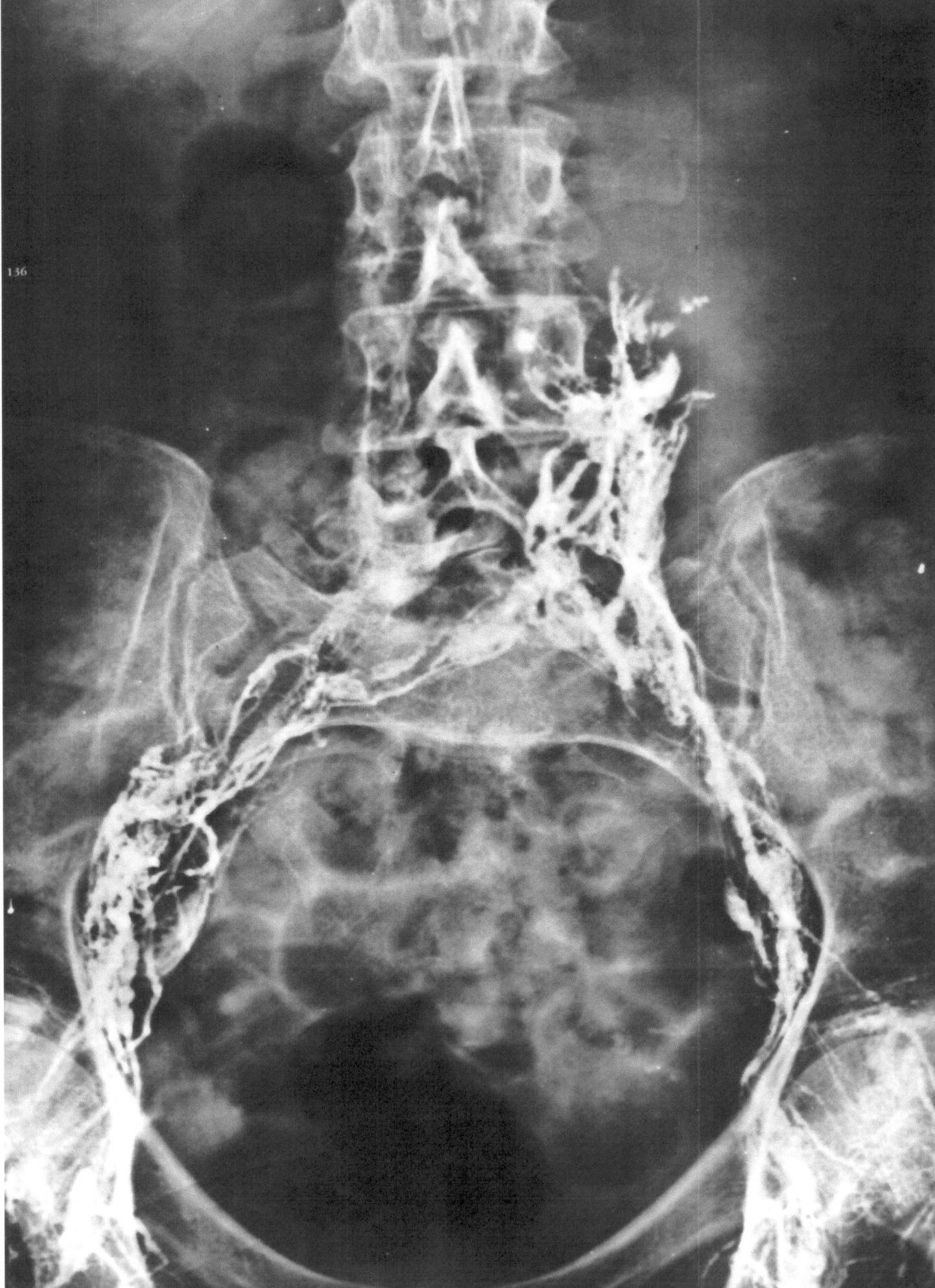

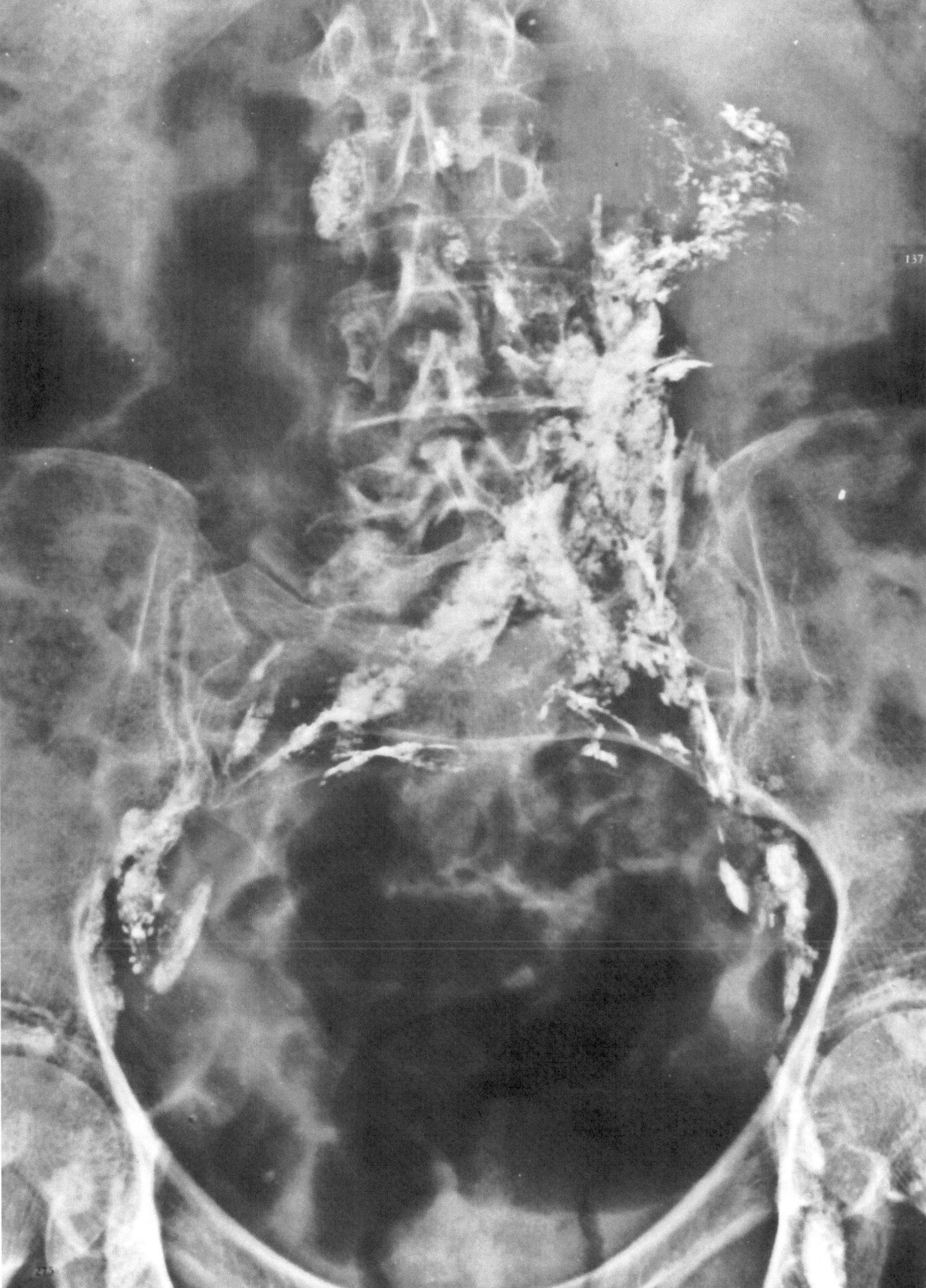

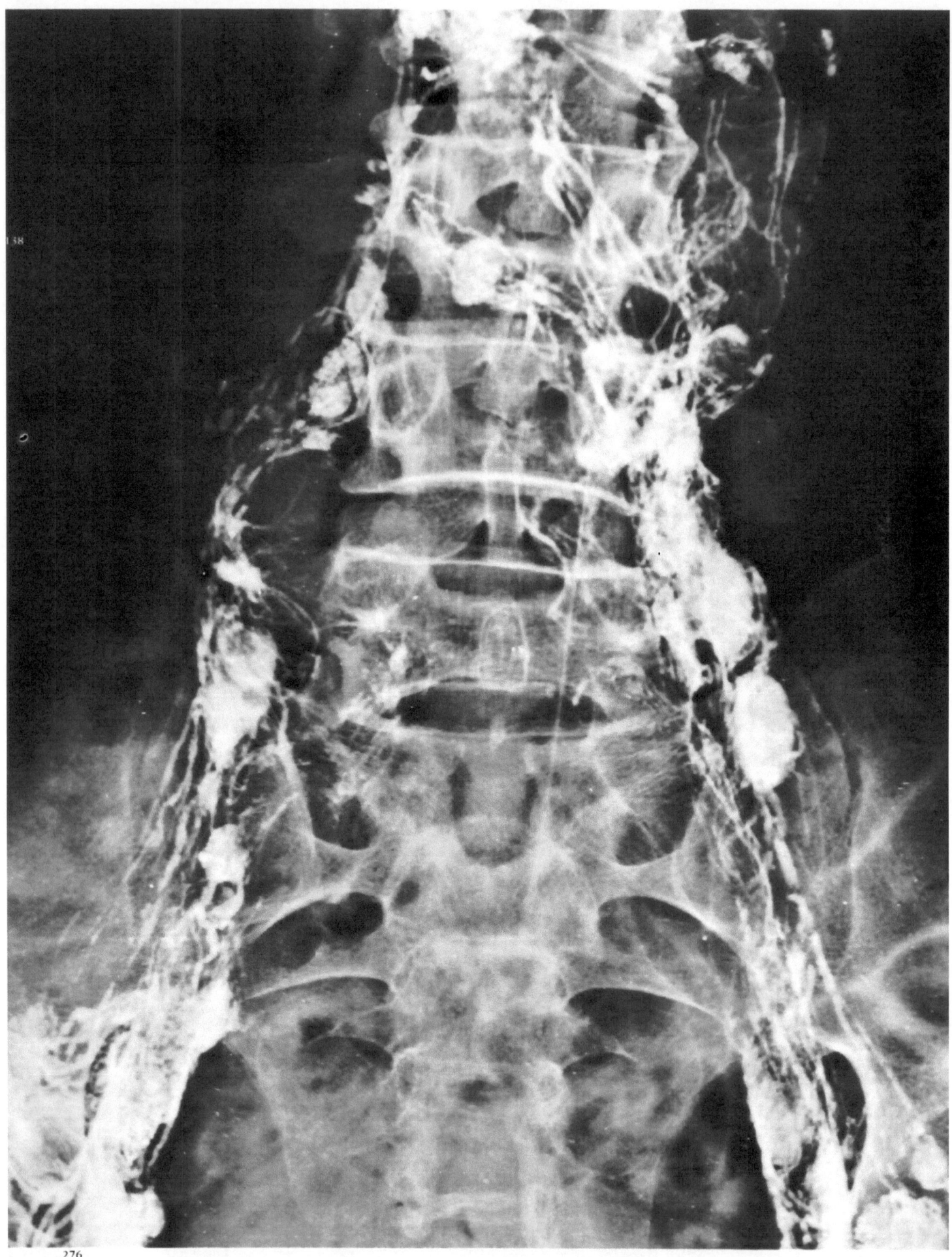

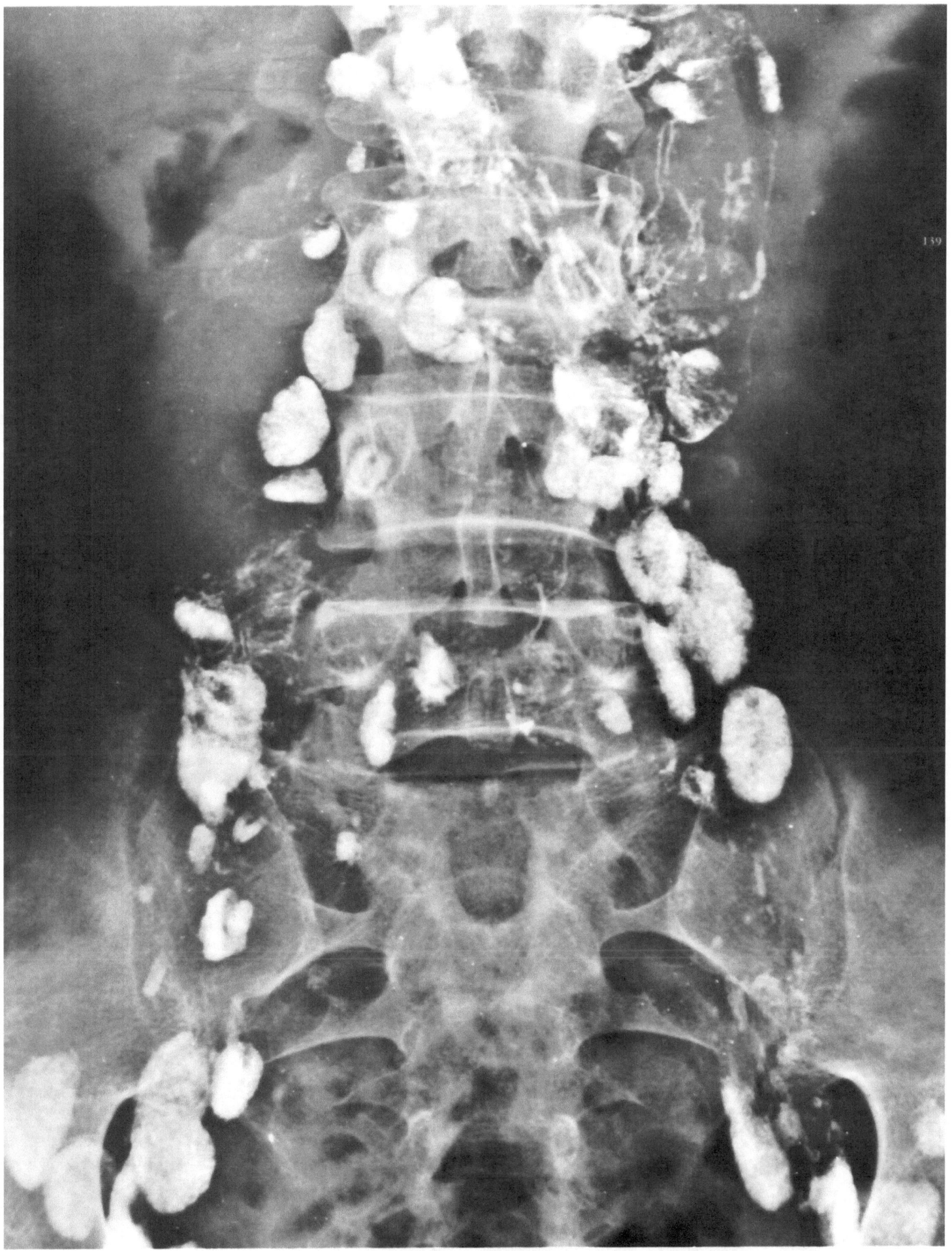

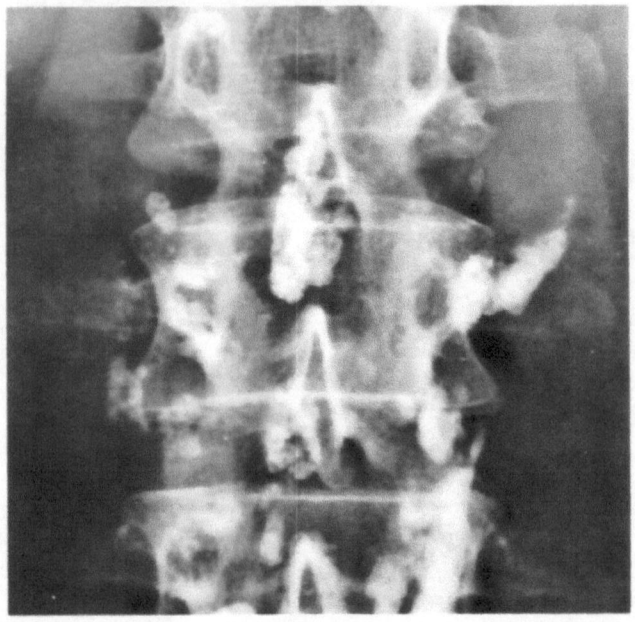

279

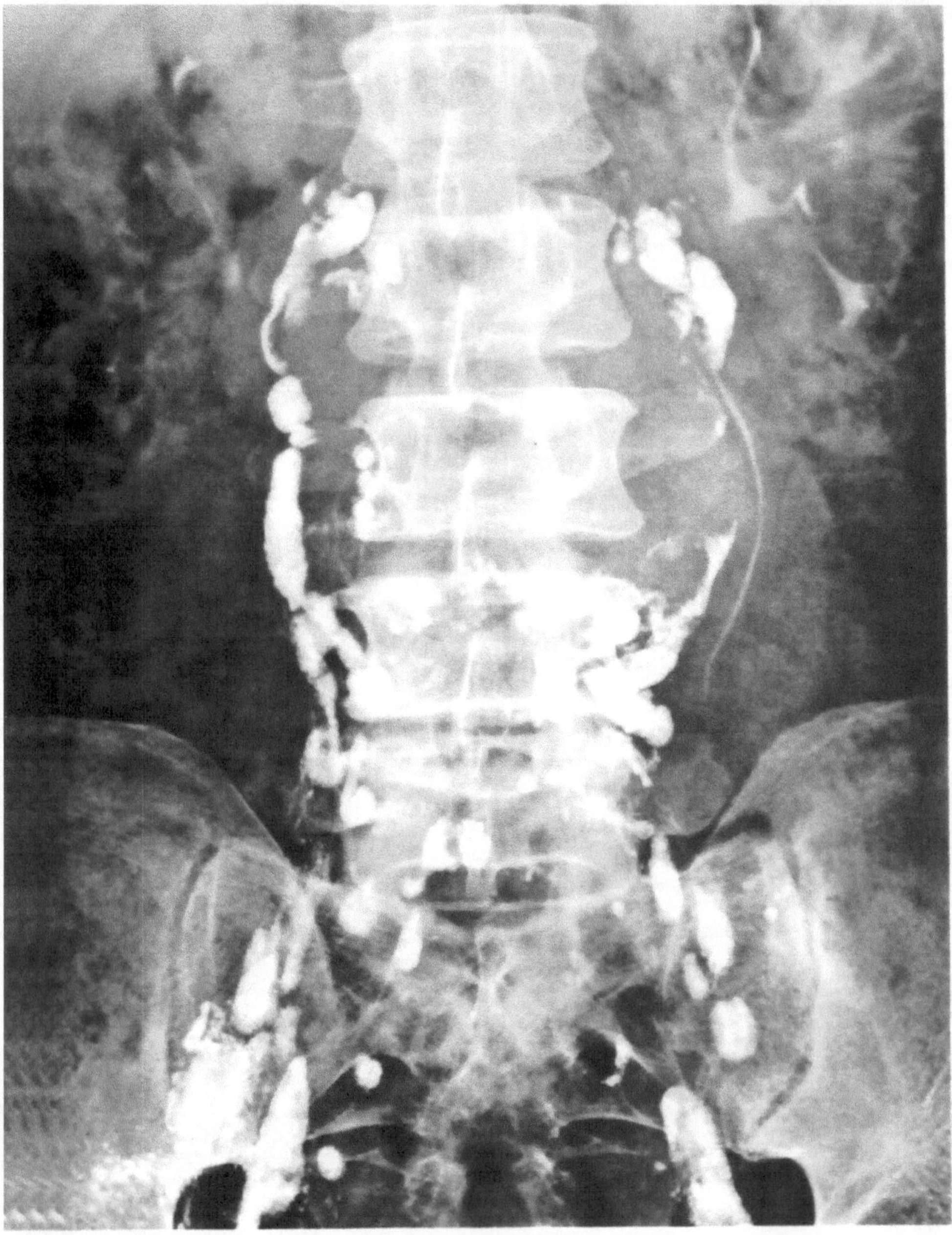

fig. 278 Tumour of the right testicle (seminoma). Lymphadenogram and intravenous pyelogram: extensive formation of metastases to the left and right of L2-L4 with displacement of the still normal lymph nodes and arching of the ureters. Lymph nodes affected by inflammation especially in the right para-iliac region.
Comment: Although anatomically a lymphatic channel runs directly from the testicle to the iliac lymph nodes, metastases are very seldom seen there. Lymph nodes affected by inflammation are found regularly.

figs. 279-281 Tumour of the left testicle (teratoma). If at the typically preferred location of metastases formation (L2-L3), the lymphadenogram (fig. 279) shows lymph nodes displaced several cm. from the medial line – then metastases are to be seriously suspected. Because of the anatomical location of the vena cava, the cavogram is not useful in demonstrating or excluding pathological lymph node masses to the left of the lumbar vertebral column. To establish the diagnosis of metastases, care is however required and roentgenological follow-up studies can be helpful (no change in the picture on follow-up radiograms 3 weeks (fig. 280) and 3 months later (fig. 281)).

fig. 282 Tumour of the left testicle (seminoma); lymphadenogram, intravenous pyelogram and cavogram: extensive pathological lymph node mass to the left L2-L4. Although the pathological lymph node mass extends over the median line, only a slight arching of the vena cava is seen due to its anatomical position.

278

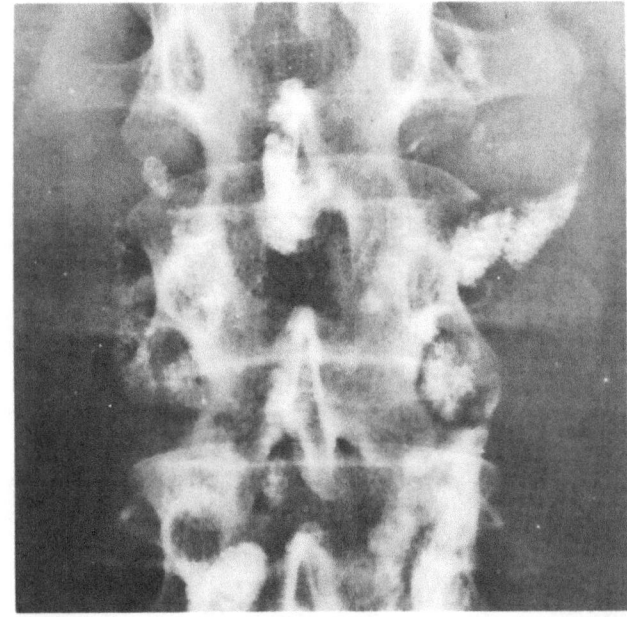

280

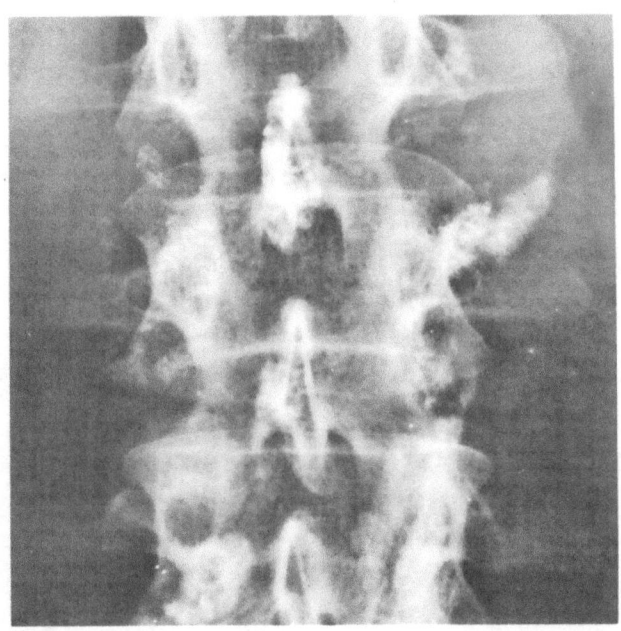

281

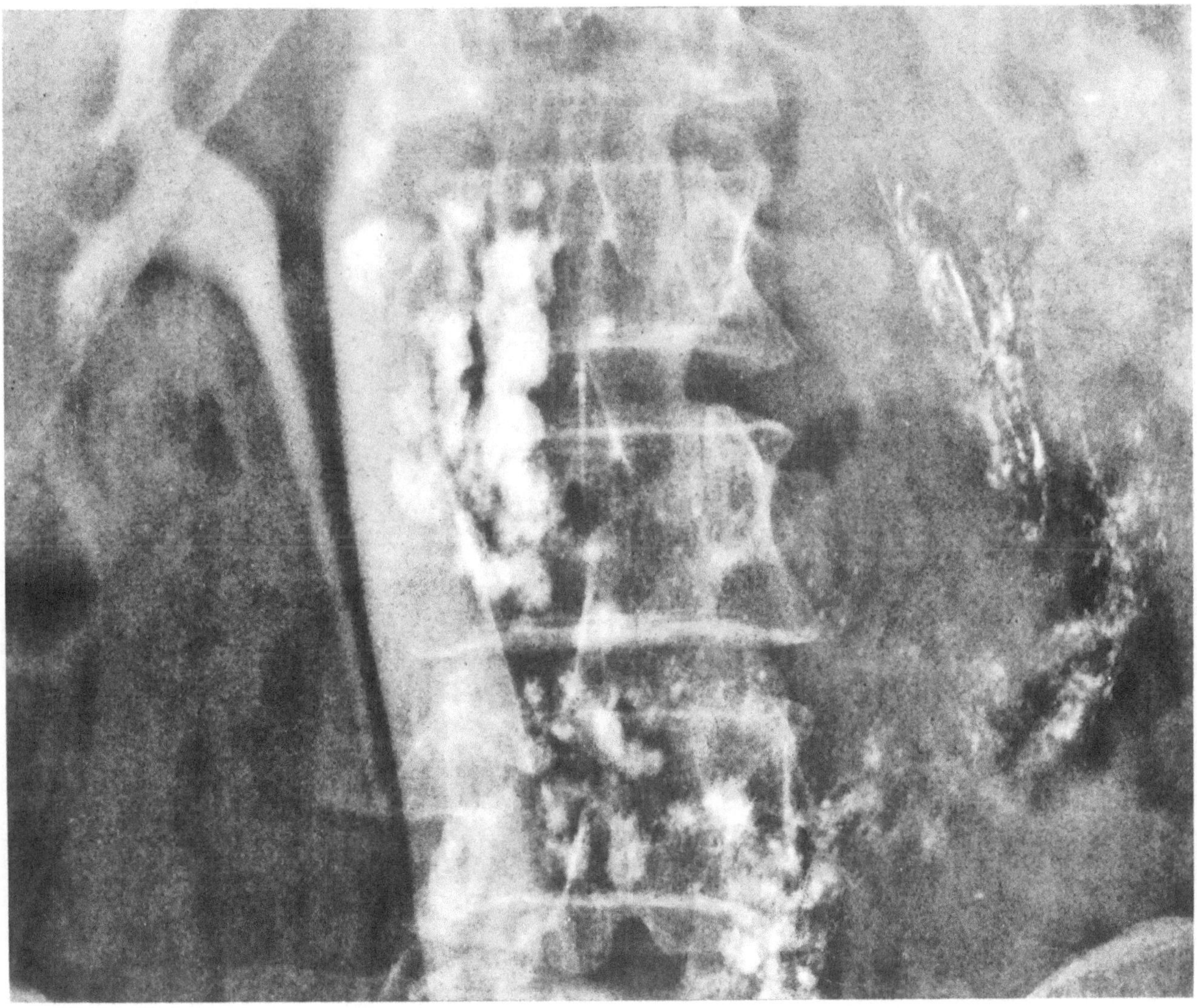

282

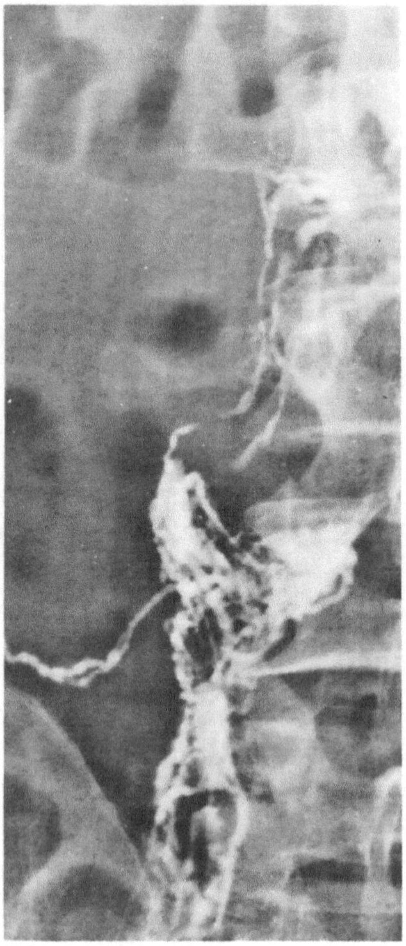

283

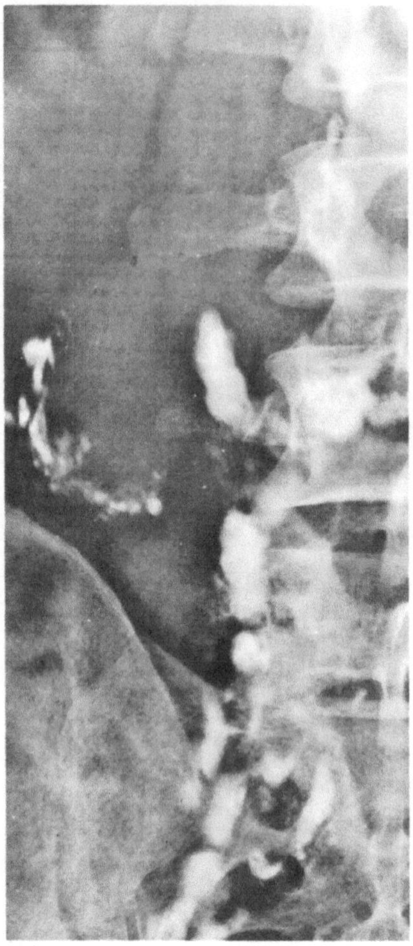

284

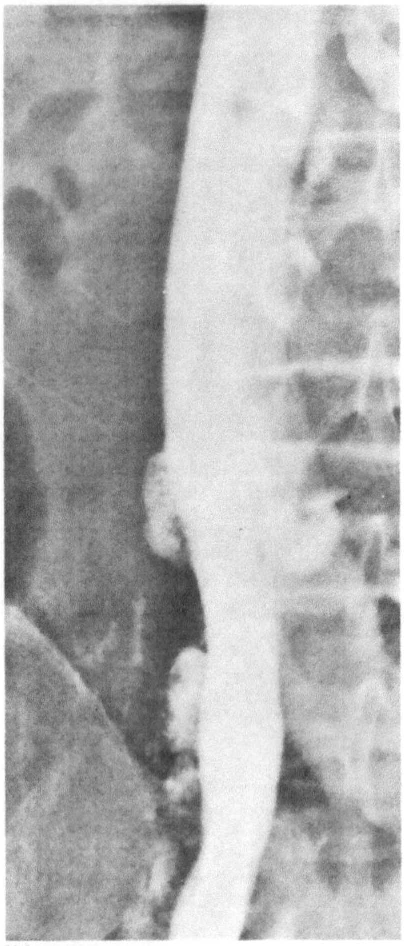

285

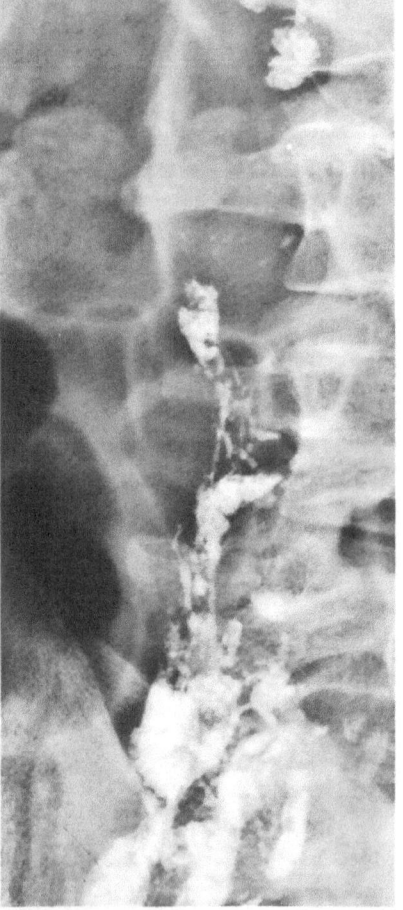

287

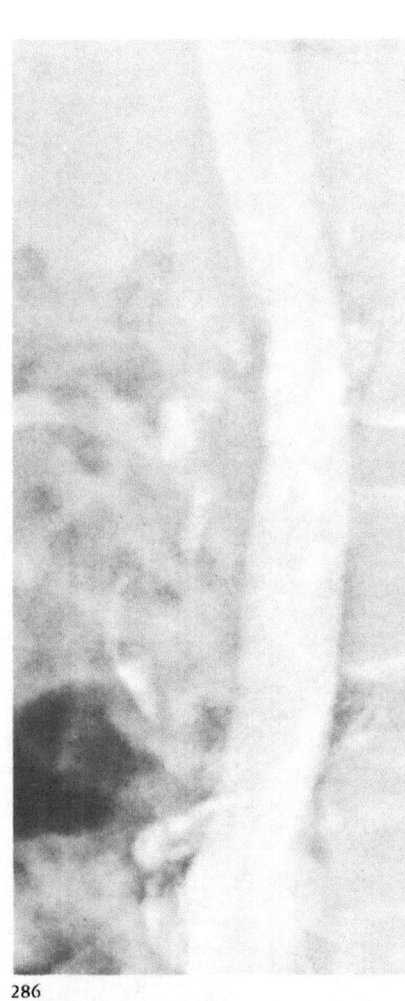

286

figs. 283-290 Tumour of the right testicle (seminoma). Two patients with a suspect right paralumbar region on the lymphogram (figs. 283, 287) and lymphadenogram (figs. 284, 288). The films for these patients are almost identical. However supplementary phlebocavography showed no pathological lymph node masses in the first patient (figs. 285, 286: anteroposterior and lateral phlebocavogram) and extensive lymph node masses in the second patient (figs. 289, 290: anteroposterior and lateral phlebocavogram).

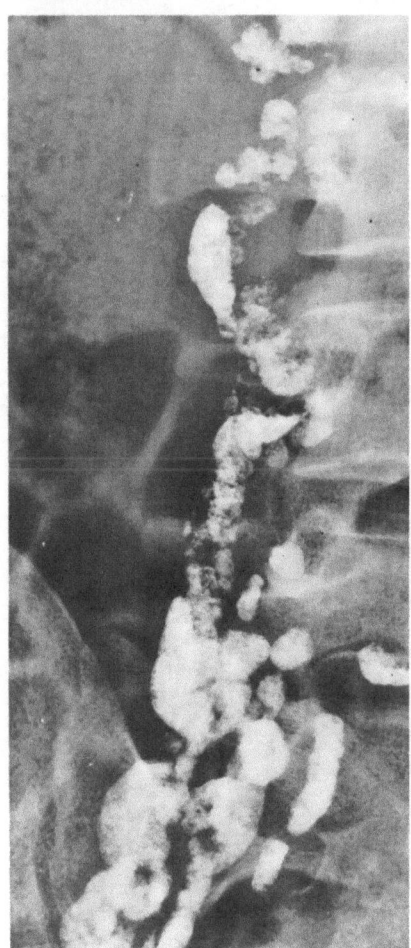

288

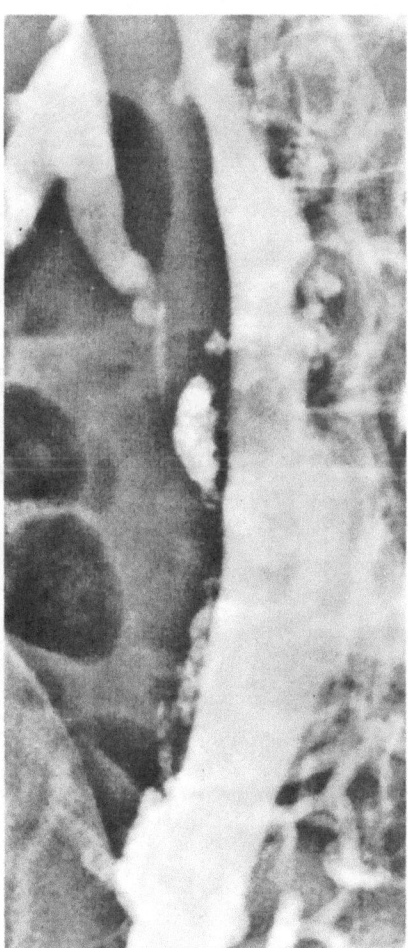

289

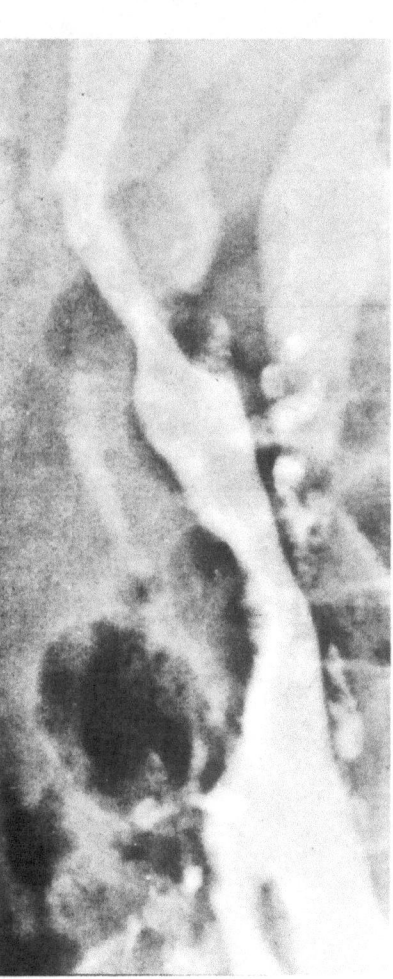

290

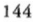

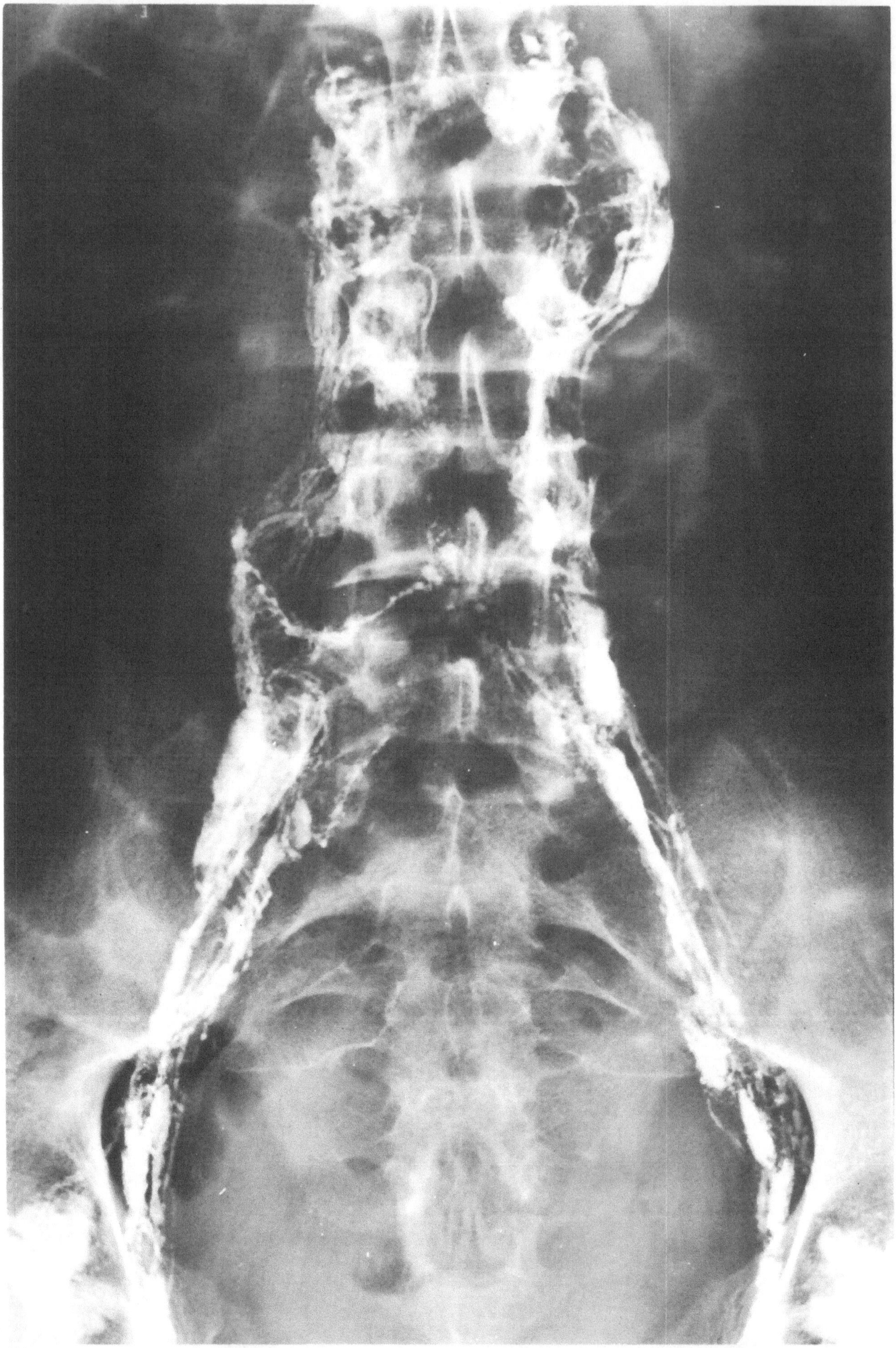

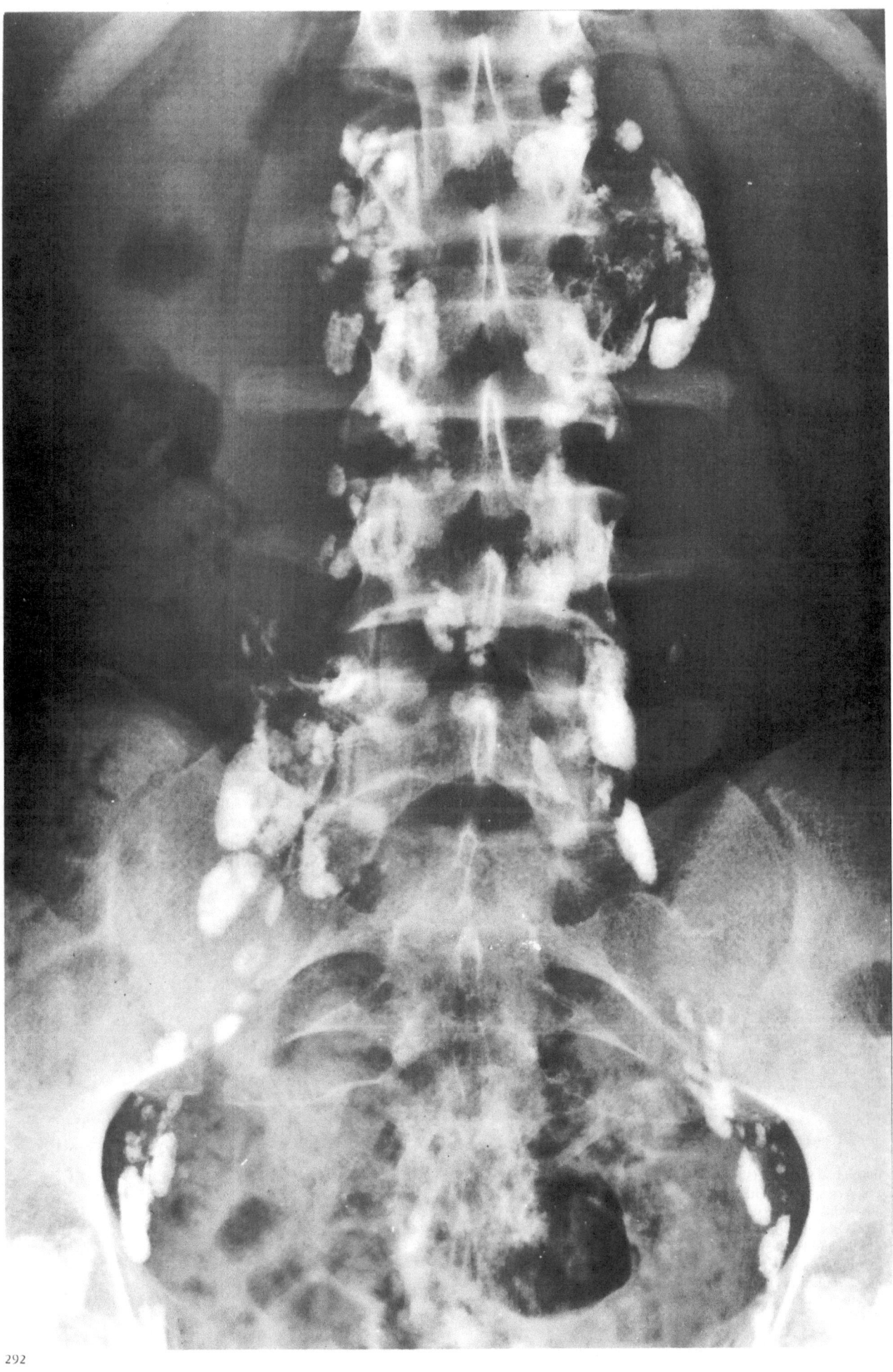

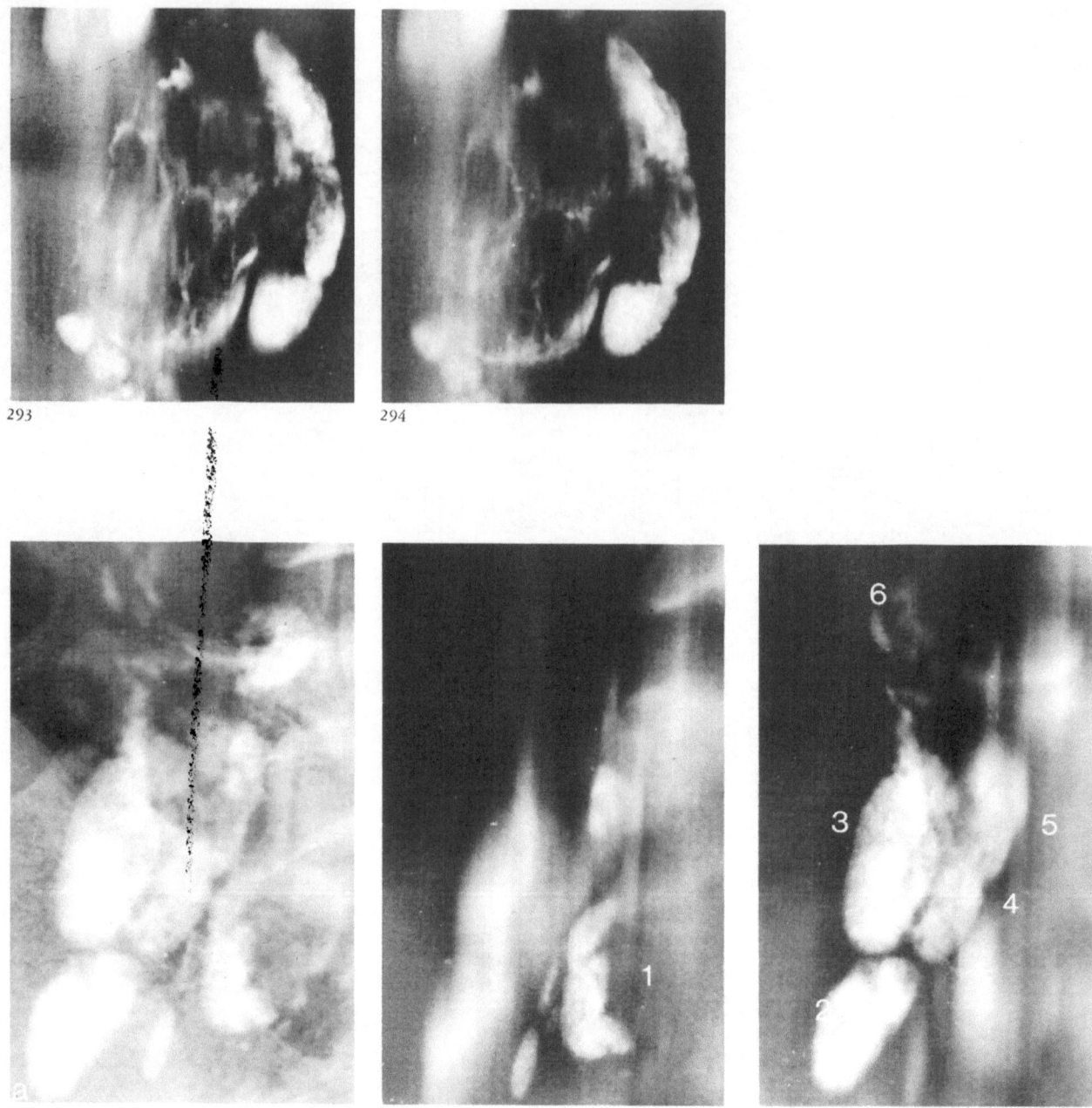

293

294

295

296

297

figs. 291-300 Tumour of the right testicle consisting of teratoma and embryonal carcinoma. Extensive formation of metastases in left paralumbar L2-L3 region (lymphogram: fig. 291, lymphadenogram: fig. 292 and tomograms: figs. 293, 294): highly suspicious right paralumbar L5 region on lymphogram and lymphadenogram. Tomograms (figs. 296, 297, 298) reveal normal lymph nodes and nodes affected by inflammation (1), (2), (3), (4), (5) and (7) as well as several spots of contrast medium which cannot be differentiated (6). On the phlebocavogram (figs. 299, 300), especially the lateral exposure, a considerable indentation is seen at this location due to a pathological lymph node mass. Confirmed after surgery and pathological examination.

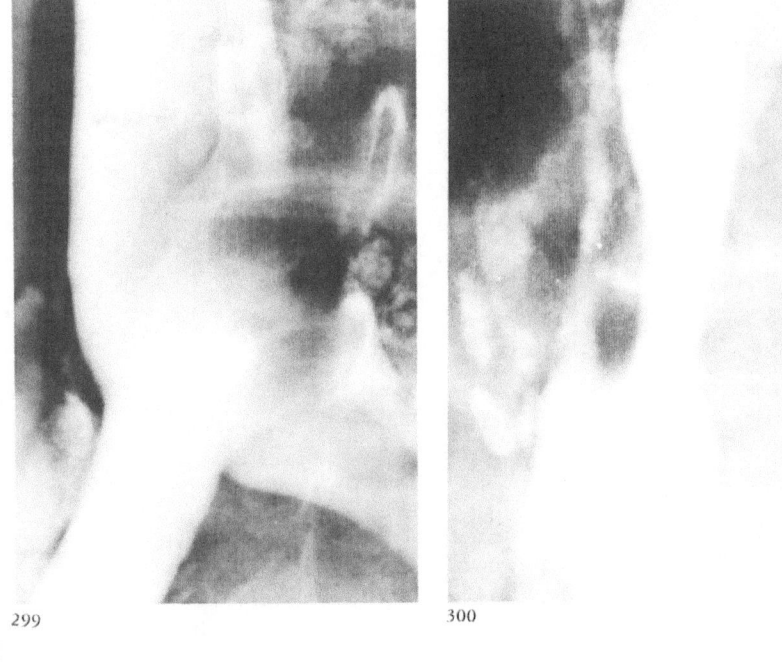

299

300

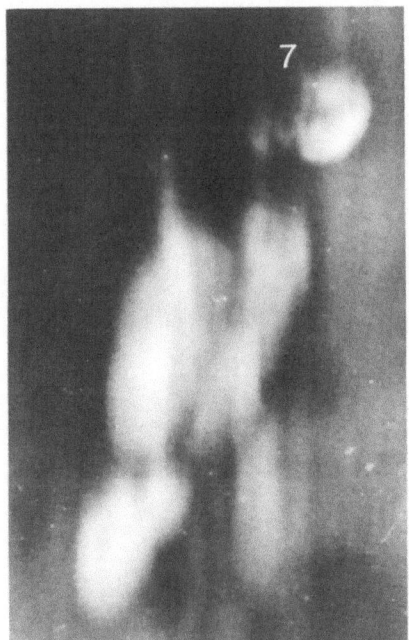

298

figs. 301 and 302 Tumour of the left testicle (embryonal carcinoma). A large lymph node involved by metastases in the inguinal region on the tomograms.
Comment: Metastases in the inguinal region from a tumour of the testicle only occur after previously performed operations in this region (see also fig. 303).

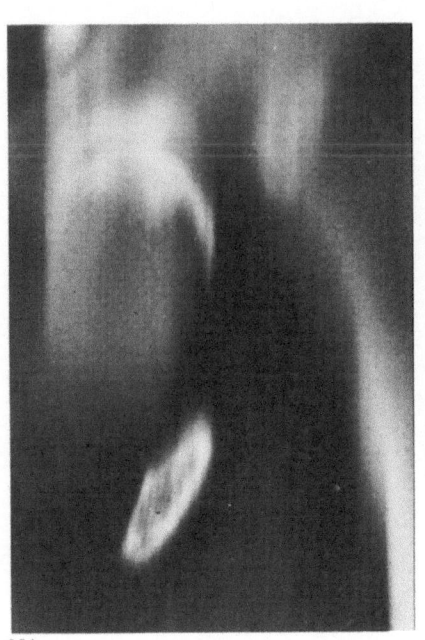

301

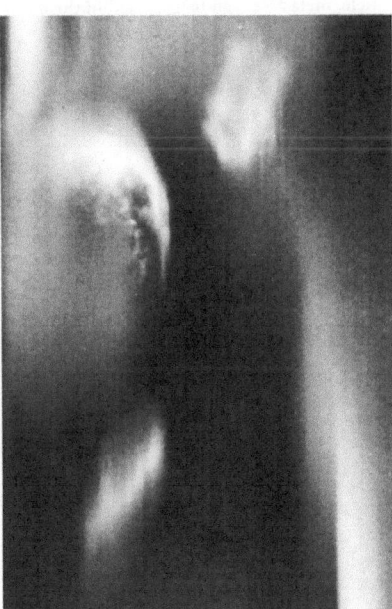

302

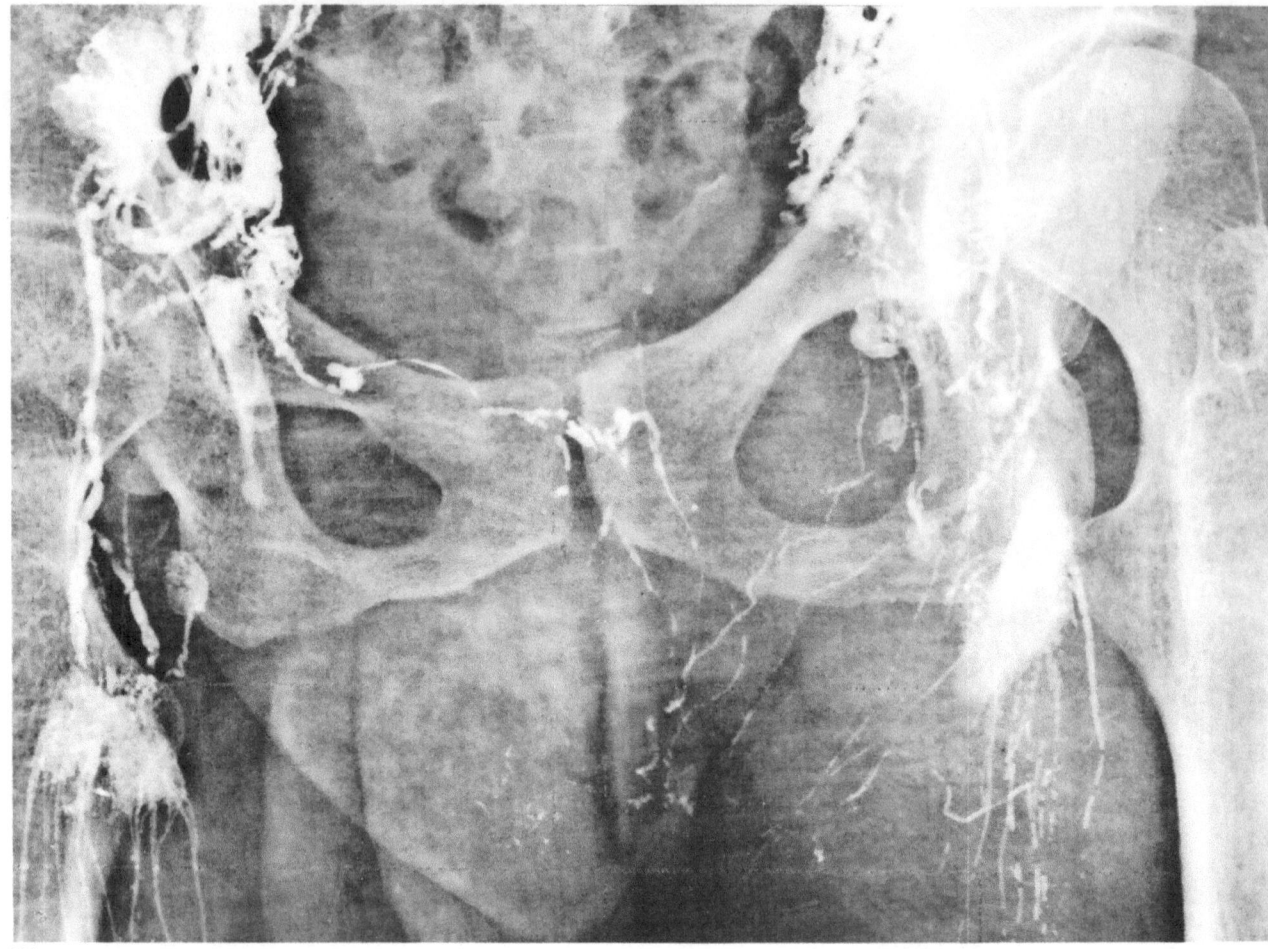

303

fig. 303 Lymphogram of a normal man opera-
ted on in his youth for a non-descended left testicle. As a result of anatomical changes after the
operation, a totally new lymphatic drainage developed (left inguinal region – testicle – lower
right iliac region).

Comment: This lymphogram obviously illus-
trates that should a tumour develop in this testicle, metastases can be expected in the left inguinal and lower right iliac regions.

figs. 304-309 Melanosarcoma of the right leg;
lymphogram (fig. 304), lymphadenogram (fig.
305) and tomograms (figs. 306, 307, 308, 309):
metastases of melanosarcoma in subinguinal
lymph node (→); the other lymph nodes in the
groin show no abnormalities.

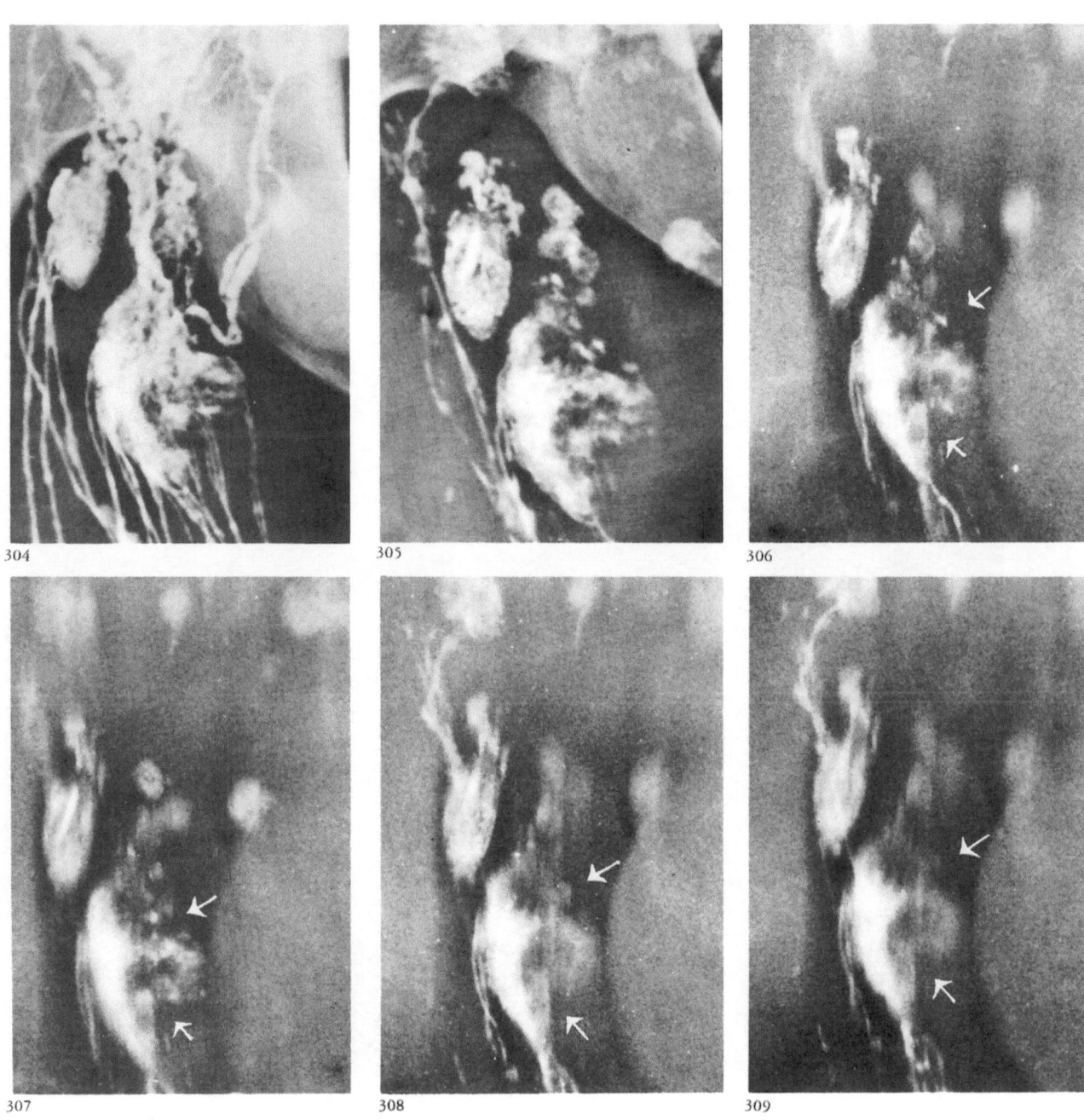

304

305

306

307

308

309

figs. 310-315 Melanosarcoma of the left heel; lymphadenogram (figs. 310, 312), tomograms (figs. 313, 314, 315) and post-operative follow-up radiogram (fig. 311): one large subinguinal lymph node affected by metastases, one small inguinal lymph node affected by metastases (→), lymph nodes in the iliac region affected by inflammation and normal lymph nodes. The follow-up radiogram shows that the total lymph node excision was not adequate. The pathological-anatomical eximination revealed that the interpretation of the lymphogram of the inguinal lymph node was incorrect; it contained fat and fibrosis and not metastases.

150

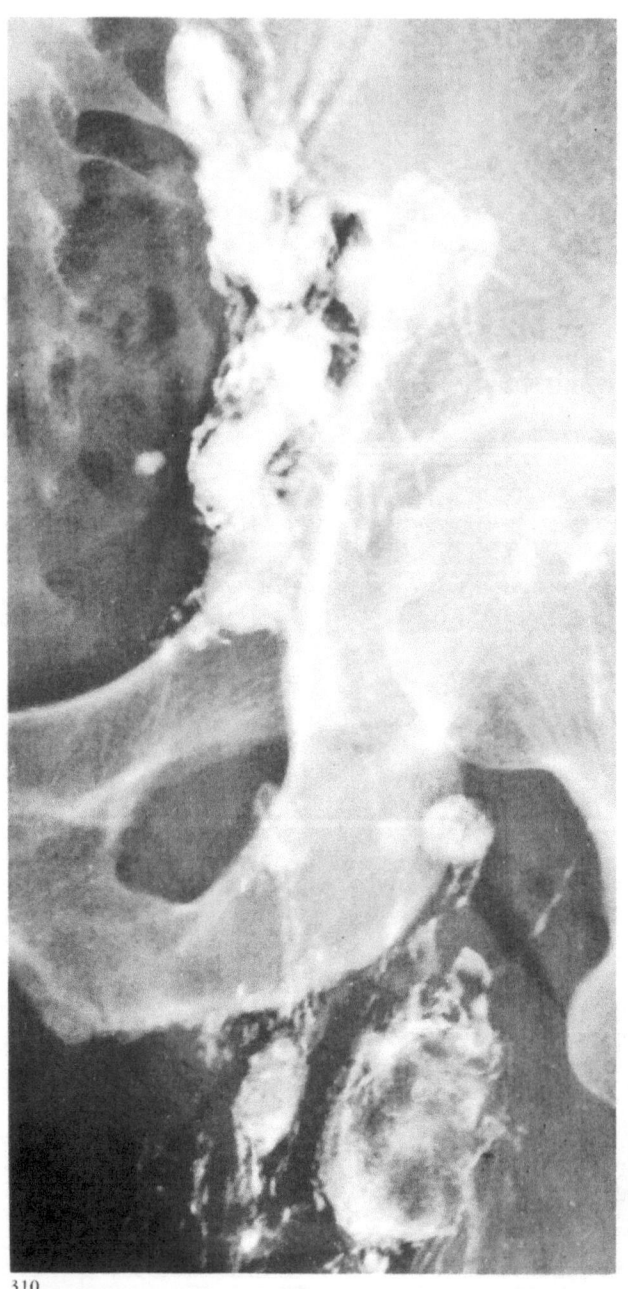

310

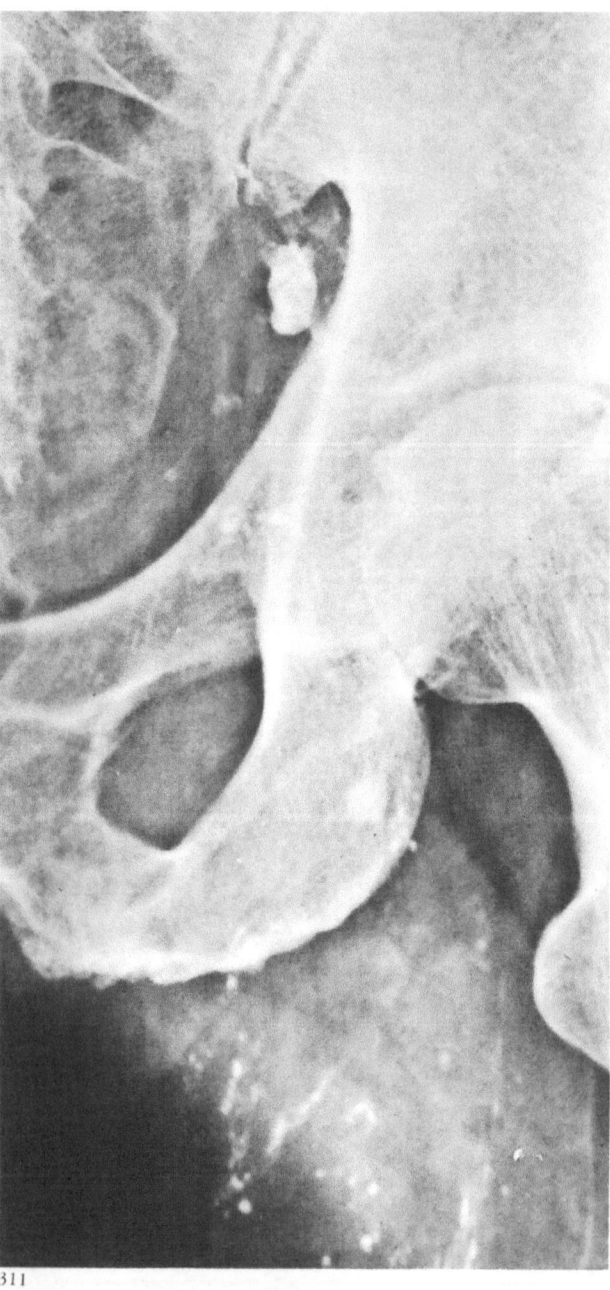

311

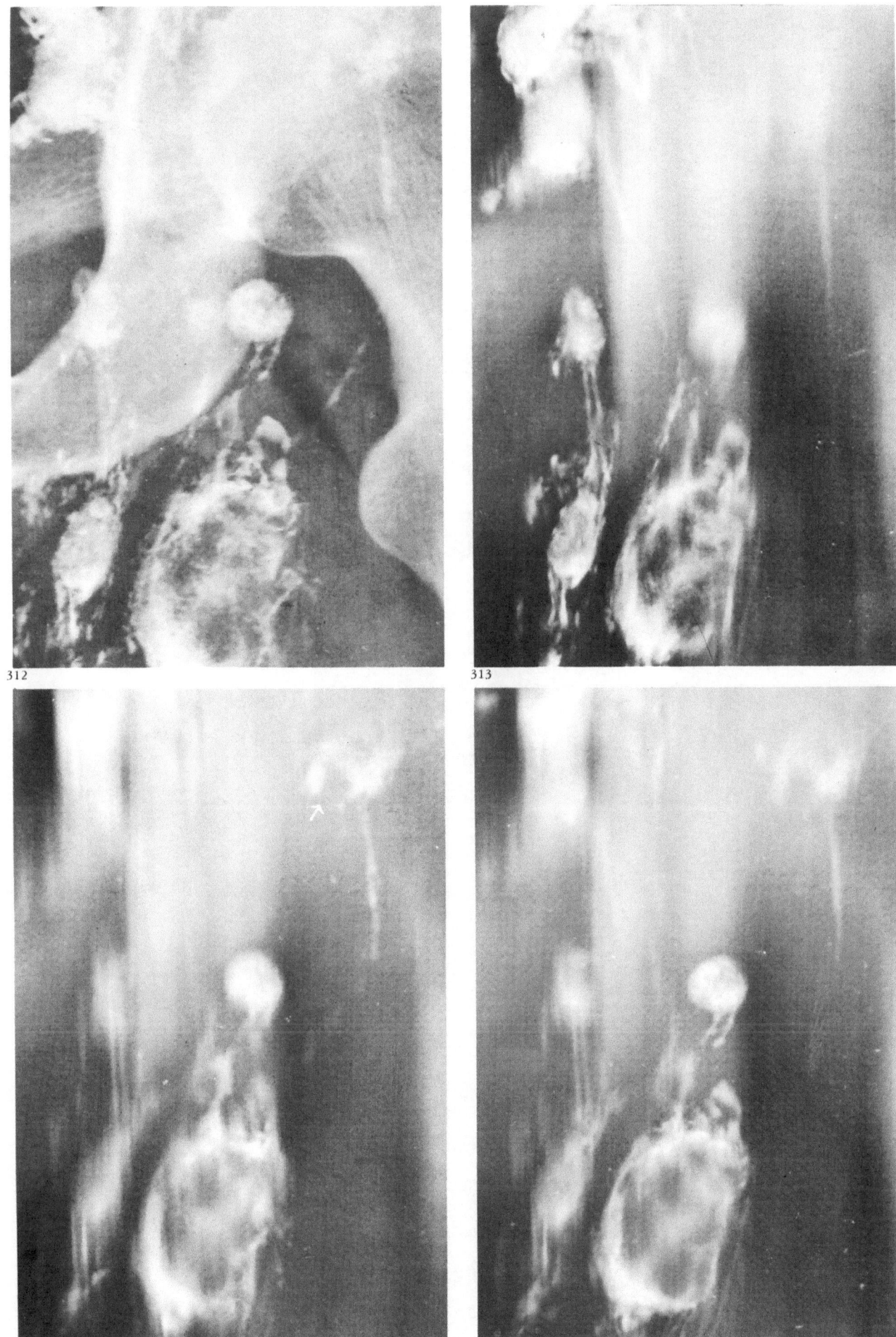

312

313

314

315

152

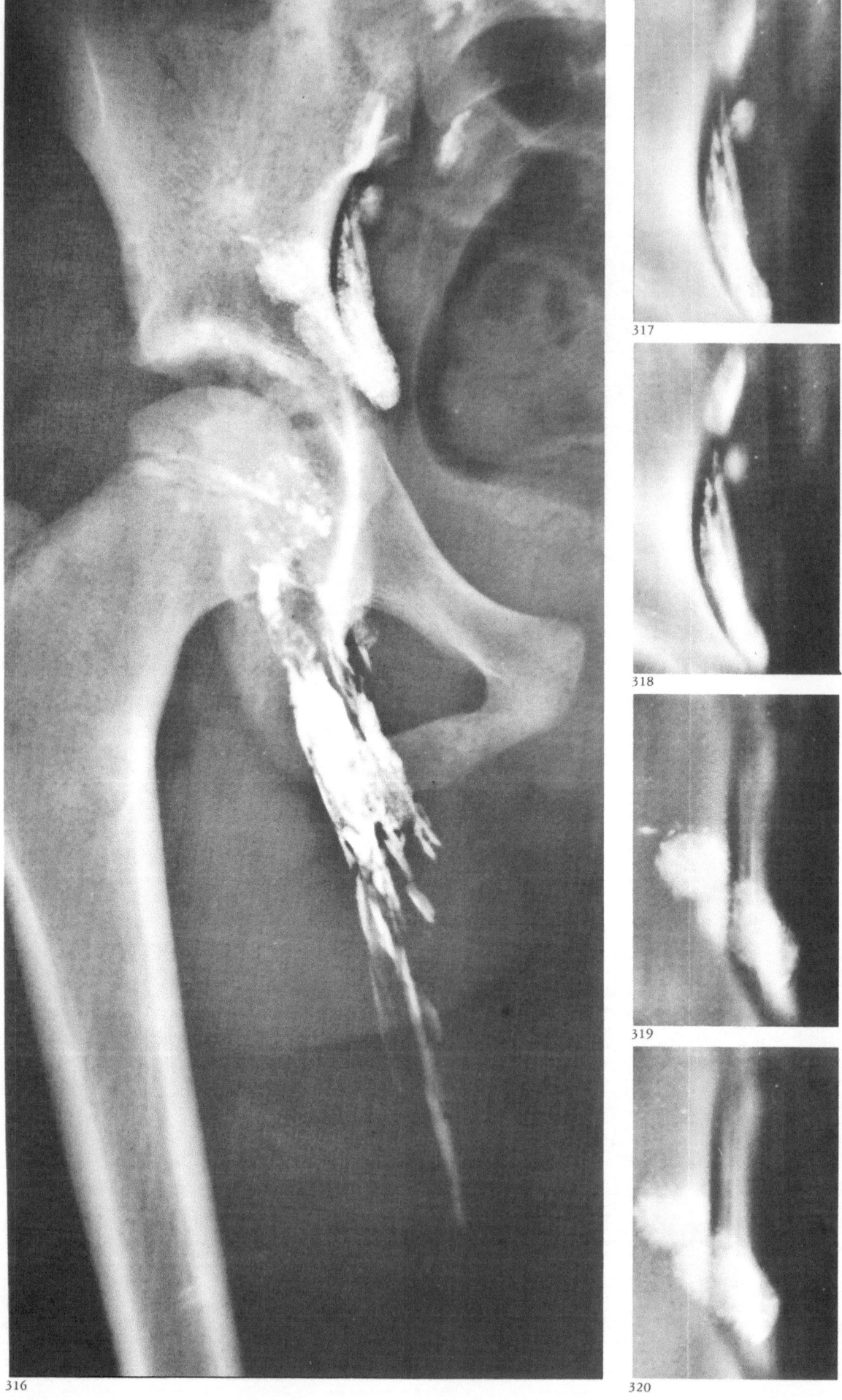

316

317

318

319

320

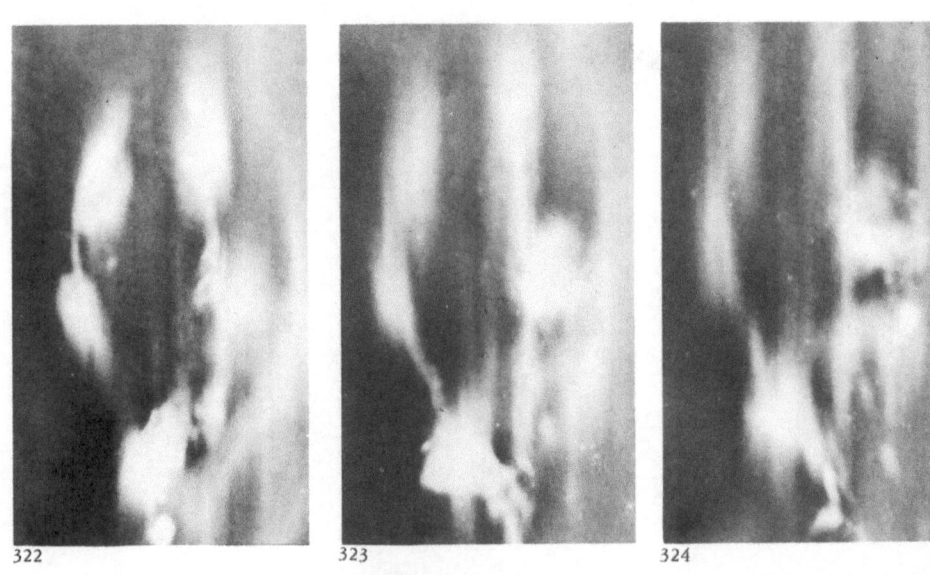

322   323   324

figs. 316-320 Melanosarcoma of the right leg; lymphography after surgery and removal of one pathological lymph node in the inguinal region. Lymphadenogram (fig. 316) and tomograms (figs. 317, 318, 319, 320) of the iliac lymph nodes: all lymph nodes are roentgenologically normal which was confirmed by pathological-anatomical examination after a second operation.

Comment: For melanosarcoma of the extremities, it is more important to evaluate the iliac lymph nodes on the lymphogram than the inguinal lymph nodes. The inguinal lymph nodes are usually removed anyway; if the iliac lymph nodes must also be excised, a more comprehensive surgical technique must be followed.

figs. 321-324 Melanosarcoma of the left lower leg; lymphography after excision and removal of all nodes in the groin. Lymphadenogram (fig. 321) and tomogram (figs. 322, 323, 324) of the iliac lymph nodes; in the inguinal region, one lymph node has been left behind, the iliac lymph nodes are roentgenologically normal.

Comment: If, after total excision of the nodes in the groin, lymphoedema does not develop – irrespective of the duration – then the lymph node excision was not complete. In practice it appears to be exceedingly difficult to remove all lymph nodes adequately without a previous lymphographic examination and control radiograms during the examination.

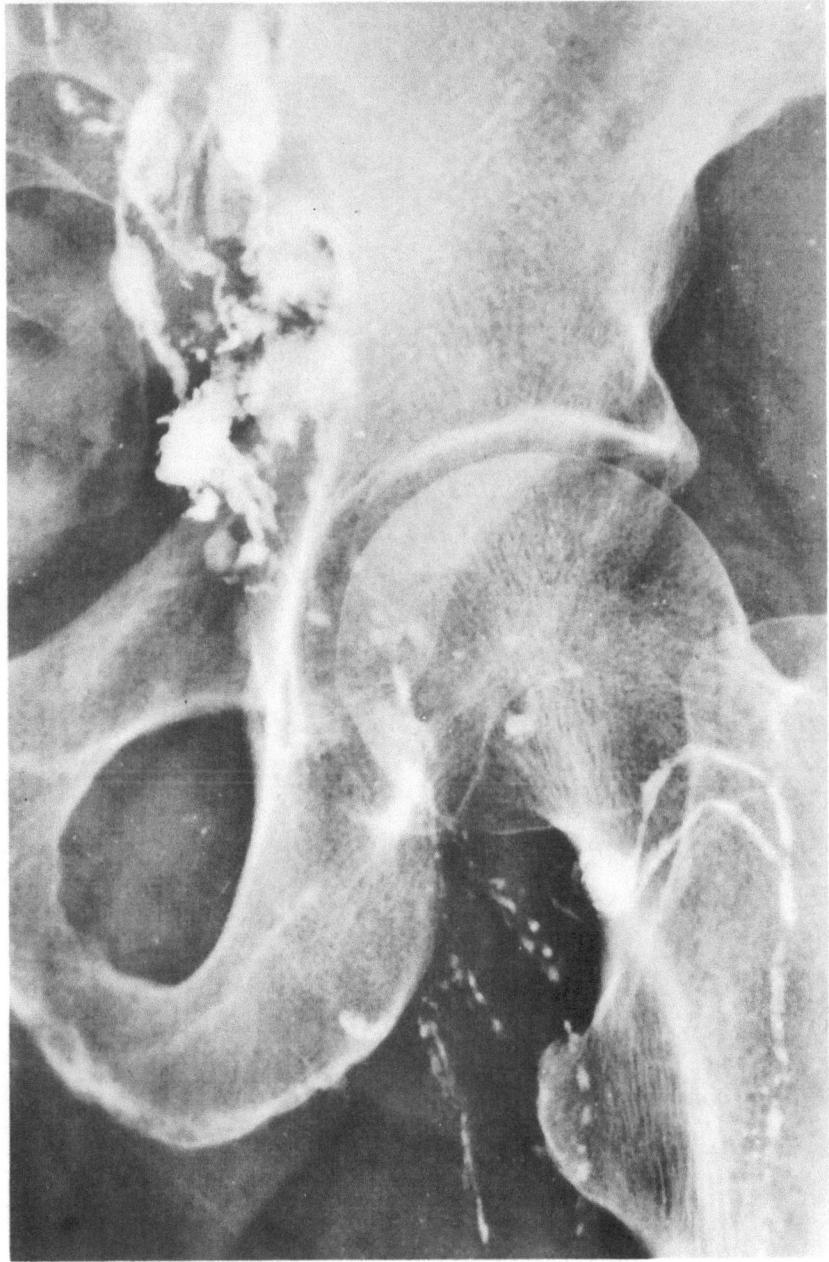

321

154

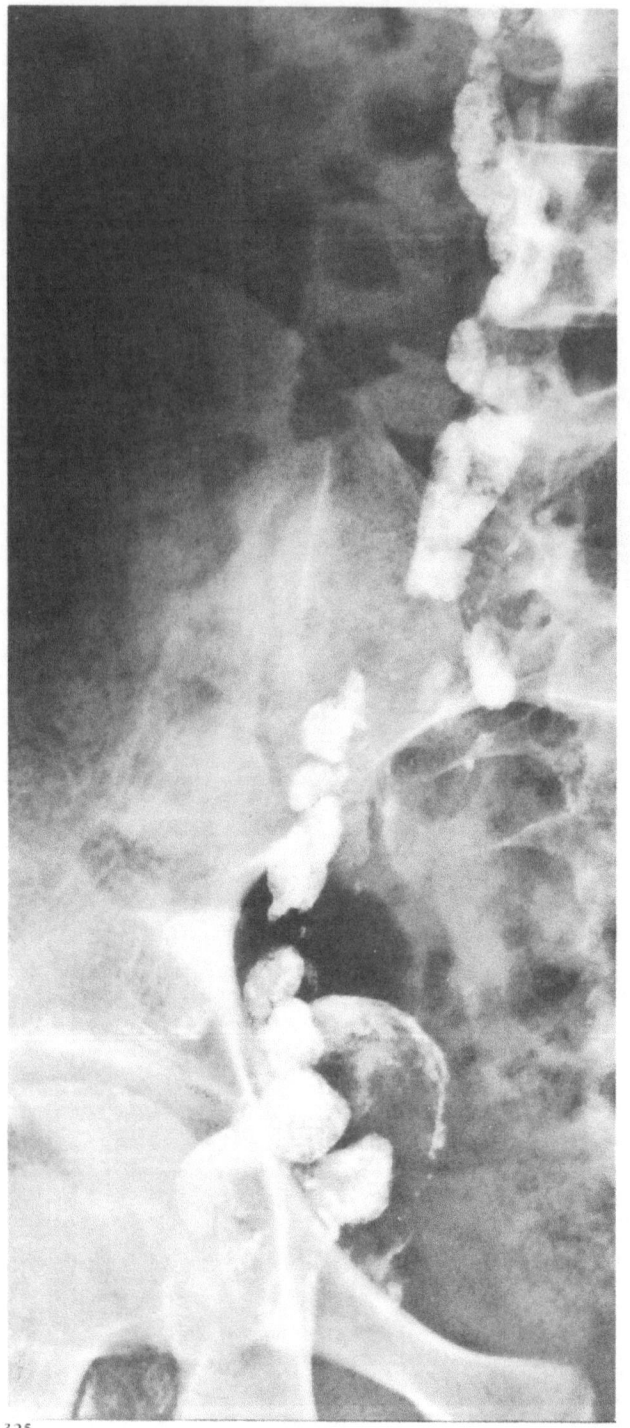

325

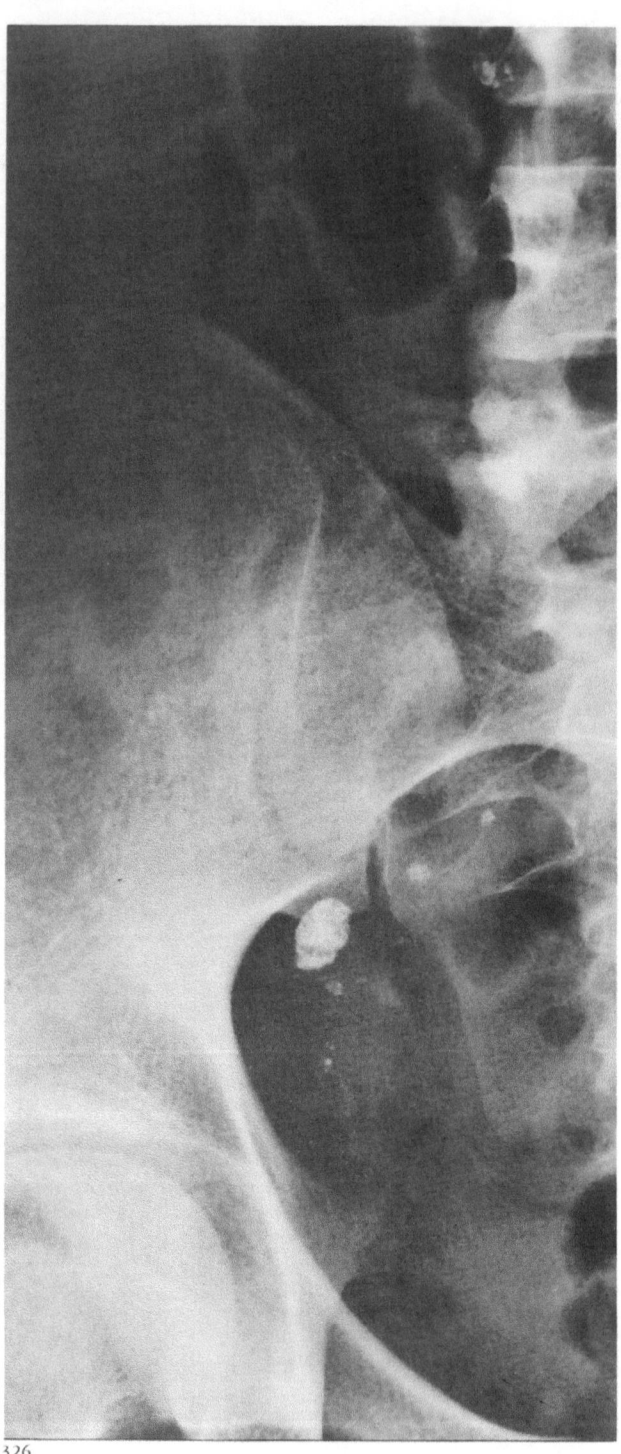

326

figs. 325-332 Melanosarcoma of the right leg.
Lymphography after excision of tumour and all
nodes in the groin. Lymphadenograms (figs.
325, 327), tomograms (figs. 328, 330, 332), follow-up radiograms after the operation (fig. 326)
and excised pathological lymph nodes (figs.
329, 331): one inguinal node (forgotten during
surgery) and 4 iliac lymph nodes roentgenologically normal, 2 large highly pathological lymph
nodes (figs. 328, 330). The follow-up radiogram
after the second operation (fig. 326) shows that
one iliac lymph node was left behind. The
roentgenological diagnosis was confirmed by
pathological-anatomical examination (figs. 329

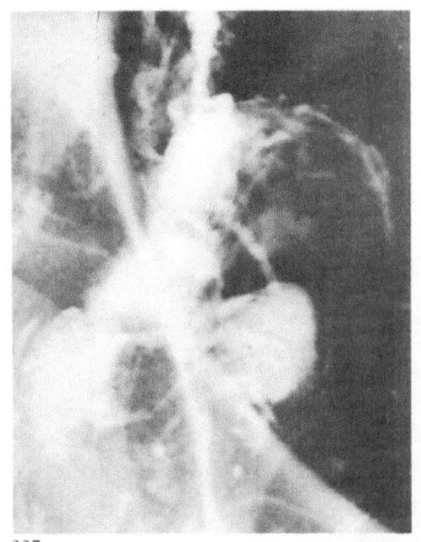

327

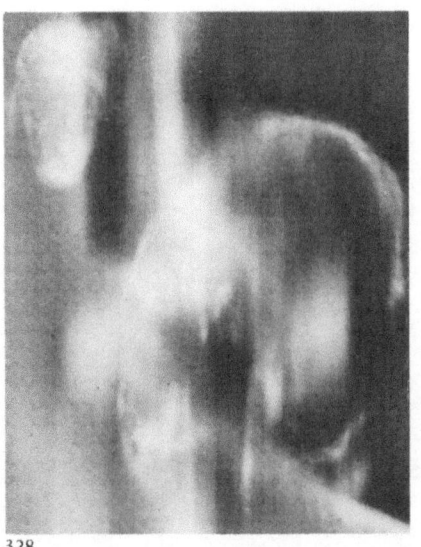

328

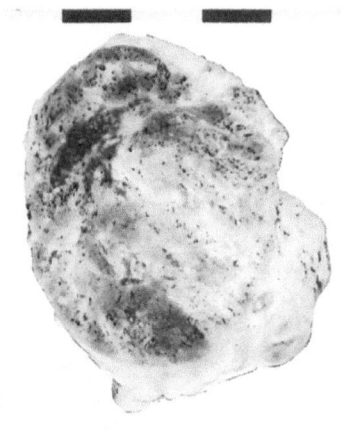

329

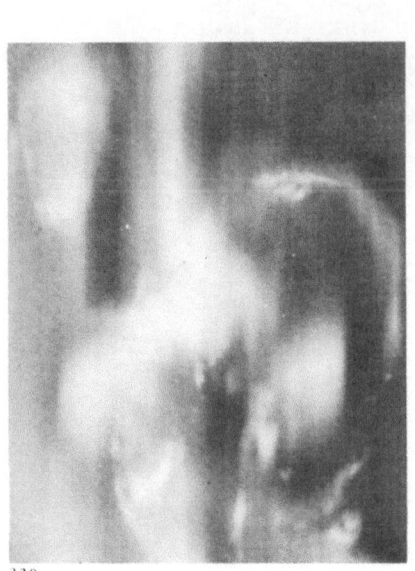

330

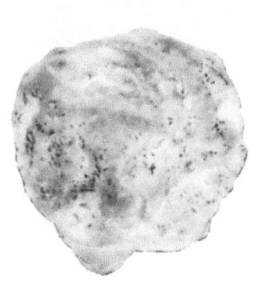

331

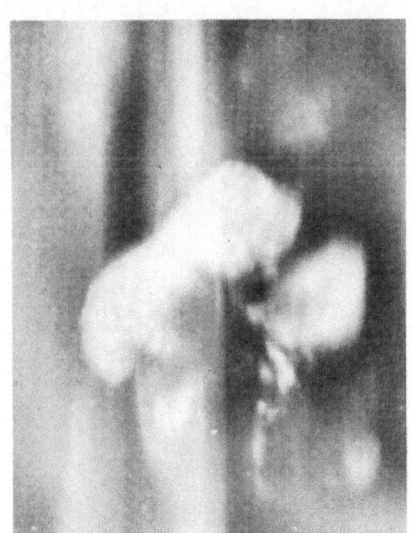

332

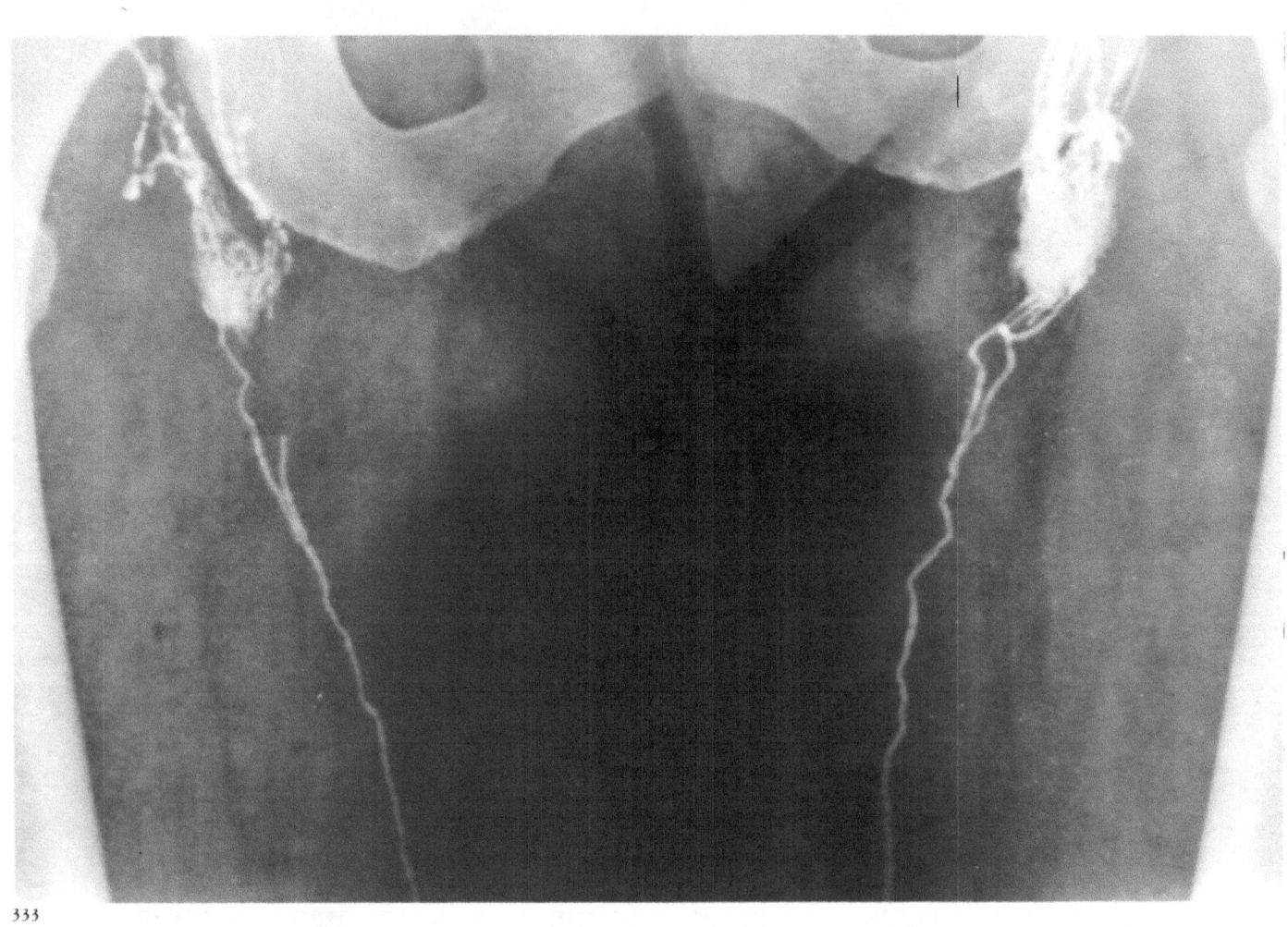

fig. 333 Primary lymphoedema of both legs. Hypoplasia of the lymphatic channels on the lymphogram.

fig. 334 Primary lymphoedema; lymphatic varices on the lymphogram.

fig. 335 Secondary lymphoedema; foot.

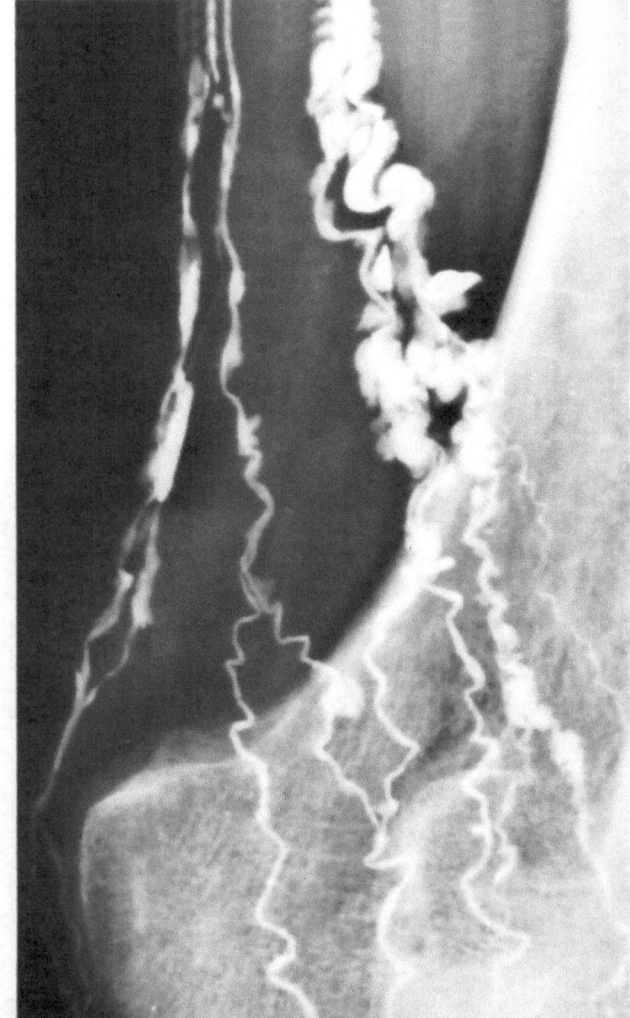

334

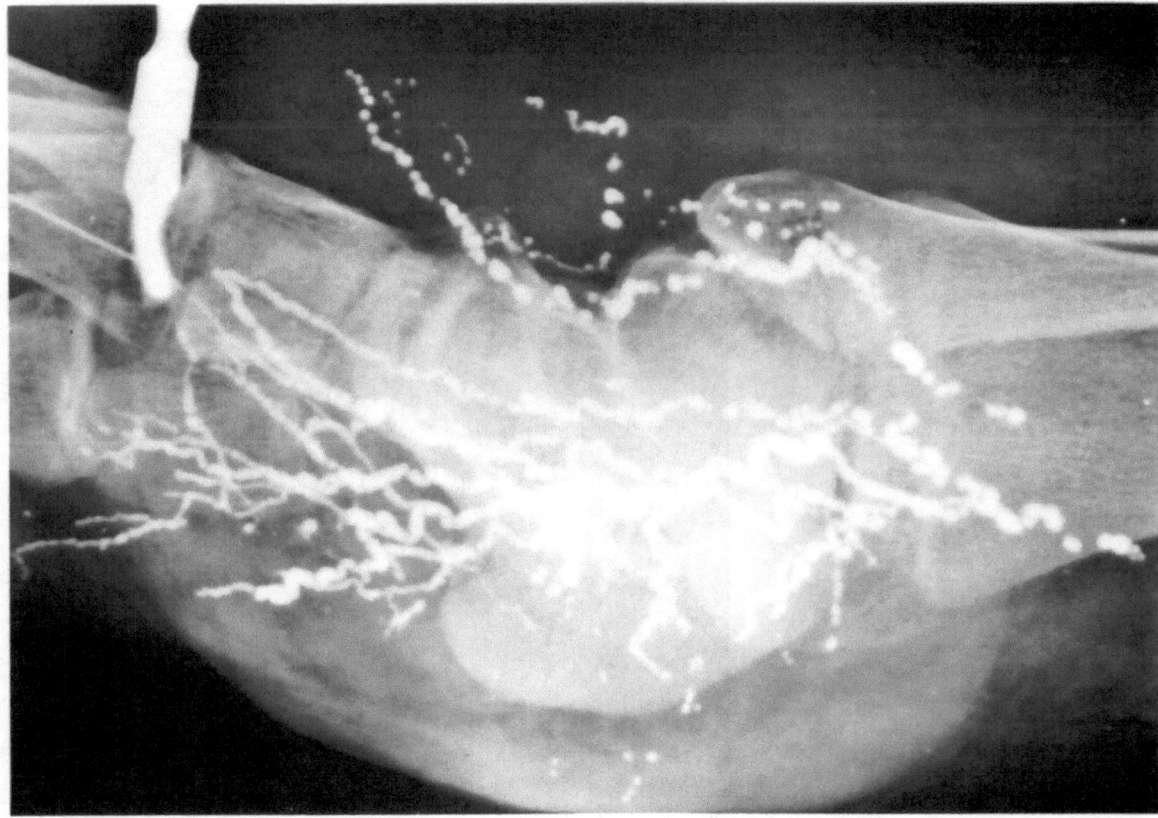

335

158   fig. 336 Secondary lymphoedema; lower leg
and ankle.

fig. 337 Secondary lymphoedema; lower leg.

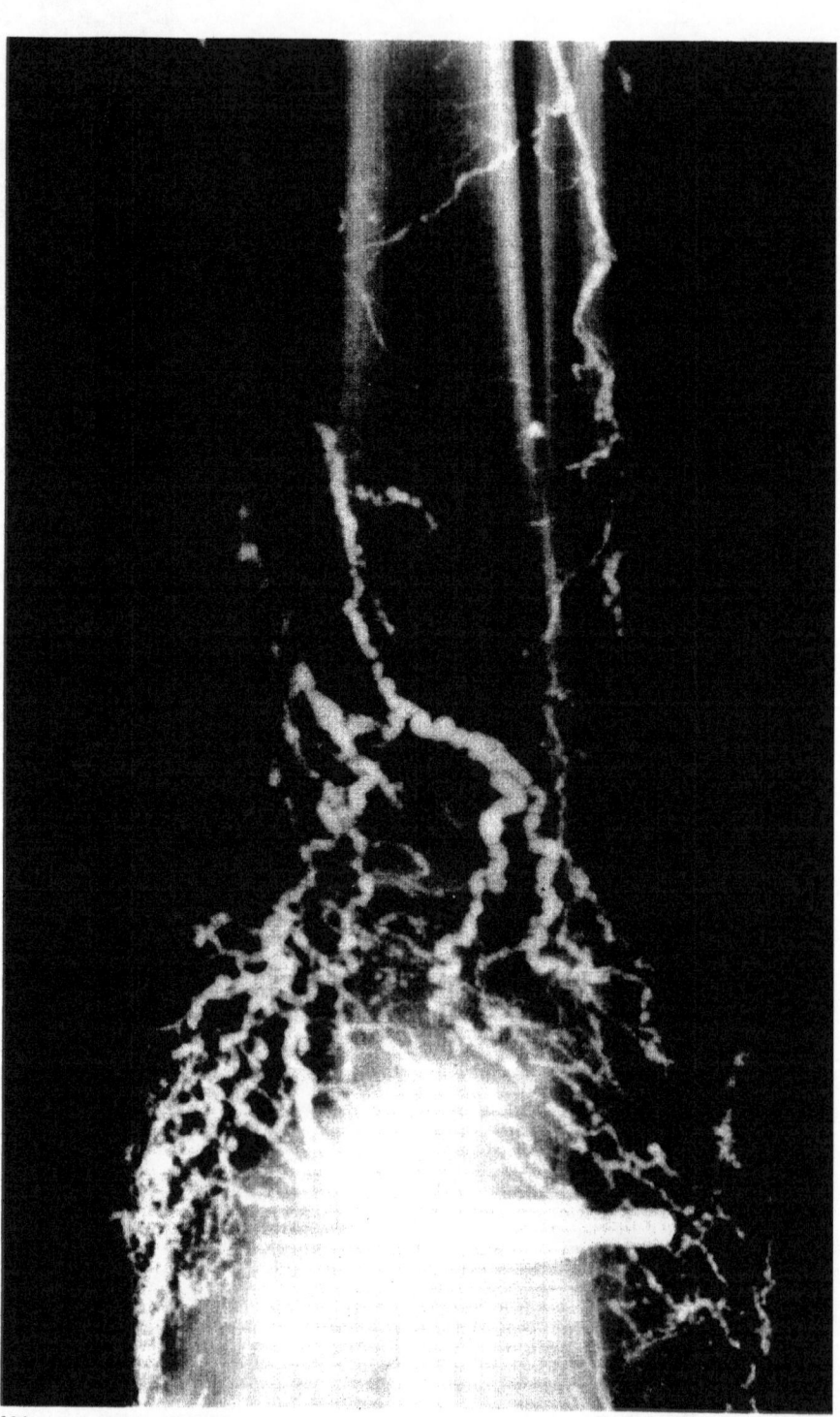

336

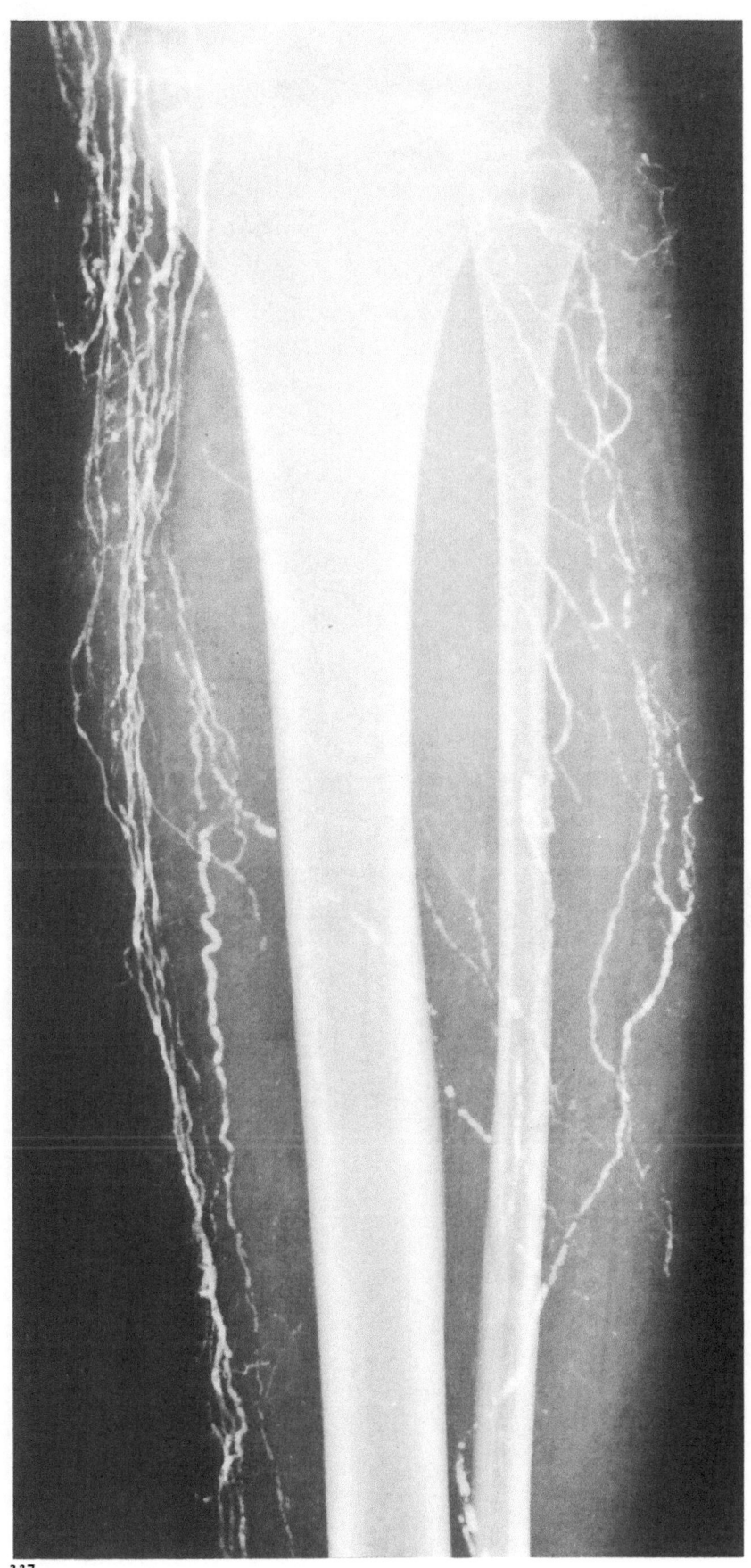

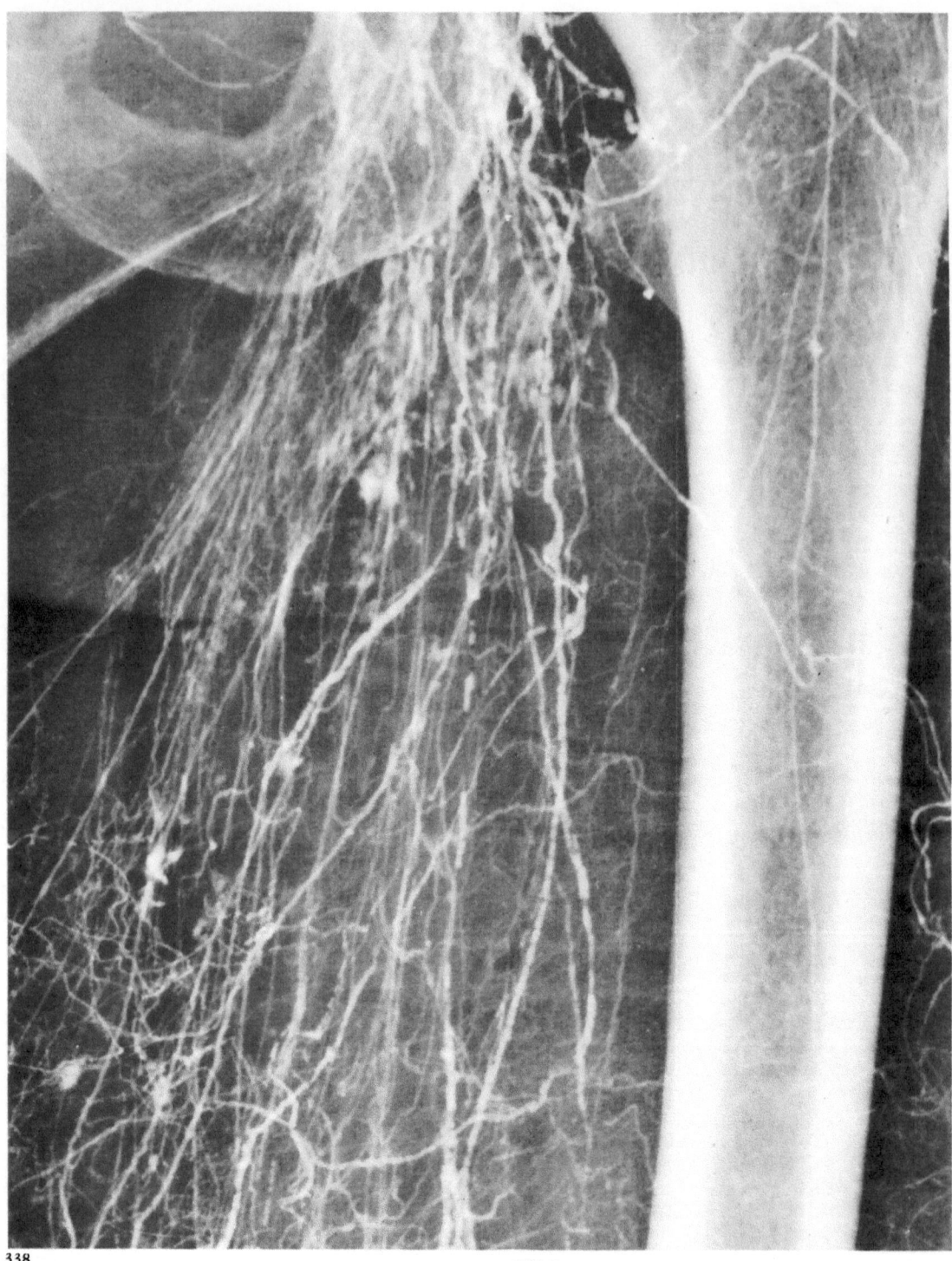

338

fig. 338 Secondary lymphoedema; thigh.

fig. 339 Secondary lymphoedema of the lower
leg as a result of a total block in the lower iliac
region.

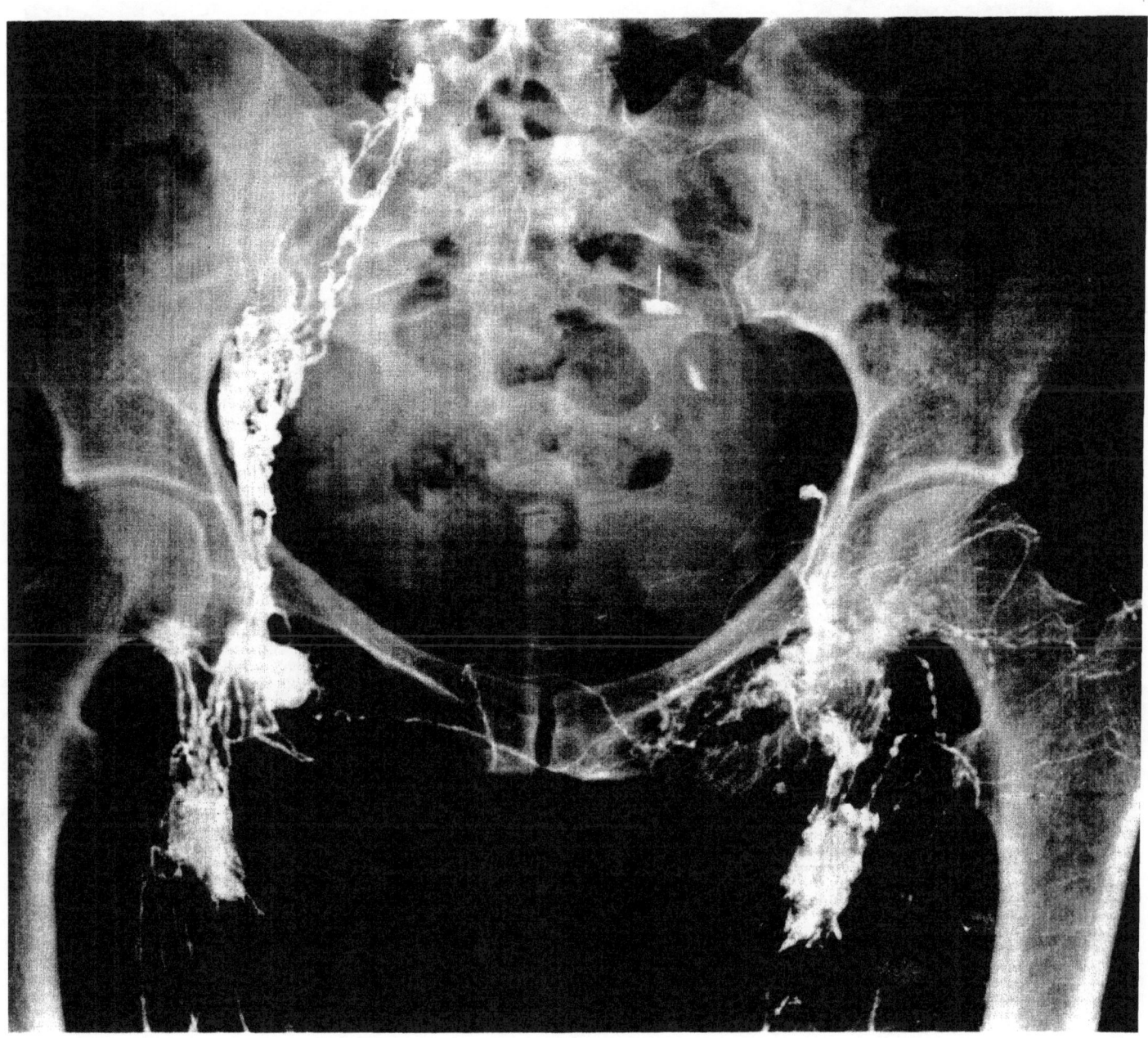

339

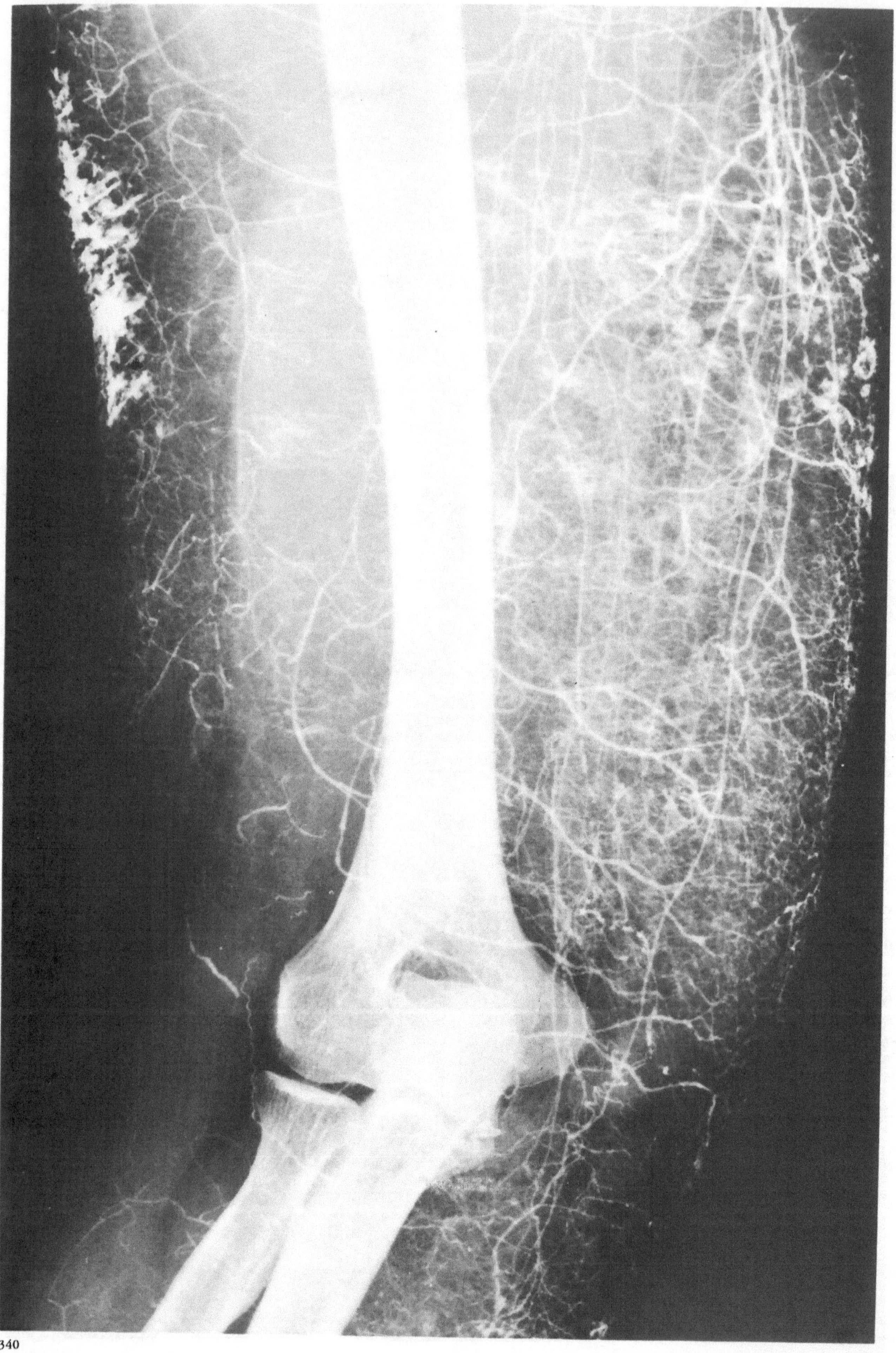

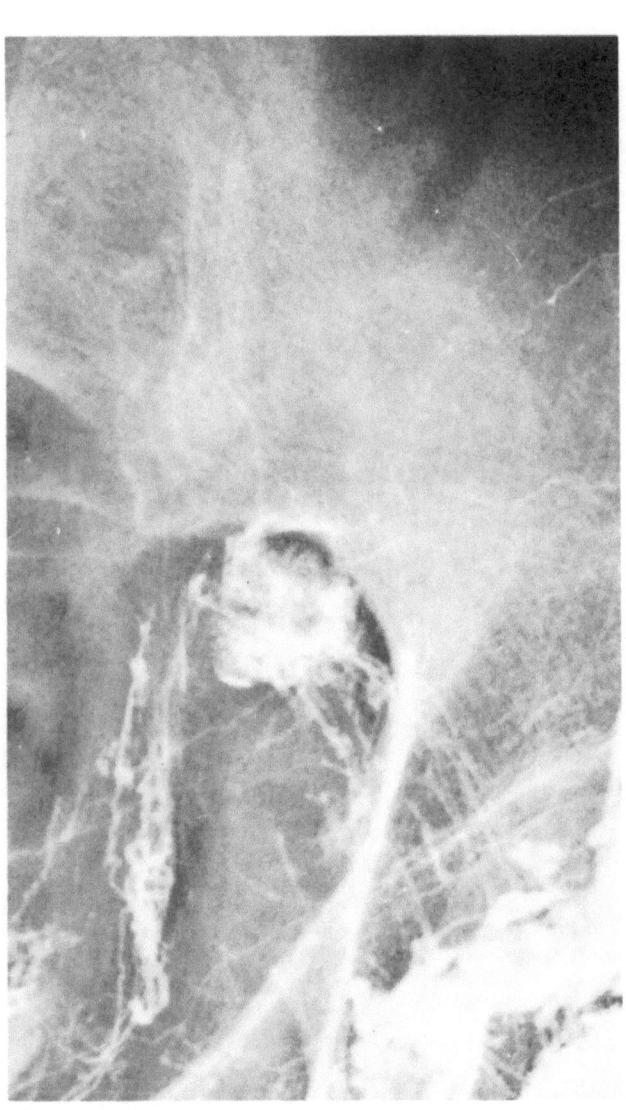

341

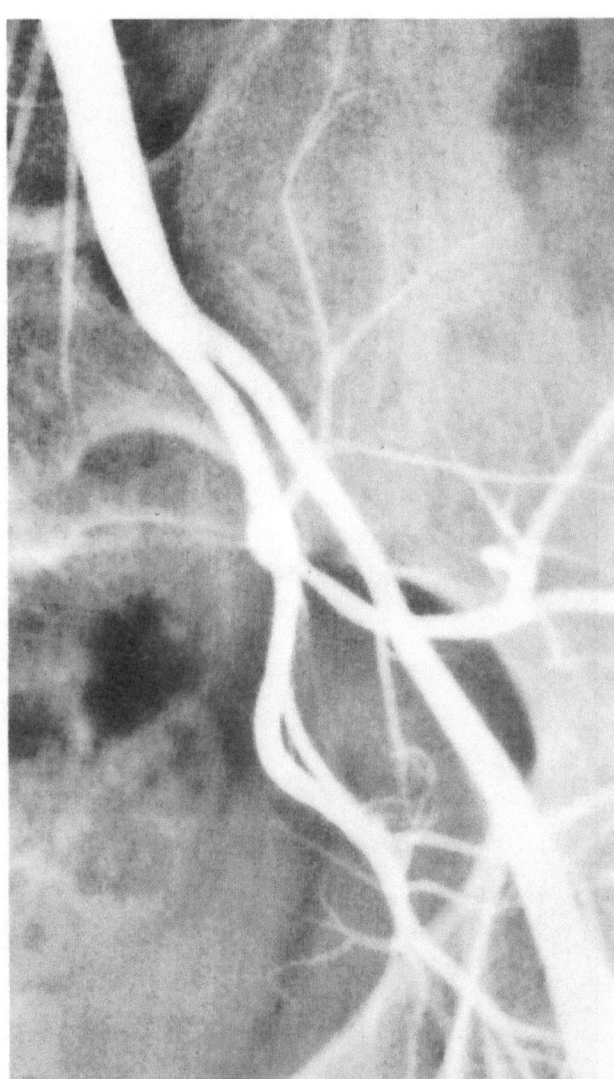

342

figs. 341 and 342 Clinical primary lymphoedema. Lymphography and arteriography were carried out during one session. Lymphadenogram (fig. 341) shows a total block in the left iliac region. The visible lymph nodes appear inflammed. Arteriogram (fig. 342) shows that the arteria iliaca externa et hypogastrica are narrowed and arch outwards to the left in the pelvis minor. Roentgenological diagnosis: secondary lymphoedema caused by pathological lymph node masses in the pelvis minor. Confirmed after surgery and histological examination.

fig. 340 Secondary lymphoedema of the arm. In addition to normal lymphatics, an increased number of small, twisting lymph vessels as well as dermal backflow.

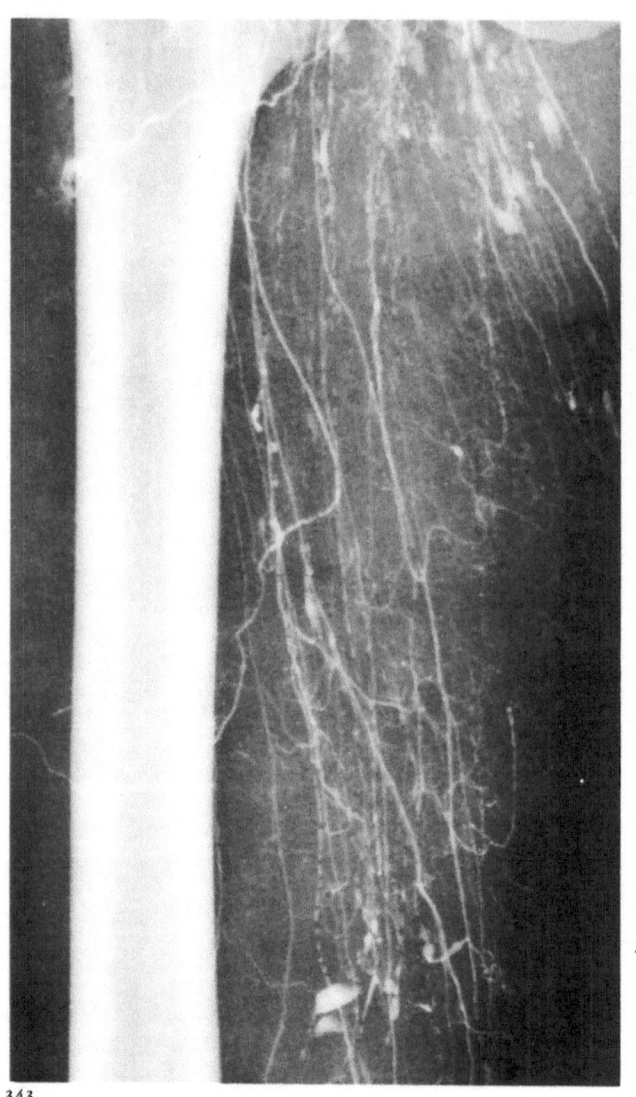

343

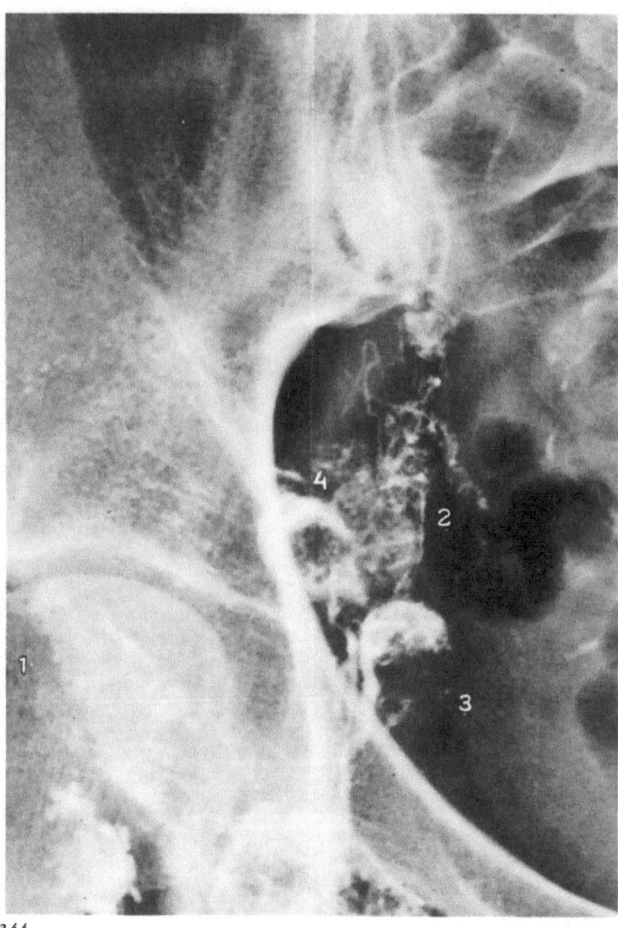

344

figs. 343-347 Clinical primary lymphoedema. The lymphogram (fig. 343) shows numerous, small, irregular, tortuous lymphatics in addition to normal ones. The lymphadenogram (fig. 344) reveals a total block in the right iliac region. The lymph nodes visible in the right inguinal and lower iliac regions are enlarged (1), (2), (3) and (4). Further differentiation is not possible. Supplementary tomograms (figs. 345, 346, 347) show lymph nodes to be enlarged. The marginal sinuses are interrupted and the internal structure has for the most part disappeared. Roentgenological diagnosis: secondary lymphoedema due to metastatic carcinoma. Confirmed by histological examination.

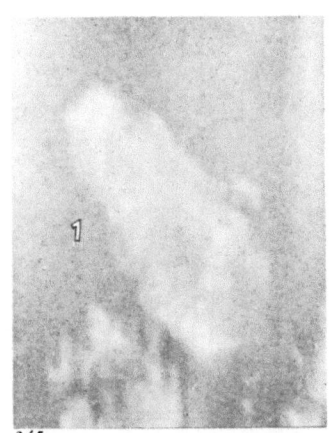

345

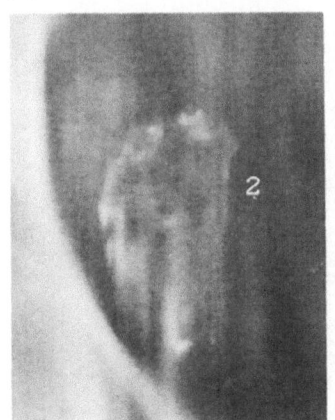

346

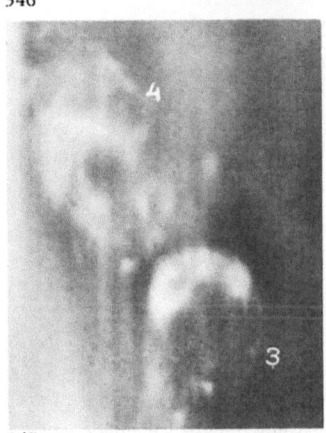

347

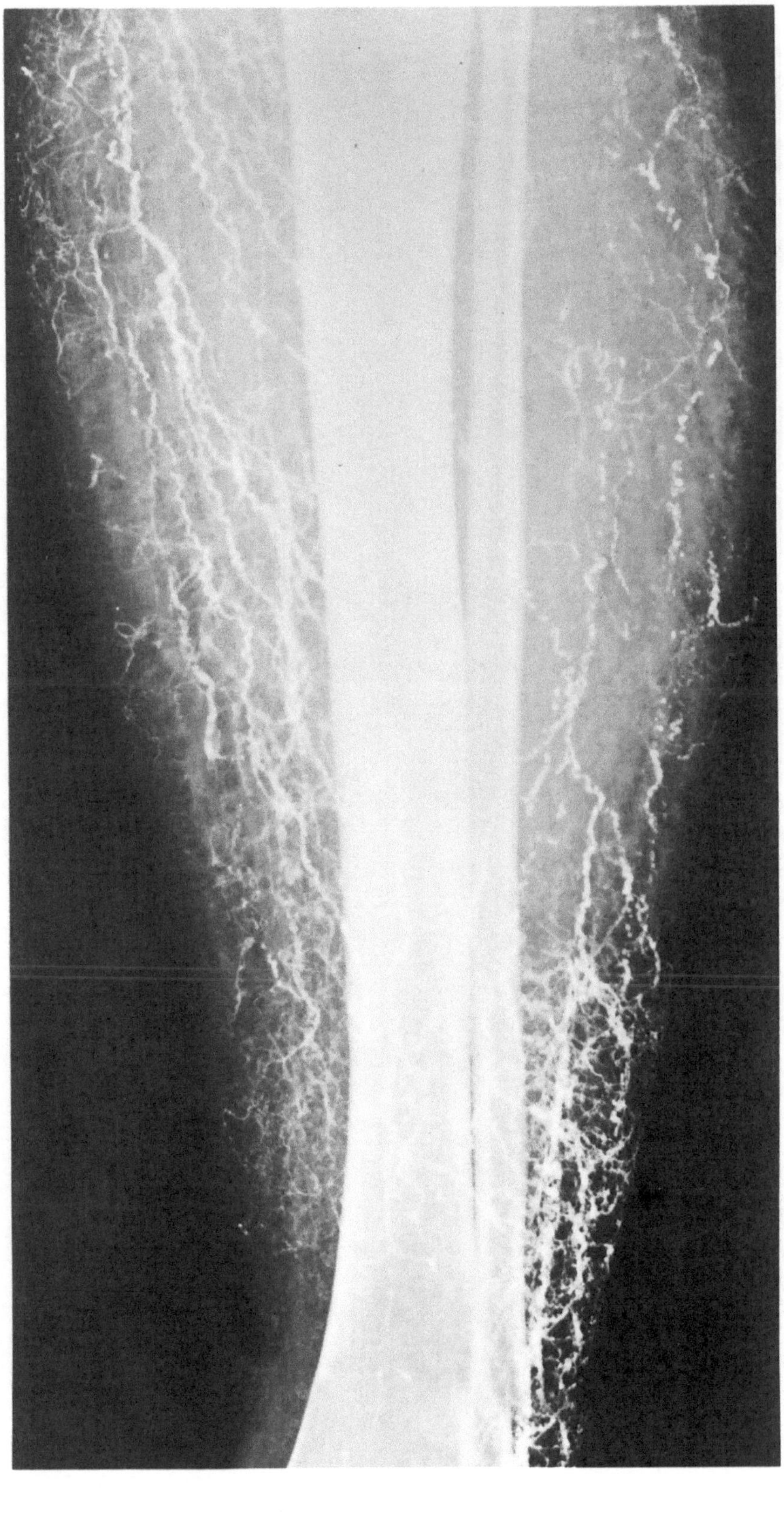

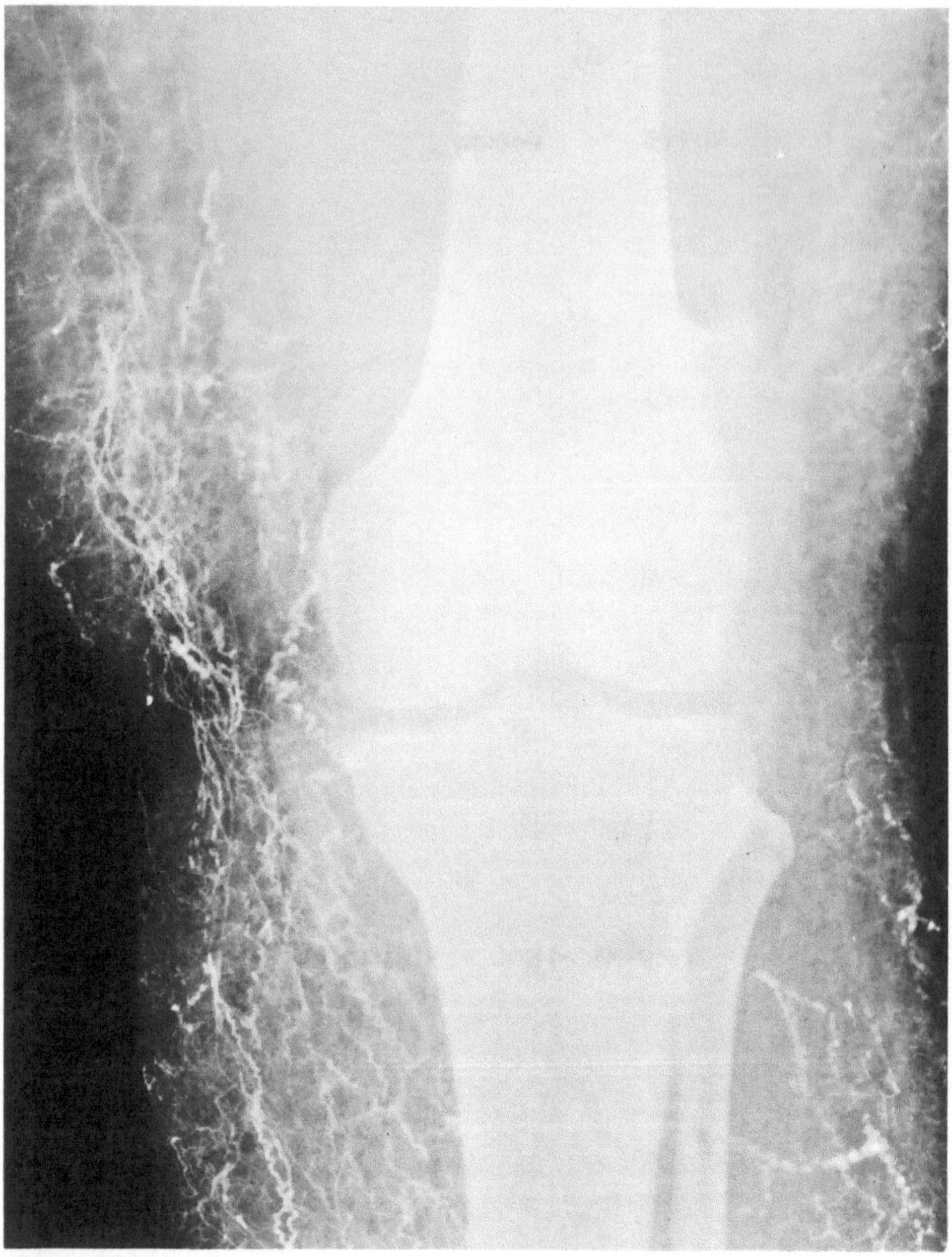

349

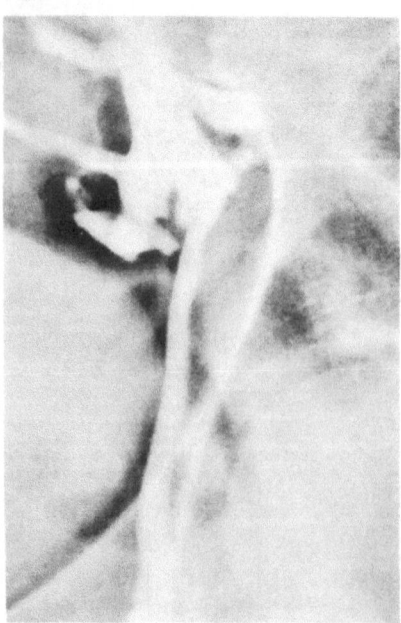

350

figs. 348-350 Clinical primary lymphoedema. Roentgenological diagnosis: secondary lymphoedema (figs. 348, 349) with a total block in the lower left iliac region. Phlebography (fig. 350) gave a highly abnormal picture of the vena iliaca. Laparotomy was now justified. The patient however refused and did not return for further examination. This happens often. Although the patients have a swollen leg, they feel otherwise healthy and find the long series of examinations extremely unpleasant.

figs. 351 and 352 Secondary lymphoedema of the left arm caused by a lymph node mass in the axilla. Histological examination of the lymph node puncture: non-specific inflammation. On the lymphadenogram (fig. 351) and tomogram (fig. 352), the lymph nodes are enlarged and show involvement by a malignant disease. Pathological-anatomical diagnosis after excision of a lymph node: mycosis fungoides.

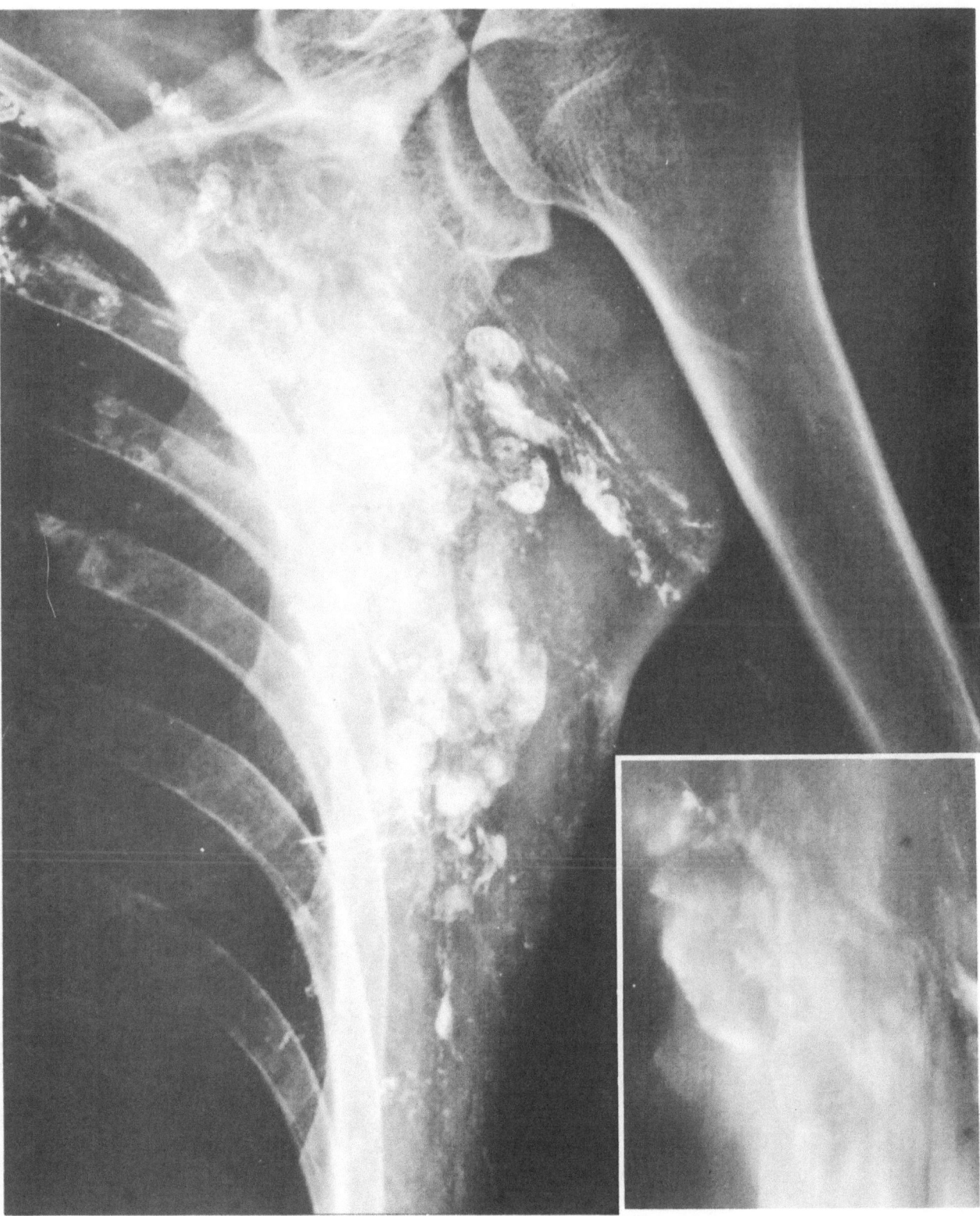

351

352

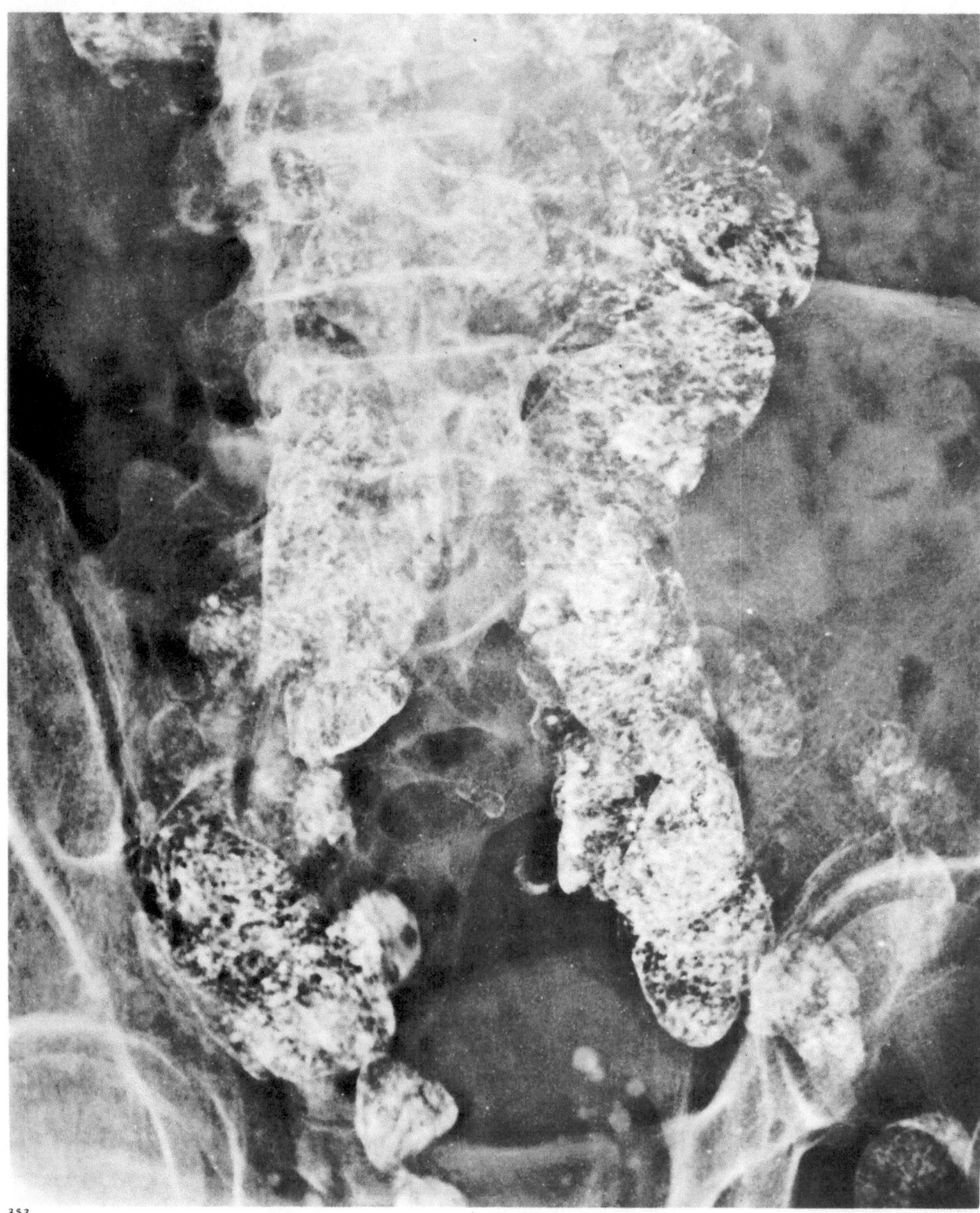

figs. 353-356 Secondary lymphoedema. Lymphadenogram of 4 patients with chronic lymphatic leukaemia (fig. 353), Hodgkin's disease
(figs. 354, 355) and carcinoma of the bladder
with metastases (fig. 356). Only the last patient
had lymphoedema.
Comment: Metastatic carcinomas are more likely to cause a stop or lymphatic obstruction and
thus lymphoedema than extensive lymph node
masses due to malignant reticulosis. In malignant reticulosis, there is usually drainage via the
thoracic duct; development of lymphoedema is
then rare. (see fig. 357-363).

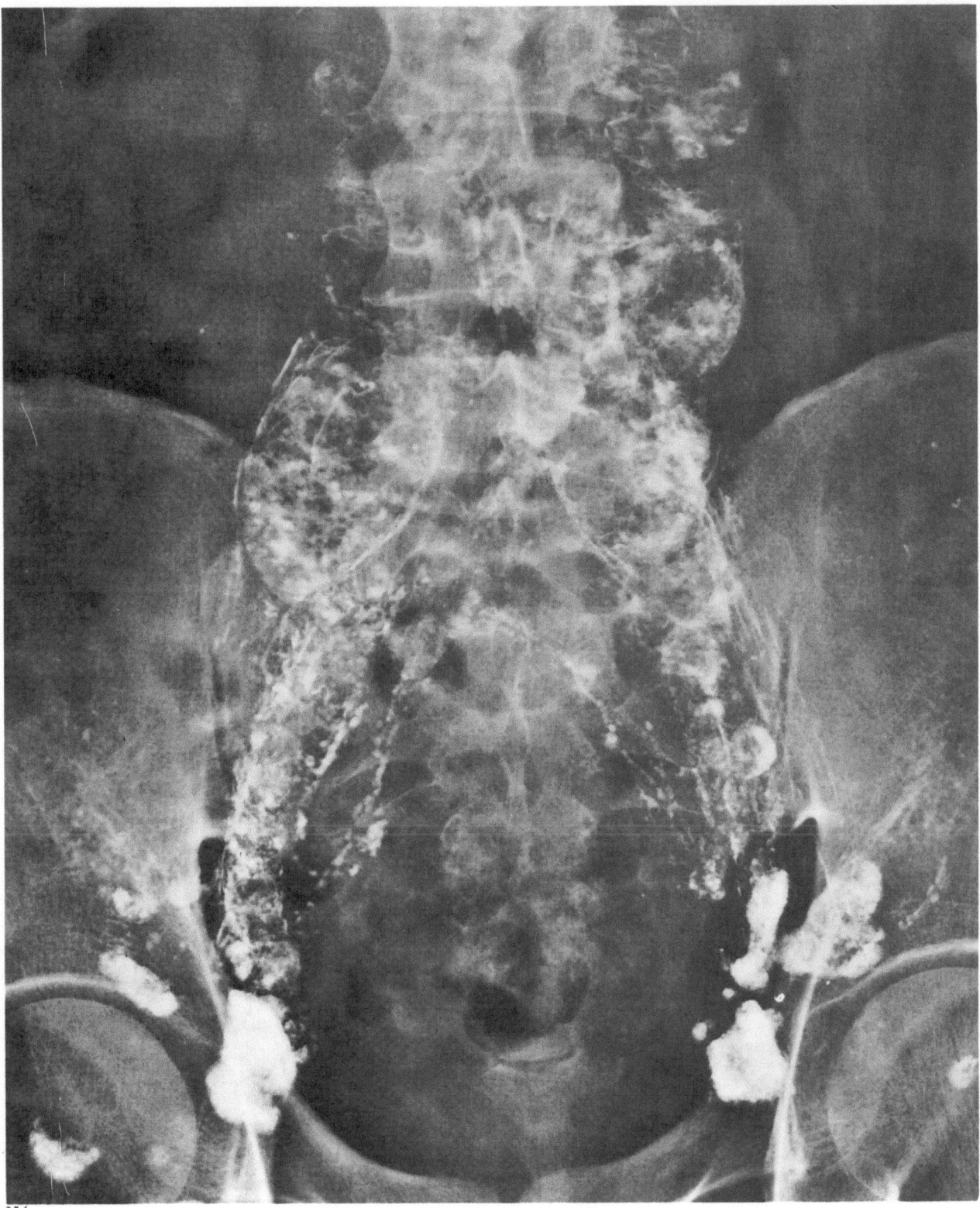

354

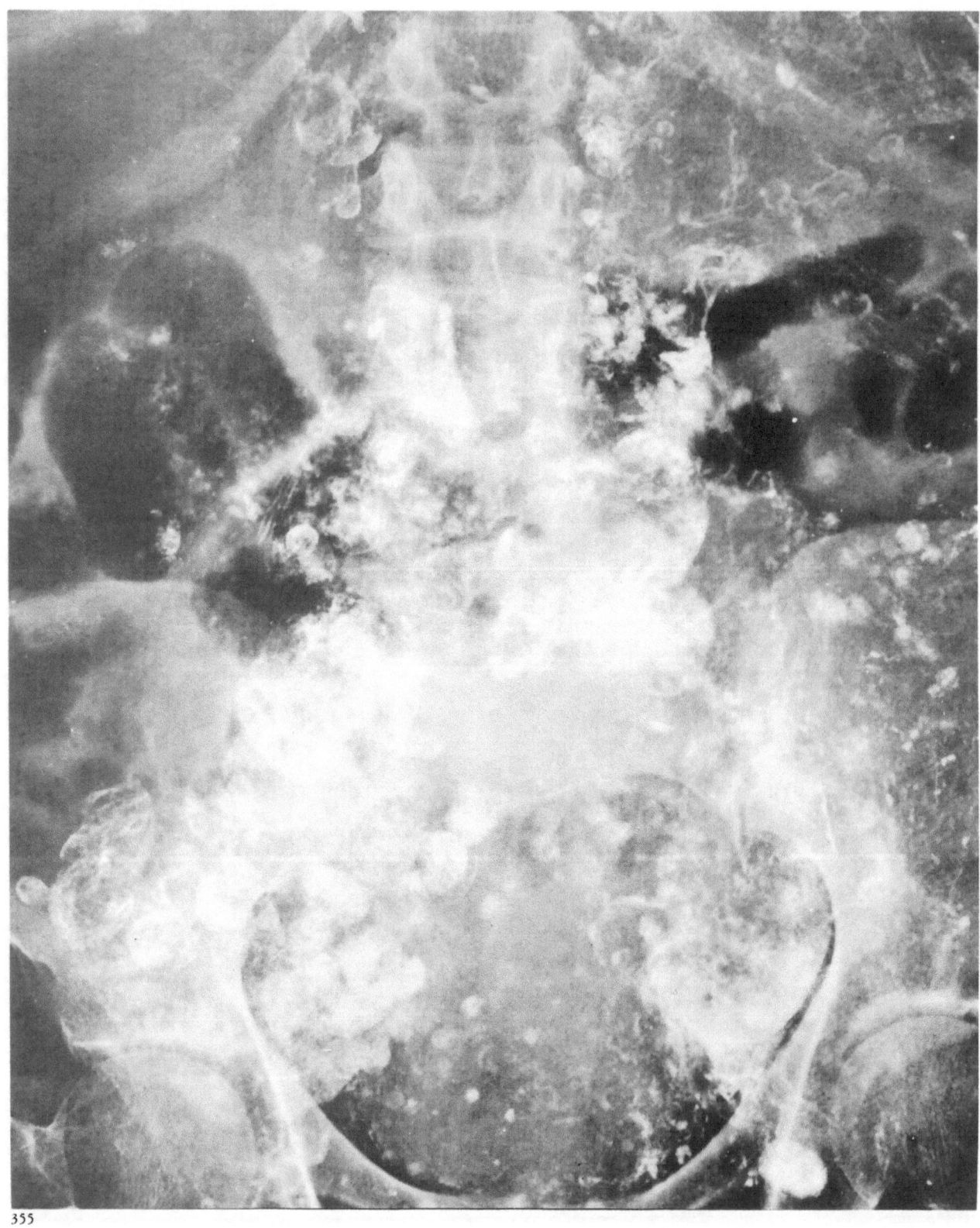

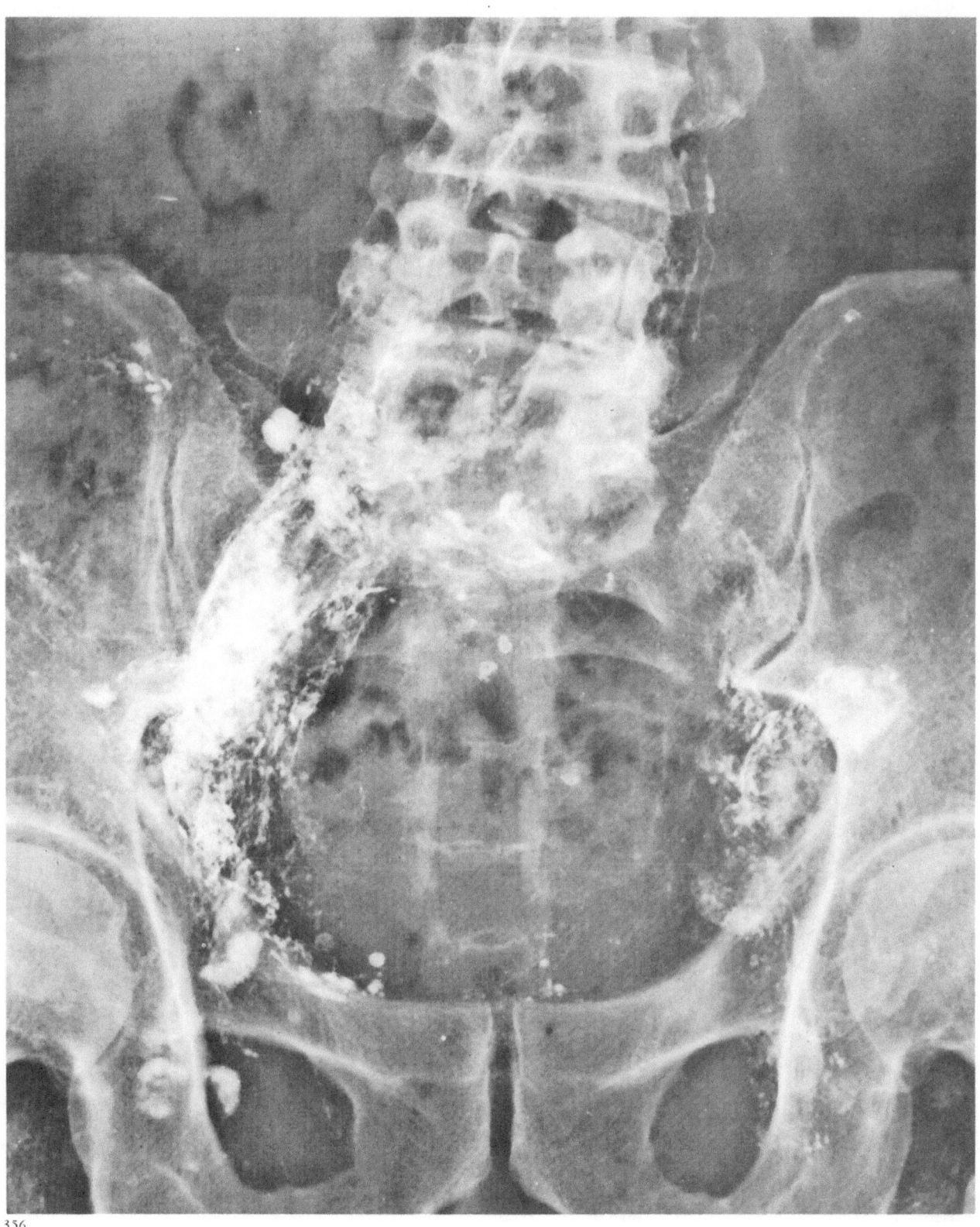

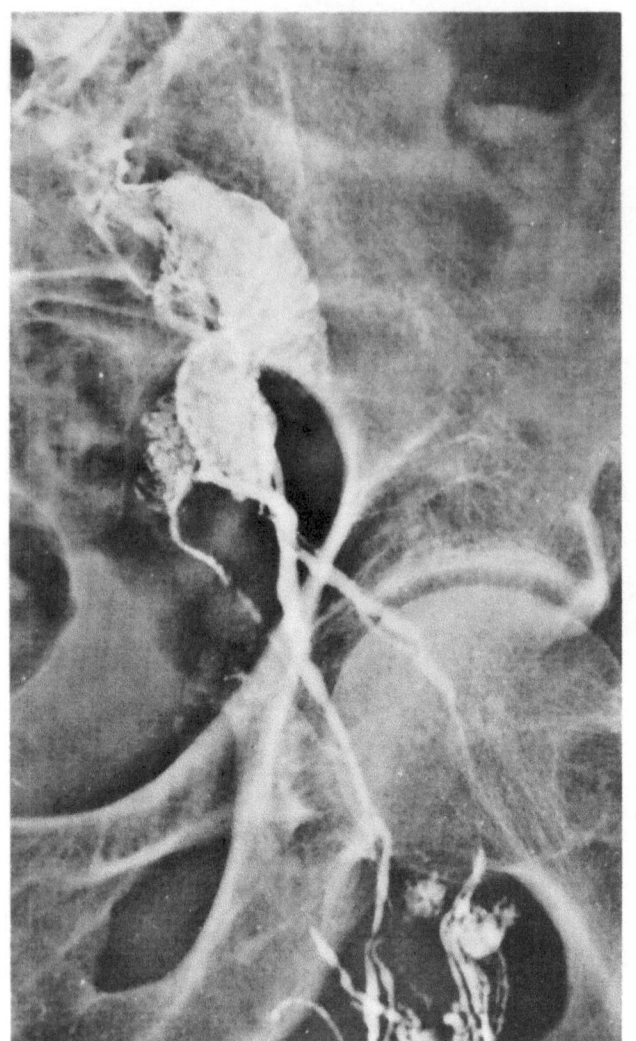

357

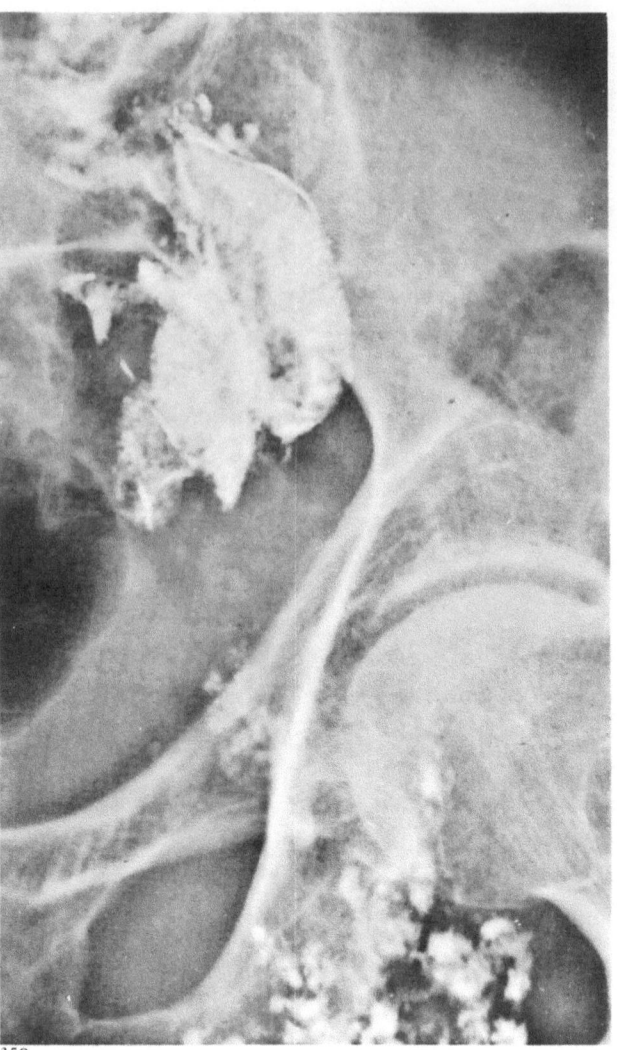

358

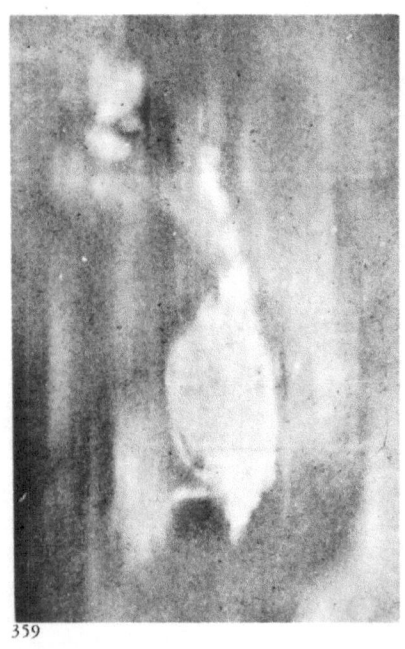

359

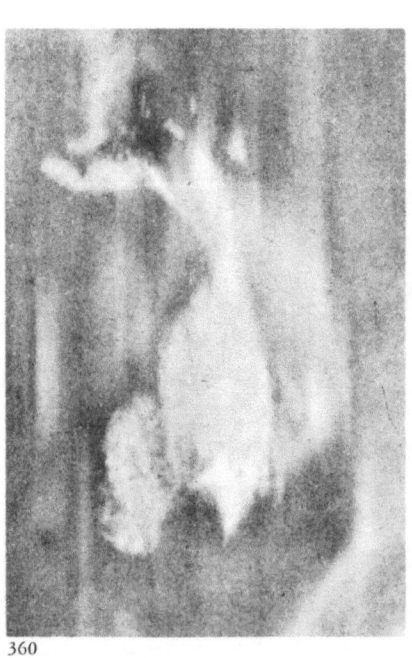

360

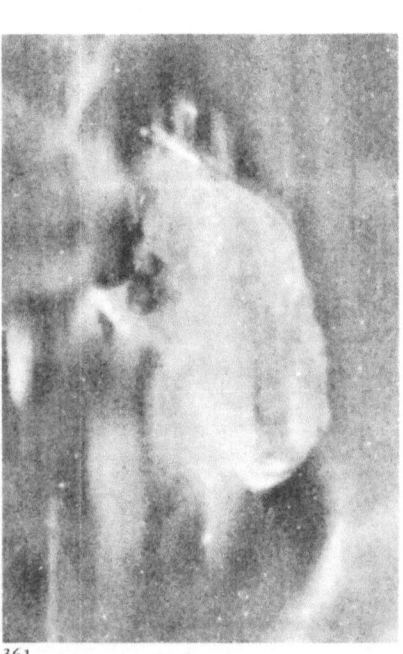

361

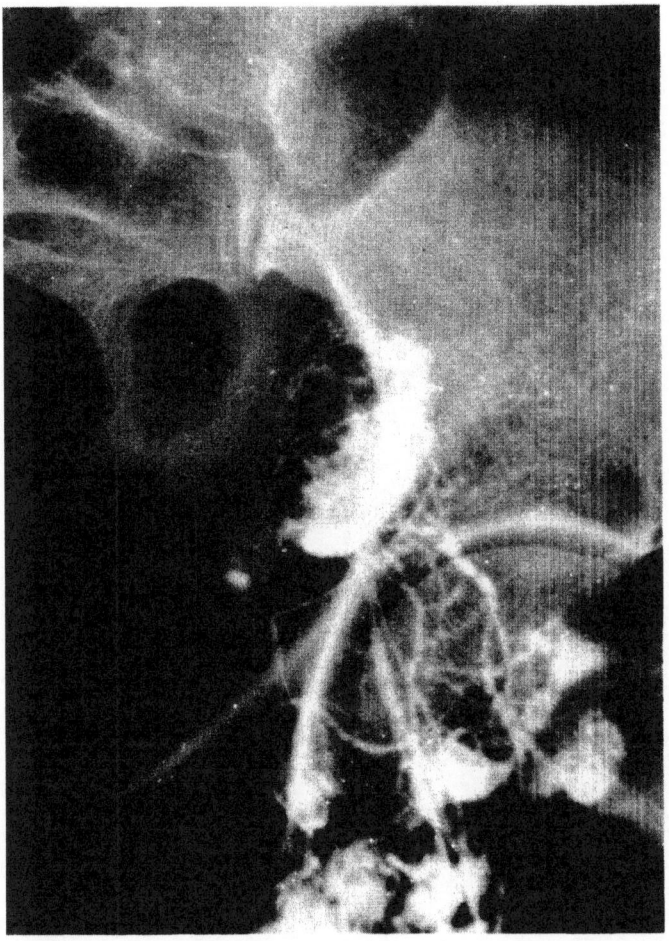

362

figs. 362 and 363 Secondary lymphoedema of 173
the left leg. Clinical and pathological-anatomical diagnosis: Hodgkin's disease. On the lymphogram (fig. 362) and lymphadenogram (fig.
363), a total block is visible in the left iliac region; below the block is an enlarged involved
pathological lymph node. Because of the roentgenological picture and the fact that a lymphoedema due to malignant reticulosis is rare,
the roentgenological diagnosis was lymphoedema as a result of a total block by metastatic carcinoma. Confirmed after revision of pathological-anatomical examination.

figs. 357-361. Secondary lymphoedema of the
left leg caused by a matted lymph node mass
due to lymphosarcoma; above, a block is visible
on the lymphogram. Lymphogram (fig. 357),
lymphadenogram (fig. 358) and tomograms
(figs. 359, 360, 361). This is one of the rare cases
of lymphoedema caused by a lymph node mass
due to a malignant reticulosis.

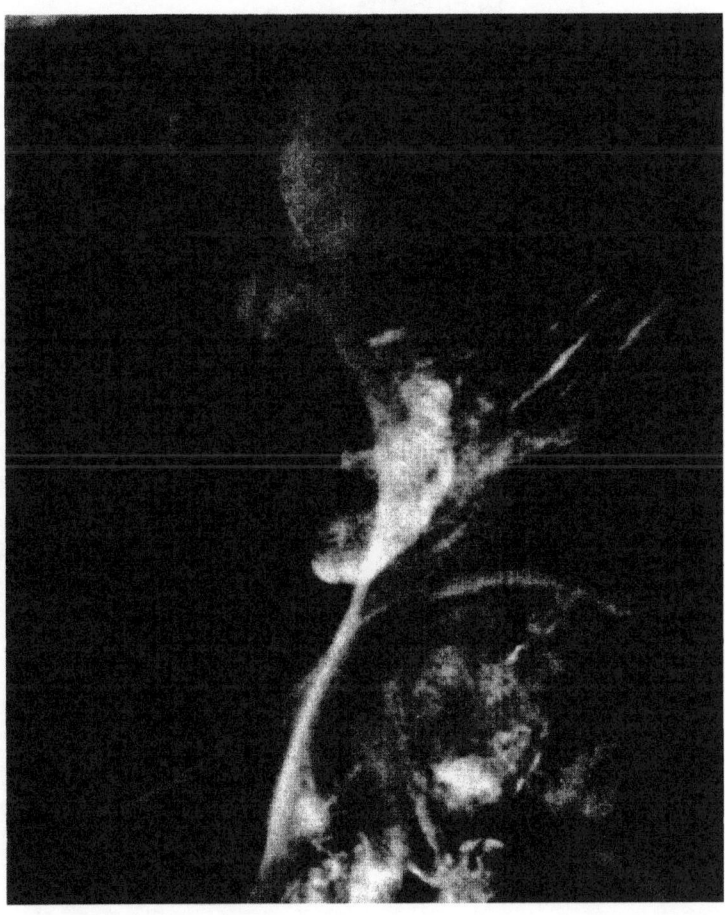

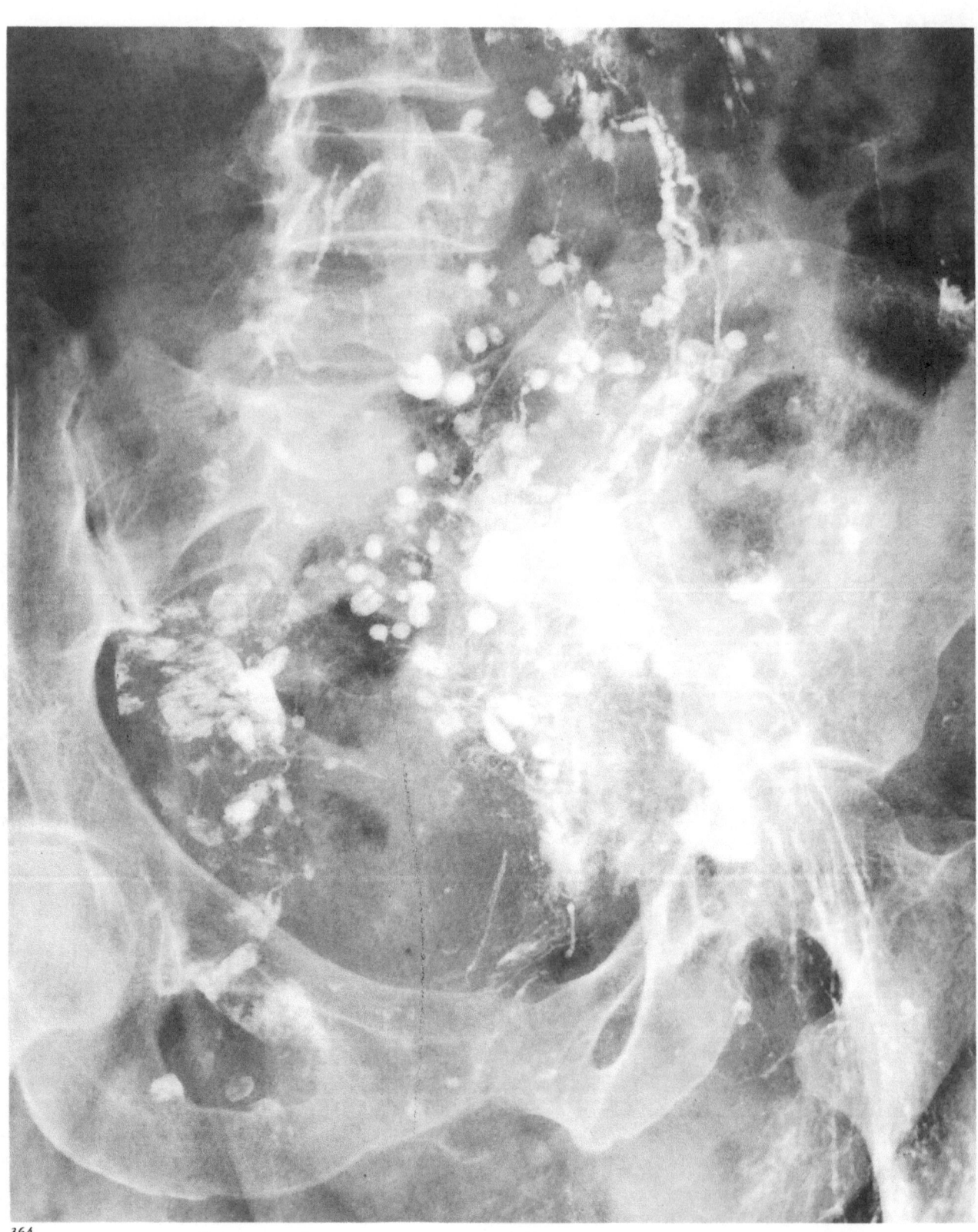

fig. 364 Secondary lymphoedema of both legs. On the lymphadenogram, the internal architecture of a number of small and several large pathological lymph nodes cannot be interpreted. Collateral lymphatic channels are filled with contrast fluid. Before the lymphographic examination, the patient had already been treated extensively with cytostatics, radiation therapy and repeated surgery. In the course of time, there were three different pathological-anatomical diagnoses: Hodgkin's disease, lymphosarcoma and reticulum cell sarcoma.

Comment: These patients in the terminal stage are no longer benefitted by lymphography and for this reason the examination should not be executed.

fig. 365 Secondary lymphoedema of the left arm as a result of extensive metastases of a melanosarcoma in the axilla. Lymphadenogram.

figs. 366 and 367 Mamma amputation with excision of the axillary and subclavicular lymph nodes as well as radiation therapy. In all patients with lymphoedema of the arm, there was a block in the lymphatic drainage of the axilla (lymphogram: fig. 366). If lymphoedema does not develop, drainage is visible via the collateral lymphatic channels (lymphogram: fig. 367).

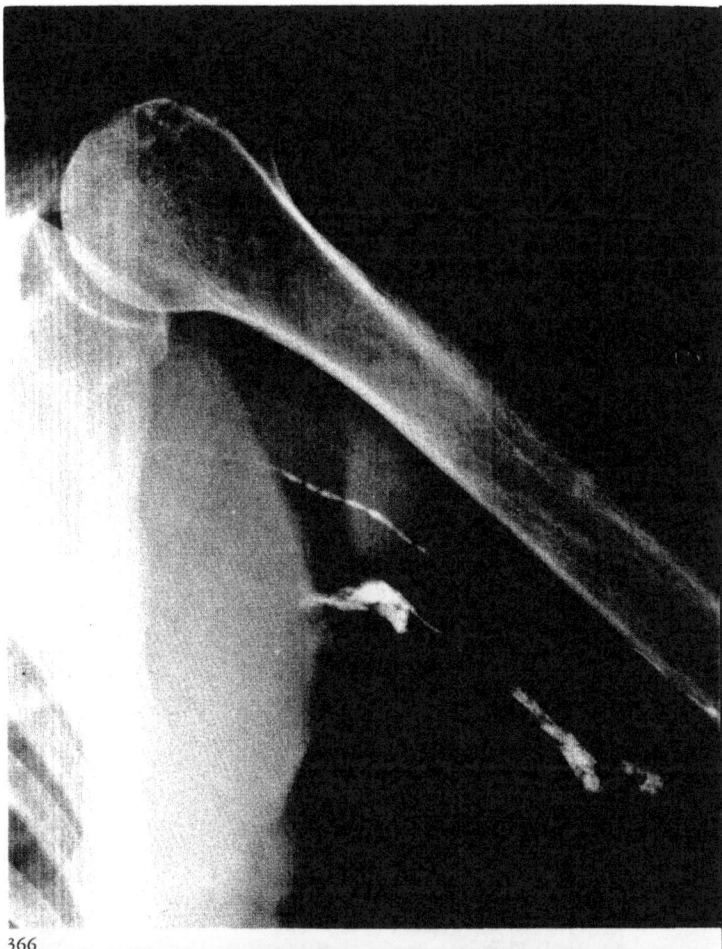

366

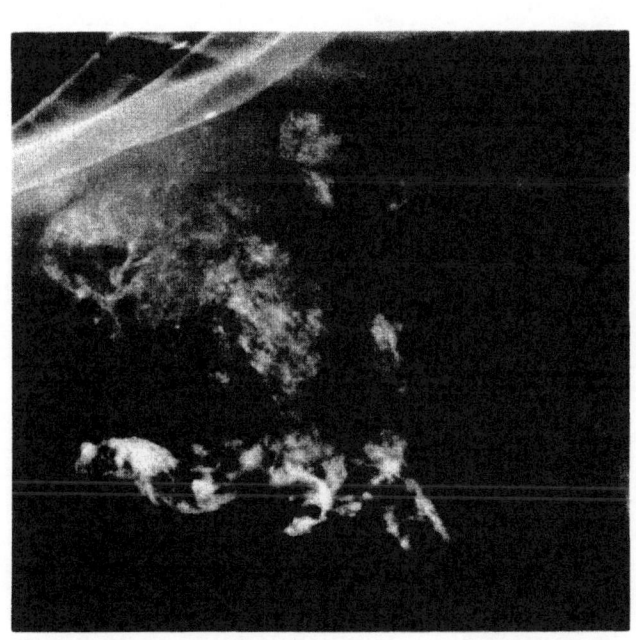

365

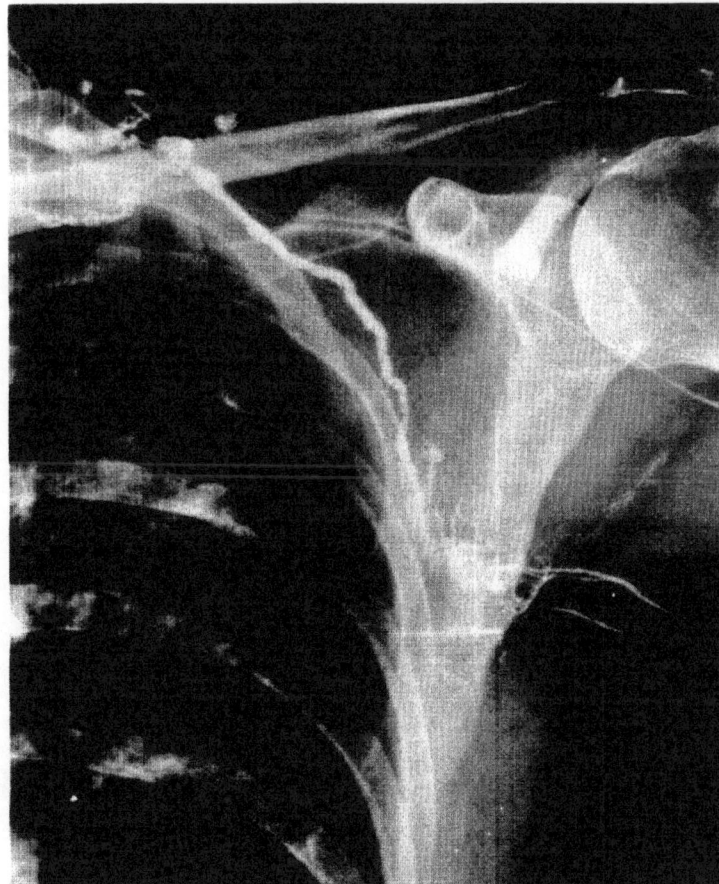

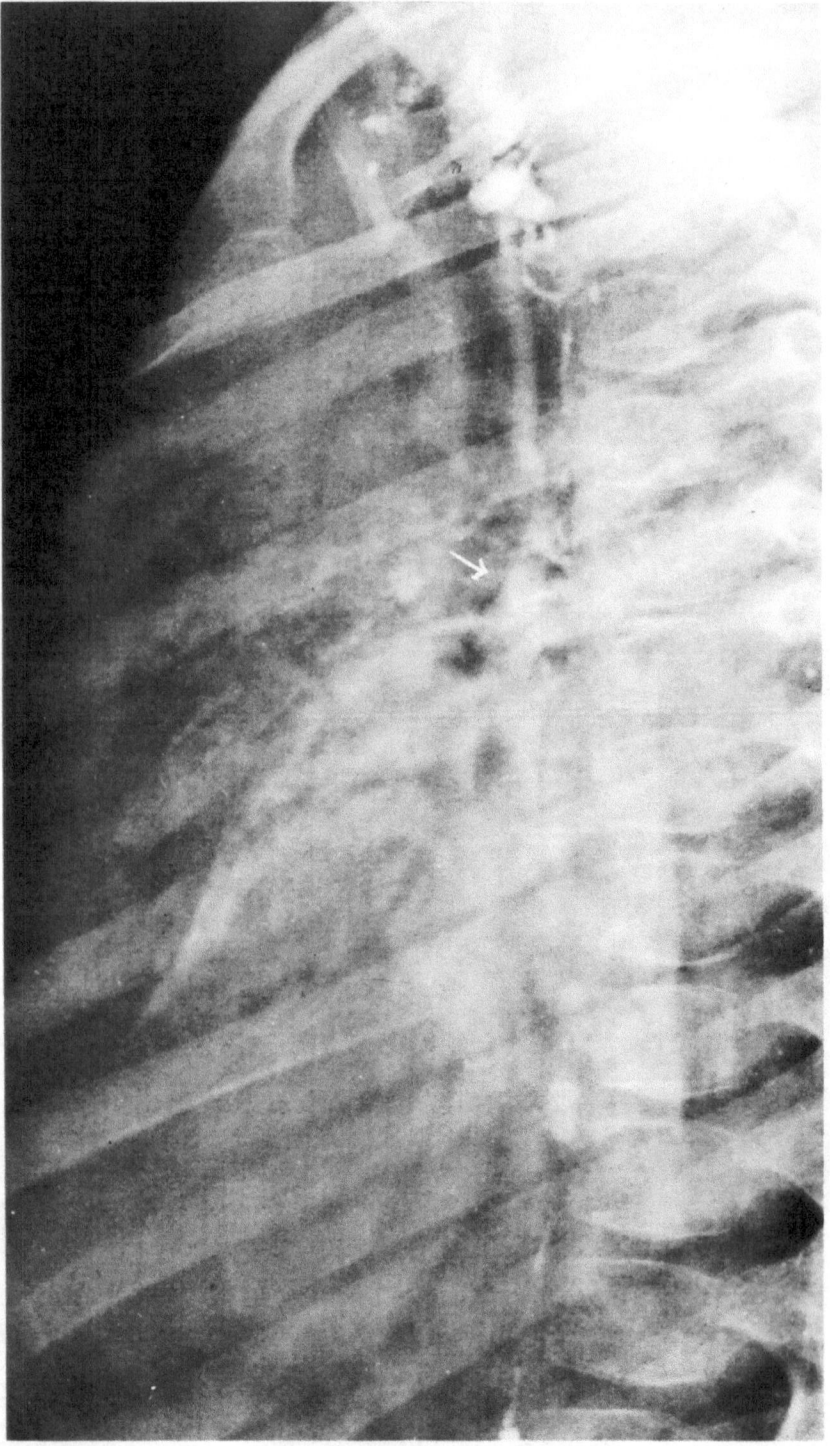

fig. 368 Chylothorax; lymphogram: lesion of the thoracic duct after Blalock's operation. Effusion of contrast fluid (→) from the thoracic duct.

figs. 369-372 Filaria with chyluria. Lymphogram (fig. 369); numerous, twisted and varicose lymph vessels in the iliac and para-aortic regions. Distended lymph vessels in the kidney and around calyces (fig. 370), the latter even more clearly seen on the supplementary intravenous pyelogram with tomogram (figs. 371, 372).

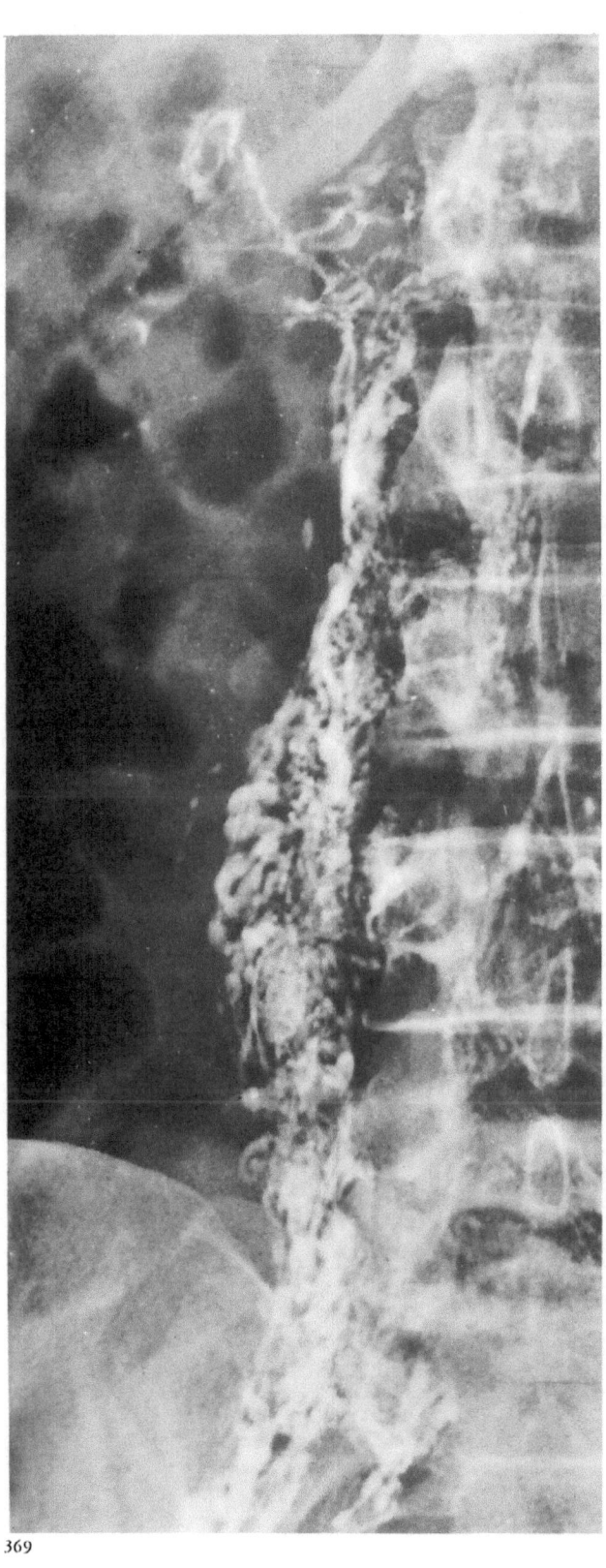

369

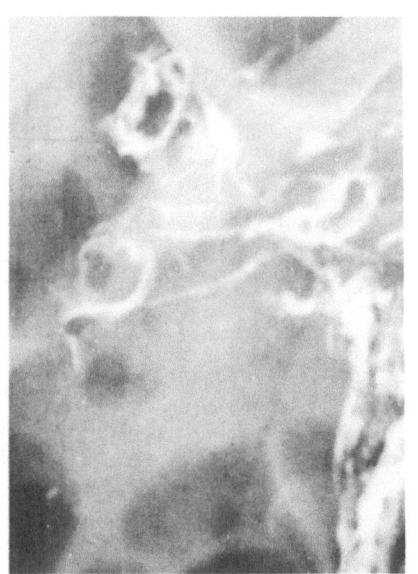

370

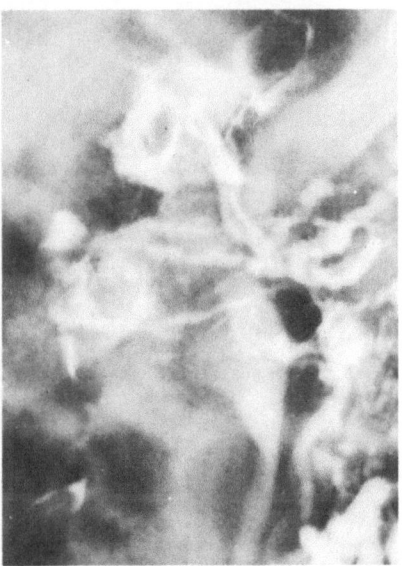

371

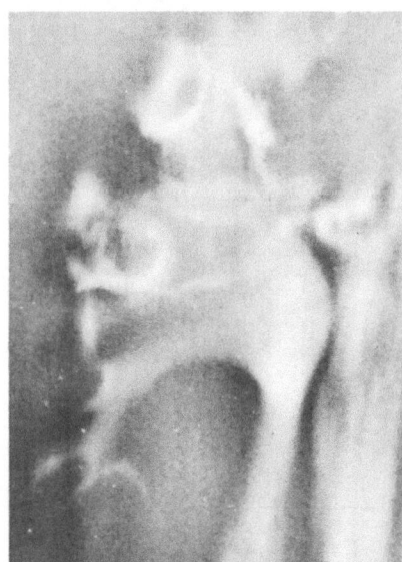

372

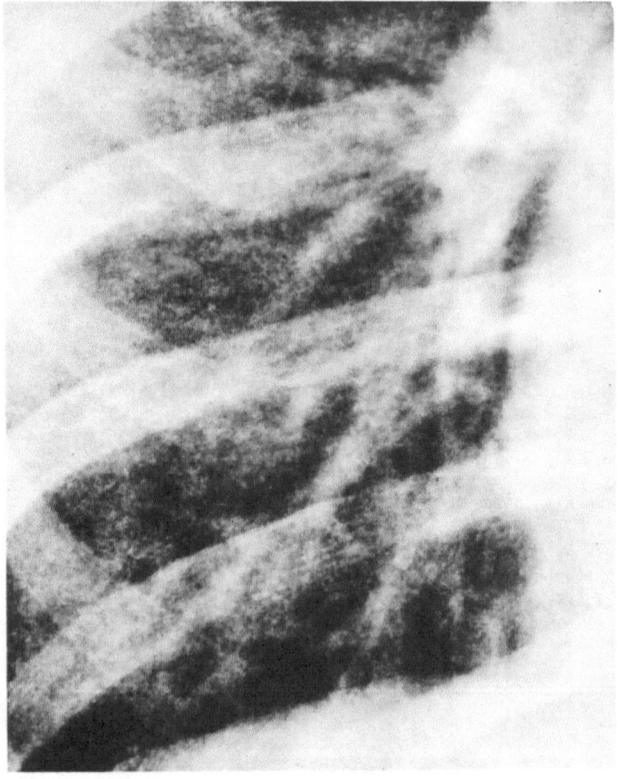

373

fig. 373 Fine stipples on the chest film as a result of multiple small lung emboli.

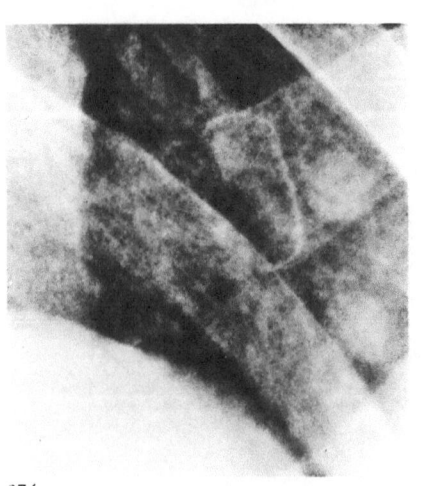

374

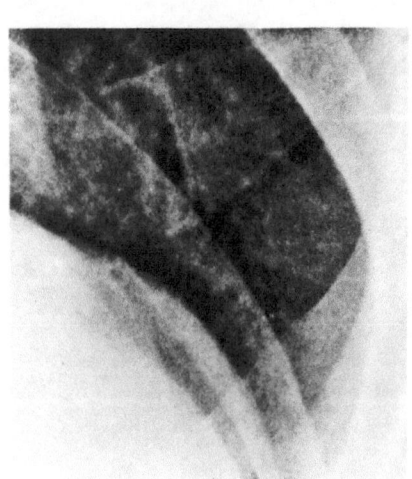

375

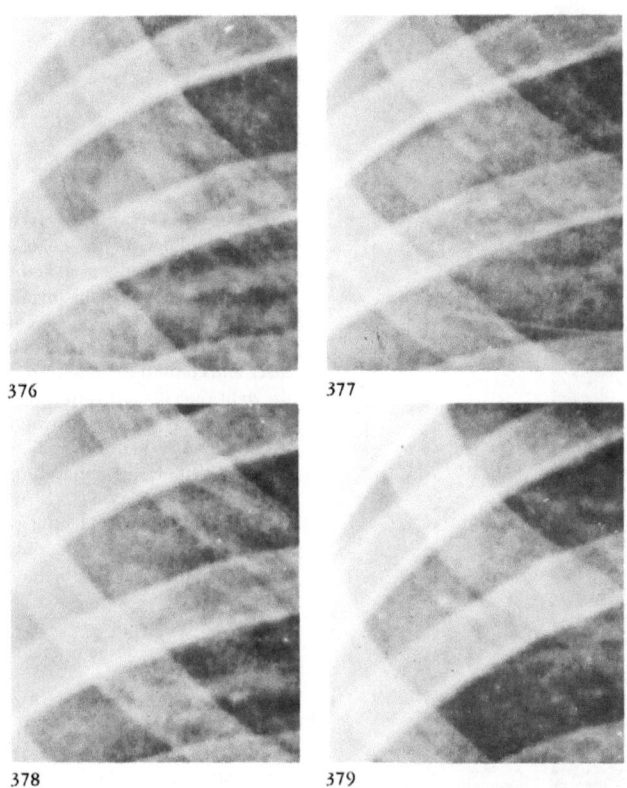

376

377

378

379

figs. 374-379 Rare occurrence of accumulation of lipiodol in the lung, which is visible on the chest film as sharply defined, spherical opacities; suggests the presence of lung metastases. Two lipiodol accumulations resembling metastases (fig. 374) had disappeared 3 weeks later on follow-up radiogram (fig. 375). One lipiodol accumulation in the lung after lymphographic examination resembling metastases (fig. 376) decreased and finally disappeared: 2 days (fig. 377), 3 days (fig. 378) and 4 days (fig. 379). *Comment:* Although this phenomenon is rare, it is necessary that a chest film be made before lymphographic examination for comparison purposes.

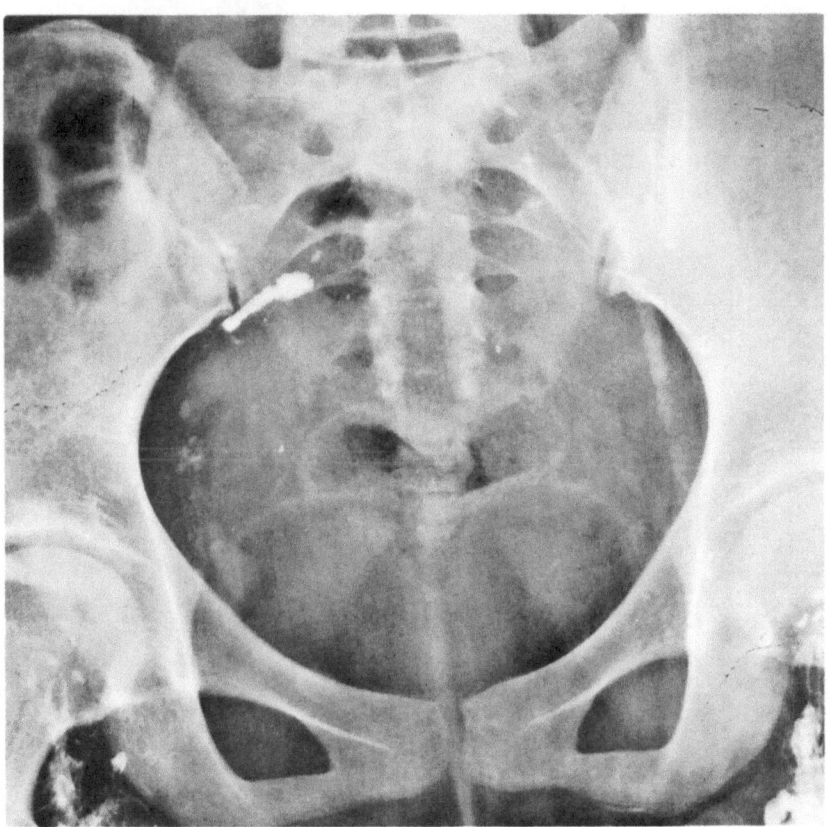

380

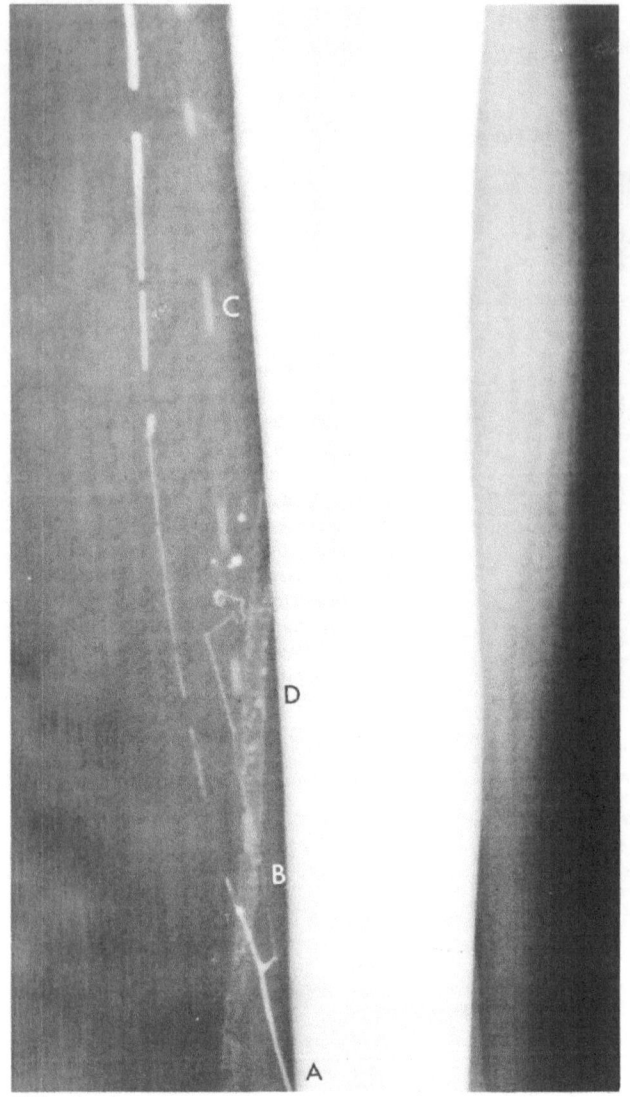

381

figs. 380 and 381 Lymphaticovenous anastomoses; lymphogram (fig. 380) of a young patient with lymphoedema and other congenital abnormalities. Beyond the inguinal region, on both sides, the lymph nodes are no longer visible but lipiodol is clearly visible in the left vena iliaca and contrast accumulations are seen in the right vena iliaca. Lymphogram (fig. 381) of the lower leg of an older patient: lymph vessel (A) with branch (B) near lymphaticovenous communication and contrast drops in vein (C). Arteriosclerotic artery (D).

Comment. Pathological lymphaticovenous anastomoses can develop not only when obstruction of the lymphatic system is expected but also in patients known to have congenital anomalies and in older patients with degenerative abnormalities of the vessels.

figs. 382-385 Complications. Rupture of lymph vessels because contrast fluid injection was too rapid (figs. 382, 383). Rupture of lymph nodes as a result of too rapid injection (fig. 384). Accidental injection of contrast fluid into a vein (fig. 385).

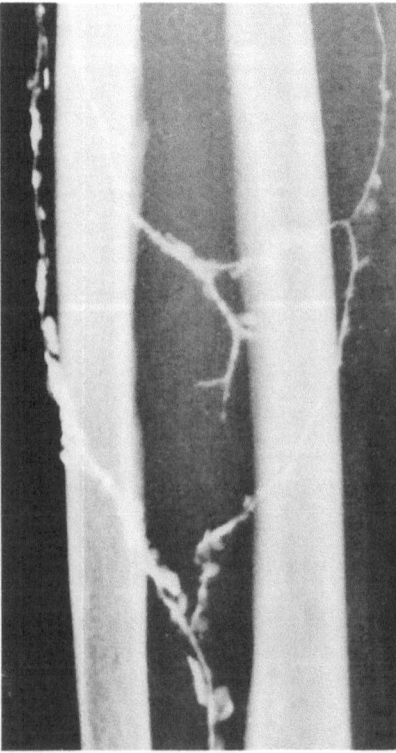

382

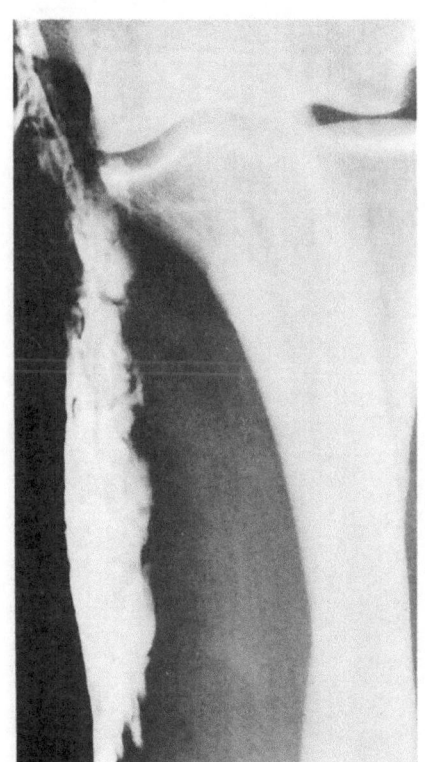

383

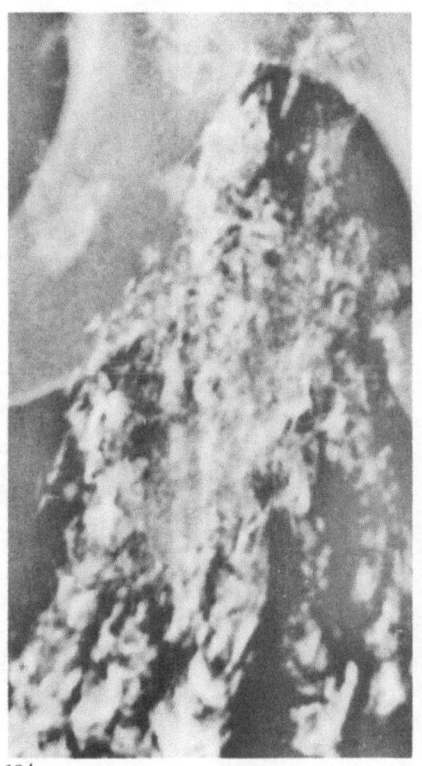

384

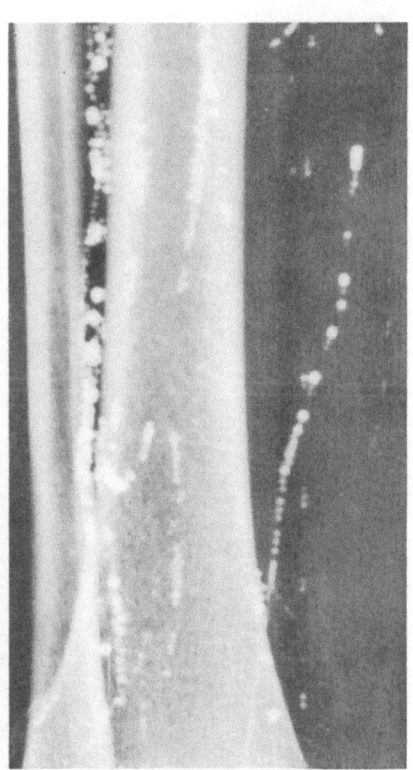

385

figs. 386 and 387 Complication. Secondary
lymphoedema of the left arm (fig. 386). Six
weeks later the oily contrast fluid is still clearly
visible in the oedematous tissue (fig. 387).

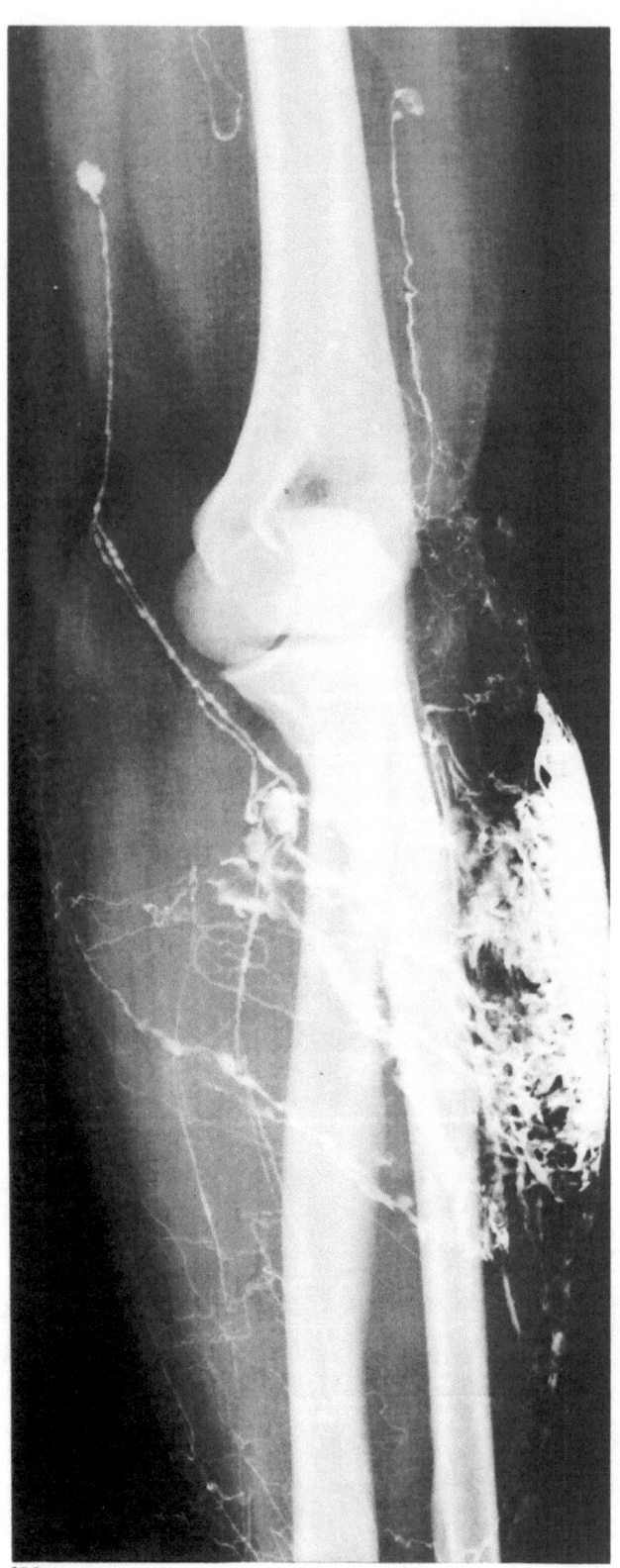

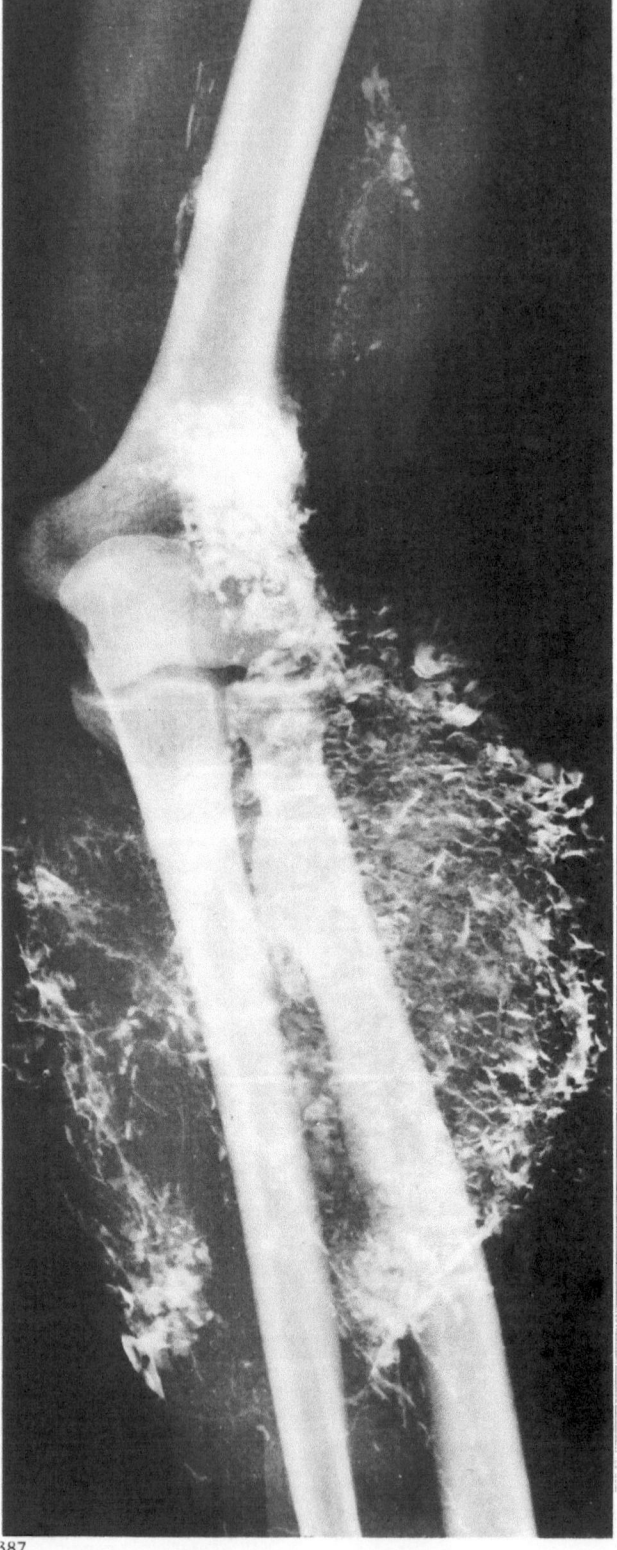

386

387

References

Abbes, M., Martin, E., Paschietta, V., Pellegrino, A., and Prat, P. P. La Lymphographie en cancérologie. Exp. Sc. Francaise, Paris (1964).

Abbes, M. La visualisation des anastomoses lymphatico-veineuses par la lymphographie. Presse méd. 74, 1374 (1966).

Acconcia, A., Technica per la linfangiografia degli arti inferiori. Rass. Ital. chir. med. 6, 59 (1957).

Akisada, M., and Tani, S. Filarial chyluria in Japan: lymphography, etiology and treatment in 30 cases. Radiology 90, 311 (1968).

Alessandri, R., Biaginī, C., e.a. Comparaison entre les tableause radiologiques et les pièces anatomiques et histologiques dans les adénopathies néoplasique. J. Belge Rad. 3, 323 (1965).

Allen, E. V. Lymphedema of the extremities. Arch. int. med. 54, 606 (1934).

Altaras, J., Haas, R., Tahalele, E. Harnblasen veränderungen im Röntgenbild bei pelvinen Lymphomen. Proc. 3′ Int. Congr. of Lymphology. Brussels 172 (1970).

Altman, D., Shaver, W. and Viamonte, M. Lymphangiography in children. Amer. j. dis. child. 104, 335 (1962).

Ariel, I. M., Resnick, M. J. Lymphodynamics in metastatic melanoma from the extremities. Arch. Surg. 94, 117 (1967).

Arnulf, G. La lymphographie au lipiodol ultra fluide. Lyon chir. 58, 307 (1962).

Arnulf, G., Benichoux, R. et Morin, G. Documents expérimenteaux et cliniques sur la lymphographie. Presse méd. 62, 1631 (1954).

Arnulf, G., et Boely, C. Physiopathologie des lymphatiques et du canal thoracique. I. Aspect, fonctionnement, moyens d'étude des lymphatiques normaux et pathologiques. Presse méd. 69, 2381 (1961). II. Les lymphatiques dans les oedèmes chroniques chirurgicaux des membres. Presse méd. 69, 2505 (1961).

Arts, V. An injection apparatus for lymphography. Am. J. Roentg. 100, 2, 466 (1967).

Arvay, N., et Picard, J. D. L'exploration radiologique des voies lymphatiques. Presse méd. 70, suppl. nr. 31 (1962).

Arvay, N., et Picard, J. D. La lymphographie en hématologie. Rev. prat. 12, 1695 (1962).

Arvay, N., Picard, J. D. et Manlot, G. Technique de lymphographie abdominothoracique. Rev. Franc. étud. clin. biol. 7, 435 (1962).

Askar, O. M., Kassem, K. A. The lymphatics of the leg in deep venous thrombosis. Brit. J. Radiol. 42, 122 (1969).

Askar, O. M. Communicating lymphatics and lymphovenous communications in relation to deep venous occlusion of the leg. Lymphology 2, 56 (1969).

Averette, H. E., Hudson, R. C., Viamonte, M. I. a. o. Lymphangioadenography (lymphography) in the study of female genital cancer. Cancer 15, 769 (1962).

Banfi, A., Bonadonna, G., Carnevali, G. e.a. Preferential sites of involvement and mode of spread in malignant lymphomas. Eur. J. Cancer 4, 319 (1968).

Banfi, A., Bonadonna, G. e.a. Malignant lymphomas: further studies on their preferential sites of involvement and possible mode of spread. Lymphology 2, 130 (1969).

Bao-Shan Jing. Improved technique of lymphangiography. Am. J. Roentg. 98, 952 (1966).

Barnes, M. R., de Poto, D. W. The use of polaroid film in lymphography. Lymphology 1, 25 (1969).

Bartels, P. Das Lymphgefäszsystem. Bardelebens Handbuch der Anatomie des Menschen. Jena, Fischer (1909).

Baum, S., Bron, K. M., Wexler, L. e.a. Lymphangiography, cavography and urography. Comparative accuracy in the diagnosis of pelvic and abdominal metastases. Radiology 81, 207 (1963).

Beltz, L., Esser, G., Greuzmann, M. Zur Lymphdynamics in Portal Hypertension, Fortschr. Röntgenstr. 111, 1 (1964).

Beltz, L., and Thurn, P. Das Lymphogramm beim tumorösen, retroperitonellen Lymphblock. Fortschr. Röntgenstr. 102, 278 (1965).

Beltz, L., and Thurn, P. Zur verlaufskontrolle des Lymphadenograms bei retroperitonealen Lymphknotentumoren. Fortschr. Röntgenstr. 104, 1 (1966).

Beltz, L., Linzbach, Ch., Thelen, M., and Hermanutz, D. Lymphografische Metastasen Kriterien im Lymphangiogram- und Diagnose und Differentialdiagnose. Rad. Diagn. 5, 604, (1972).

Beltz, L. Die Lymphangiografie in der Diagnostik primärer maligner Lymphome. Dtsch. med. Wschr. 97, 124 (1972).

Blaudo, K. Kavografie und Re-lymphografie als wichtige Zusatzuntersuchungen bei Hodentumoren, und gynäcologischen Karzinomen. Radiol. diagn. 5, 674 (1972).

Blom, J. M. H. and Oort, J. Een experimenteel onderzoek naar de invloed van lipiodol op de versleping van deeltjes en op de filterfunctie van lymphklieren. Ned. tijdschr. geneesk. 112, 35, 1571 (1968).

Blom, J. M. H. and Oort, J. The effect of lymphography with lipiodol ultrafluide in the barrier function of the lymph node. Radiol. clin. biol. 39, 317 (1970).

Bonadonna, G., Banfi, A. e.a. Preferential sites and mode of spread of Hodgkin's disease and lymphoreticular sarcomas on the basis of clinical evaluation of 500 cases. Tumori, 53, 551 (1967).

Bonadonna, G., Fossati-Bellani, F. The spread of malignant lymphomas in children. Tumori, 54, 311 (1968).

References

184

Borisser, M. G. Les accidents de la lymphographie. Sem. Hop. 68, 1658 (1968).

Botreau-Roussel. Elephantiasis arabum. Lymphangite éléphantiasique à rechutes. J. chir. 49, 821 (1937).

Brichner, T. J., Boyer, C. W. and Perry, R. H. Limited value of lymphography in Hodgkin's disease. Radiology 90, 52 (1968).

Brody H. S., Helff, J. R., and Bujdoso, L. Lymphangiography: an aid in urological surgery. J. Urol. 91, 606 (1964).

Bron, K. M., Baum, S. and Abrams, H. L. Oil embolism in lymphangiography: incidence, manifestations and mechanism. Radiology 80, 194 (1963).

Bruce, P. T., Hare, W. S. C. Failure of metastatic nodes to fill during lymphography. Chir. Radiol. 18, 88 (1967).

Bruun, S. and Engeset, A. Lymphadenography. Acta radiol. 45, 389 (1956).

Buono, M. S. Del, and Rüttimann, A. Lymphographic observations in chronic secondary lymphedema (Ital). Minerva chir. 17, 655 (1962).

Busch, F. M., Sayegh, E. S. and Chenault, O. W. Some uses of lymphangiography in the management of testicular tumours. J. Urol. 93, 490 (1965).

Cahn, E. L. Steinfeld, J. L. (editors). Conference on lymphography. Cancer Chemother. Rep. 52, 1 (1968).

Callahan, D. H., Graf, E. C., Gersalk, J. and Turbow, A. M. Lymphangiography and simultaneous excretory urography as diagnostic aid in chyluria. J. Urol. 93, 417 (1965).

Calnan, J. S., Kountz, S. a.o. Venous obstruction in the aetiology of lymphedema praecox. Brit. Med. J. 2, 221 (1964).

Calnan, J. S. Lymphedema: the case for doubt. Brit. J. plast. Surg. 21, 32 (1968).

Carvalho, R., Rodrigues, A. and Pereira, S. Sur la méthode radiographique de mise en évidence des lymphatiques chez le vivant. J. radiol. électrol. 18, 180 (1934).

Casley-Smith, J. R. How the lymphatic system works. Lymphology 1, 77 (1968).

Celis, A. Kuthy, J. and Castillo, E. Del. The importance of the thoracic duct in the spread of malignant disease. Acta radiol. 45, 169 (1956).

Chassard, J. L. and Papillon, J. Lymphographie et maladie de Hodgkin. J. Belge Rad. 3, 295 (1965).

Chassard, J. L., Feremans, W., Kropholler, R. W., Laugier, A. and Marcovits, P., and Picard, J. D. Premiers résultats de l'examen de plus de 300 lymphographies de maladies de Hodgkin vues par le groupe des Lymphographistes OERTC. Abst. 3' Int. Congr. of Lymphology Brussles, 6 (1970).

Chavez, C. M., Beeroug, L. G. and Evers, C. G. Hepatic oil embolism after lymphography: role of systemicoportal lymphaticovenous anastomosis. Am J. Surg. 110, 456 (1965).

Chiappa, S., Galli, G., Guarino, M. e.a. Quelques possibilités de la radiothérapie endolymphatique dans le domaine de la gynécologie. J. radiol. électrol. 44, 157 (1963).

Chiappa, S., Galli, G., Luciani, L. and Severini, A. Consideration on the restoration of the lymphatic circulation after pelvic lymphadenectomy. Surg. Gynec. and Obstet. 120, 323 (1965).

Chiappa, S., Uslenghi, C., Bonadonna, G. e.a. Combined testicular and foot lymphangiography in testicular carcinomas. Surg. Gynec. and Obstet. 123, 1 (1966).

Clouse, M. E., Hallgrimson, J. and Wenlund, D. E. Complications following lymphography with particular reference to pulmonary oil embolisation. Am. J. Roentg. 96, 4, (1966).

Cockett, A. T. and Goodwin, W. E. Chyluria: attempted surgical treatment by lymphatico-venous anastomosis. J. Urol. 88, 566 (1962).

Cohen, L. B., Nelson, G., Wood, A. M. a.o. Lymphangiography in filarial lymphedema and elephantiasis. Amer. j. trop. med. hyg. 10, 843 (1961).

Cohen, R., Viamonte, M., Cypress, E. a.o. Lymphangiography in a patient with chylous ascites. Radiology 81, 219 (1963).

Collette, J. M. Lymphographie expérimentale et clinique. Acta chir. belg. 54, 607 (1955).

Collette, J. M. Envahissements ganglionnaires inguino-ilio-pelviens par lymphographie. Acta radiol. 49, 154 (1958).

Collette, J. M. Techniques et résultats de la lymphographie et de la lympadénographie. Acta radiol. 16, 43 (1961).

Cook, P. L., Jeliffe, A. M., Kendall, B. and Meloughlin, M. J. Role of lymphography in diagnosis and management of malignant reticulosis. Brit. J. Radiol. 39, 561 (1966).

Crile, G. The place of lymphadenectomy in cancer surgery. Lymphology 5, 89 (1972).

Damascelli, B., Musumeci, R., and Uslenghi, C. Instruments for lymphography. Lymphology 2, 166 (1969).

Dana, M., Desprez-Curely, J. P., Bismuth, V. and Bourdon, R. La lymphographie dans les maladies de la peau. Ann. Radiol. 7, 555 (1964).

Dankmeyer, J. Petite histoire de l'anatomie de Leyde. Leiden, Ydo (1957).

Dargent, M., Chassard, J. L. et Dargent, D. La lymphographie ilio-pelvienne au lipiodol ultrafluide par voie pédieuse dans le cancer du col utérin. Ann. chir. sept. (1963).

Davidson, J. W., Clarke, E. A. and Walker, D. Radiographic appearances in chromo-lymphadenography. J. Canad. A. Radiol. 19, 316 (1967).

Davidson, J. W. Lipiod embolism to the brain following lymphography: Case report and experimental study. Am. J. Roentg. 105, 763 (1969).

Davidson, J. W., Clarke, E. A. and Reid, J. Lymphographic features and epidemiological aspects of Hodgkin's disease. Abst. 3' Int. Congr. of Lymphology. Brussels, 111 (1970).

Davidson, J. W., and Clarke, E. A. Radiographic features of Hodgkin's disease. Lymphology 5, 95 (1972).

Declève, A. and Maldague, P. Technique de confrontation radio-anatomo-histologique dans l'interpretation de la lymphographie. J. Belge Rad. 6, 301 (1966).

Desmons, M., Ramiorel, H. Essaimage néoplastique périlymphatique après lymphographie dans un cas de tumeur melanique du pied. J. Radiol. 11, 703 (1964).

Desprez-Curely, J. P., Bismuth, V., Laugier, A. e.a. Accidents et incidents de la lymphographie. Ann. radiol. 5, 577 (1962).

Desprez-Curely, J. P., et Bismuth, V. La Lymphographie. Coeur et Méd. int. 3, 369 (1964).

Desprez-Curely, J. P., Bourdon, R., Bismuth, V. e.a. Extension of malignant lymphoma to deep lying nodes. Progr. in Lymphology, ed. A. Rüttimann, Georg Thieme Verlag 136 (1967).

Dierick, W. S., and Vaerenberg, P. M. Van. Lymphographie en cancerologie. J. Belge radiol. 46, 38 (1963).

Ditchek, T. and Scanlon, G. T. Direct magnification lymphography. J. A. M. A. 199, 654 (1967).

Dodd, G. D., Rutledge, E. and Wallace, S. Postoperative pelvic lymphocysts. Am. J. Roentg. 108, 312 (1970).

Dolan, P. A. and Hughes R. R. Lymphography in genital cancer. Surg. Gynec. and Obst. 118, 1286 (1964).

Dos Santos Ferreira. Le système lymphatique de l'estomac et ses voies de drainage pour le thorax. Presse méd. 70, 950 (1962).

Dumont, A. E. Tell us... about the lymphatic system. Lymphology 1, 95 (1968).

Elema, J. D., Minden, S. H., van and Oldhoff, J. Some experience with chromolymphography. Arch. chir. neerl. 20, 291 (1967).

Eley, C. S. and Brennan, M. J. Lymphangiosarcoma: a lethal complication of chronic lymphedema. Arch. Surg. 94, 223 (1967).

Elke, M., and Hodel, C. Lipidspeicherung in Hypernephrommetastasen der Lunge nach Lymphographie. Z. Krebsforsch. 69, 253 (1967).

Elke, M. and Nidecker, A. Metastaserungswege von Hodentumoren und ihre lymphografische Metastasenmorphologie. Rad. diagn. 5, 660 (1972).

References

Engzell, U., Rubio, C., Tjernberg, B. and Zajicek, J. The lymph node barrier against Vx2 cancer cells before, during and after lymphography. Europ. J. Cancer. 4, 305 (1968).

Fabian, C. E., Nudelman, E. J. and Abrams, H. L. Postlymphangiogram film as indicator of tumor activity in lymphoma. Invest. Radiol. 1, 386 (1966).

Farrel, W. J. Lymphangiographic demonstration of lymphovenous communications after radiotherapy in Hodgkin's disease. Radiology 87, 630 (1966).

Fischer, H. W. A critique of experimental lymphography. Acta radiol. 52, 448 (1959).

Fischer, H. W. and Zimmerman, G. R. Roentgenologic visualization of lymph nodes and lymphatic channels. Am. J. Roentg. 81, 517 (1959).

Fischer, H. W., Lawrence, M. S. and Thornbury, J. R. Lymphography of the normal adult male. Observations and their relation to the diagnosis of metastatic neoplasm. Radiology 78, 399 (1962).

Fischer, H. W. Lymphography. Radiology 80, 1002 (1963).

Fraimow, W., Wallace, S., Lewis, P. e.a. Changes in pulmonary function due to lymphangiography. Radiology 85, 231 (1965).

Fraley, E. E., Clouse, M. and Litwen, S. B. Uses of Lymphography, lymph-adenography and color lymphadenography in urology. J. Urol. 93, 319 (1965).

Frischbier, H. J. Wertbestimmung der verschiedene Metastasen Kriterien. Rad. diagn. 5, 591 (1972).

Fuchs, W. A., Rüttimann, A. und Del Buono, M. S. Klinische Indikationen zur Lymphographie. Schweiz. med. Wschr. 89, 755 (1959).

Fuchs, W. A., Rüttimann, A. und Del Buono, M. S. Zur Lymphographie bei chronischen sekundären Lymphödemen. Fortschr. Röntgenstr. 92, 608 (1960).

Fuchs, W. A. Complications in lymphography with oily contrast media. Acta radiol. 57, 427 (1962).

Fuchs, W. A. Lymphographie und Tumordiagnostik. Springer Verlag Berlin (1965).

Fuchs, W. A. and Hartel, M. P. Die Prognose des Morbus Hodgkin auf Grund der Lymphknotenstruktur im Lymphogramm. Fortschr. Röntgenstr. 109, 553 (1968).

Fuchs, W. A. Davidson, J. W. and Fischer, H. W. Recent results in cancer research. Springer, Berlin (1969).

Fuchs, W. A. Frage der artspezifischen lymphografischen Metastasen Kriterien bei bestimmte Organtumoren. Rad. diagn. 5, 627 (1972).

Gergely, R., and Zsebök, Z. De la lymphangiographie. Press. méd. 64, 2200 (1956).

Gergely, R., Zsebök, Z. and Földi, M. Die diagnostischen Anwendungsmöglichkeiten der Lymphangiographie. Fortschr. Röntgenstr. 85, 175 (1956).

Gergely, R. Die Bedeutung der Lymphangiographie in der Chirurgie. Chirurg 29, 49 (1958).

Gerteis, W. Die Lymphographie beim Genitalcarcinoom der Frau. Arch. Gynäk. 200, 109 (1964).

Gerteis, W., Kindermann, G., Weishaar, J. Die kleine Metastase im Lymphogramm. Abst. 3' Int. Congr. of Lymphology. Brussels 167 (1970).

Gold, R. H. Lymphangiographic manifestations of Whipple's disease simulating malignant neoplasm. Abst. 3' Int. Congr. of Lymphology Brussels 114 (1970).

Gough, J. H., Gough, M. H. and Thomas, M. L. Pulmonary complications following lymphography with note on technique. Brit. J. Radiol. 37, 416 (1964).

Gould, R. J. and Schaffer, B. The surgical applications of lymphography. Surg. Gynec. Obst. 114, 683 (1962).

Grandval, C. M. Lymphography in Gastro-enterology. Abst. 3' Int. Congr. of Lymphology. Brussels 134 (1970).

Gregl, A., Eydt, M. e.a. Chromolymphographies of the upper extremities. Fortschr. Röntgenstr. 108, 565 (1968).

Hafner, E., Fuchs, W. A. and Kuffer, F. Lymphangiography in lymphangiomatosis of bone. Lymphology 5, 129 (1972).

Hashimoto, E. Studies on diagnosis and treatment of lymphatic diseases. Jap. Circulat. J. 31, 1361 (1967).

Hass, A. C. The value of exploratory laparotomy in malignant lymphoma. Radiology 101, 151 (1971).

Herman, P. G., Benninghoff, D. L., Nelson, J. H. e.a. Roentgenatomy of the ilio-pelvic-aortic lymphatic system. Radiology 80, 182 (1963).

Herman, P. G., Benninghoff, D. L. and Schwartz, S. A physiologic approach to lymph flow in lymphography. Am. J. Roentg. 6, 1207 (1964).

Herzog, W. Bedeutung der Lymphographie für die Allgemeinchirurgie. Abst. 3' Int. Congr of Lymphology. Brussels 120 (1970).

Hilweg, D., Wieners, H. Die Bedeutung der Lymphographie für die Erfassung des retroperitonealen Metastasierungswegen maligner Hodentumoren. Urologe 3, 143 (1969).

Hilweg, D., Novak, D., Wieners, H., e.a. The role of lymphography in the staging of malignant tumors of testis and the urinary bladder. Abst 3' Int. Congr. of Lymphology, Brussels 125 (1970).

Hliniak, I, and Vorbrodt, J. The use of lymphangiography in the cervical cancer. Rad. diagn. 5, 655 (1972).

Hodari, A. A., Hodgkinson, C. P. Lymphangiogram of Meig's Syndrome. Obstet. Gynec. 32, 477 (1968).

References

186

Hopf, M. A. La cavographie, méthode complémentaire de la lymphographie. Radiol. clin. biol. 39, 177 (1970).

Hreshchyshyn, M. M., Sheehan, F. R. and Holland, J. F. Visualization of retroperitoneal lymph nodes. Lymphangiography as an aid in the measurement of tumor growth. Cancer 14, 205 (1961).

Humber, P. and Zaharian, S. Les chylo-thorax. Am. Chir. 6, 386 (1967).

Iriarte, P. Jagasia, H., and Thurman, W. G. Lymphangiography for malignant diseases in children. J. A. M. A. 188, 501 (1964).

Ishida, O., Uchida, H. e.a. Lymphography in malignant tumors, chyluria and chyloperitoneum. Med. J. Osaka Univ. 15, 417 (1965).

Jackson, L. G., Wallace, B., Schaffer, B. e.a. The diagnostic value of lymphangiography. Ann. int. med. 54, 870 (1961).

Jackson, R. J. A. Complications of lymphography. Brit. Med. J. 1, 1203 (1966).

Jacobssons, S. and Johansson, S. Normal roentgen anatomy of the lymph vessels of upper and lower extremities. Acta radiol. 51, 321 (1959).

Jacobsson, S. and Johansson, S. Lymphography in lymphedema. Acta radiol. 57. 81 (1962).

Jacobsson, S. Blood circulation in lymphedema of the arm. Brit. J. plast. Surg. 20, 355 (1967).

Jing, B. S. and Mc Grow, J. P. Lymphangiography in diagnosis and management of malignant lymphomas. Cancer 19, 565 (1966).

Johnson, R. E. and Cook, P. L. Hodgkin's disease: the negative lymphogram in guiding radiotherapy. Amer. J. Roentg. 102, 883 (1968).

Jossifow, G. M. Das Lymphgefäszsystem des Menschen. Jena, Fischer (1930).

Kaindl, F. Zur Pathologie der Lymphbanen in menschlichen Extremitäten. Dtsch. med. J. 8, 209 (1957).

Kaindl, F., Mannheimer, E. e.a. Lymphangiographie und Lymphadenographie der Extremitäten. Stuttgart, Thieme (1960).

Kaplan, H. S. Clinical evaluation and radiotherapeutic management of Hodgkin's disease and the malignant lymphomas. New Engl. J. med. 278, 892 (1968).

Keinert, K. Erfahrungen mit der zytologischen Punktion lymphografisch angefärbte Lymphknoten in verschiedenen Regionen. Rad. diagn. 5, 680 (1972).

Keiser, D. V., Frischbier, H. J. Die Wert der Lymphographie bei der Metastasen suche. Fortschr. Röntgenstr. 100, 299 (1964).

Kenyon, N. M., Soto, M., Viamonte, M. e.a. Improved techniques and results of lymphography. Surg. Gynec. and Obstet. 114, 677 (1962).

Ketterings, C. Lymphedema of penis and scrotum. Brit. J. plast. Surg. 21, 381 (1968).

Kikkawa, K. and Nagle, W. C. Displacement of lymphatic vessels by an abnormal vein. Radiology 102, 329 (1972).

Kinmonth, J. B. Lymphangiography in man. Clin. sc. 11, 13 (1952).

Kinmonth, J. B. Lymphangiography in clinical surgery and particularly in the treatment of lymphedema. Ann. roy. coll. surg. England 15, 300 (1954).

Kinmonth, J. B. and Taylor, G. W. Lymphatic circulation in lymphedema. Ann. surg. 139, 129 (1954).

Kinmonth, J. B., Taylor, G. W. e.a. Primary lymphedema. Clinical and lymphangiographic studies of a series of 107 patients in which the lower limbs were affected. Brit. J. surg. 45, 1 (1957).

Kittredge, R. D., Hashim, S. e.a. Demonstration of lymphatic abnormalities in a patient with chyluria. Amer. J. Roentgen. 90, 159 (1963).

Kittredge, R. D. and Finley, N. Lymphangiography in lymphoma. Amer. J. Roentgen. 4, 935 (1965).

Klinkhamer, A. C., Bosman, G. and Houtappel, H. C. E. M. Lymphografie in de urologische diagnostiek bij chylurie. Ned. tijdschr. geneesk. 23, 1033 (1967).

Koehler, P. R., Wayne, A., Meyers, M. S. e.a. Body distribution of ethiodol following lymphography. Radiology 82, 866 (1964).

Koehler, P. R., Wohl, G. T. and Schaffer, B. Lymphangiography: a survey of its current status. Amer. J. Roentgen. 6. 1216 (1964).

Koehler, P. R., and Salmon, R. B. Lymphographic patterns in lymphoma, with emphasis on the atypical form. Radiology 87, 623 (1966).

Koehler, P. R. and Schaffer, B. Peripheral lymphaticovenous anastomosis. Circulation 35, 401 (1967).

Koehler, P. R. Complications in lymphography. Lymphology 1, 4, 116 (1968).

Koehler, P. R., Tze-Chun Chiang e.a. Lymphography in chyluria. Amer. J. Roentgen. 102, 455 (1968).

Koehler, P. R. Roentgenologic aspects of lymphoma as seen on the lymphogram. Cancer Chem. Rep. 52, 171 (1968).

Koehler, P. R., Rodriquez, H. A. Visualization of substernal lymph nodes after intraperitoneal injections of radiopaque contrast media. Lymphology (abstr.) 1, 2, 73 (1968).

Koehler, P. R., Kyano, M. M. Lymphatic complications following renal transplantation. Radiology 102, 539 (1972).

Kralova, A., Cernoch, A. und Ubrich, J. Indication und Wert der Lymphografie in der gynácologischen Onkologie. Rad. Diagn. 5, 658 (1972).

Kropholler, R. W., Blom, J. M. H. and Irto, J. Lymphografie met behulp van een polytheenkatheter. Ned. tijdschr. geneesk. 15, 696 (1968).

Lachapèlle, A. P., Hugnes, A. and Lagarde, Cl. De l'étude anatome-radiologique du canal thoracique d'après 60 opaccifations sur l'être humain vivant. J. de Radiol., d'électrol. et de Méd. nucleaire 45, 1 (1964)

Lagneau, P. Physiopathologie et chirurgie du canal thoracique. J. Chir. 96, 59 (1968).

Lamarque, J. L., Pages, A., e.a. Anatomie radiologique et valeur sémiologique des images ganglionnaires en lymphographie. J. Radiol. Electrol. 48, 253 (1967).

Lameer, C. Retroperitoneale lymphografie. Thèsis (1965).

Lameer, C. Lymphografie en olie-embolie. Ned tijdschr. geneesk. 111, 71 (1967).

Lameer, C. Lymphography in the intensive radiological treatment of Hodgkin's disease. Radiol. clin. biol. 38, 61 (1969).

Lameer, C. Diagnostic information versus risks in lymphography. Radiol. clin. biol. 38, 329 (1969).

Larson, D. L. and Lewis, S. R. Deep lymphatic system of the lower extremity. Amer. J. Surg. 113, 217 (1967).

Lee, B. J., Nelson, J. H. and Schwarz, G. Evaluation of lymphography, inferior vena-cavography and intravenous pyelography in clinical staging and management of Hodgkin's disease and lymphosarcoma. New England J. Med. 271, 327 (1964).

Lee, B. J. Correlation between lymphangiography and clinical status of patients with lymphoma. Cancer Chem. Rep. 52, 205 (1968).

Leenhardt, P. and Colin, R. L'exploration lymphatique in vivo. Presse méd. 65, 1534 (1957).

Leenhardt, P., Colin, R. and Pourquier, H. La lymphographie pelvienne. J. Radiol. 39, 778 (1958).

Leiber, B. Der menschliche Lymphknoten. München, Urban und Schwarzenberg (1961).

Leriche, R. Traitement chirurgical des suites éloignées des phlébites et des grands oedèmes non-médicaux des membres inférieurs. Bull. soc. nat. chir. 53 (1927) nr 5; Gazette des Hôpitaux 100 (1929).

Litwin, S. B., Fraley, E. E., Clouse, M. E. e.a. Lymphography in patients with pelvic cancer. Surg. Obst. and Gynec. 24, 809 (1964).

Luning, M. and Richter, J. Standardprogram für lymphografische Zusatzuntersuchungen. Rad. diagn. 5, 672 (1972).

MacDonald, J. S., Laugier, A., Schlienger, M. Observations on the growth of tumours in lymph nodes changing from normal to abnormal while remaining opacified after lymphography. Clin. Radiol. 19, 120 (1968).

Makai, F., Bélan, A. and Málck, P. Lymphatic metastases of bone tumours. Lymphology 3, 109 (1971).

References

Malek, P. Physiologische, pathologische und anatomische Grundlagen der Lymphographie. 1X Int. congr. radiol. München, 384 (1959).

Malek, P., Bélan, A. und Kriegel, F. Lymphangio- und Lymphadenographie der untern Extremitäten bei Polyarthritis progressiva. Fortschritte Röntgenstr. 92, 620 (1960).

Malek, P., Bélan, A. und Kolc, J. Der Ductus thoracicus in der Röntgenkinematographie. Fortschr. Röntgenstr. 93, 723 (1961).

Malek, P., Bélan, A., Kolc, J. In vivo evidence of lympho-venous communications in the popliteal region. Acta Radiol. 3, 334 (1965).

Marchal, G., Bernard, J., Arvay, N. e.a. La lymphographie dans la maladie de Hodgkin. Nouv. rev. franc. hemat. 2, 4 (1962).

Markovits, P., Grellet, J., Gasquet, Ch. e.a. The place of lymphangiography in seminomas of the ovary. Rev. franc. gynéc. 4, 201 (1968).

Markovits, P., Blacje, R. A., Gasquet, Ch., e.a. Radiological appearance of lymphograms performed after radiotherapy. Am. radiol. 9, 835 (1969).

Marques, R. and Pereira, L. Superficial lymphography of the upper extremity (Sp.). Angiologia 14, 106 (1962).

Martin da Rocha, R., de Souza, A., Elias da Costa, C. and Leitao, M. Quelques aspects lymphographiques dans la pathologie tropicale. J. Belge radiol. 48, 275 (1965).

Mascagni, P. Vasorum lymphaticorum corporis humani. Historia et ichonographica. Sienna (1787).

Matorell, F. Chronical surgical edemas of the lower limbs. Minerva cardioangiol. 3, 73 (1955).

May, R. E., and Bogash, M. Lymphangiography as a diagnostic adjunct in urology. J. Urol. 87, 208 (1962).

Mayerson, H. S. Three centuries of lymphatic history - an outline. Lymphology 2, 143 (1969).

Mazy, G., Decleve, A. and Madagne, P. Radio-anatomo-histological correlation in lymphangiography. Abst. 3' Int. Congr. of Lymphology, Brussels 175 (1970).

Montagneraud, Y., Altan, D., Laluque, P. e.a. Les aspects lymphographiques des adènopathies filariennes. J. Radiol. Electrol. 50, 135 (1969).

Moskovitz, G., Chen, P. and Adams, D. F. Lipid embolization to the kidney and brain after lymphangiography. Radiology 102, 327 (1972).

Musshoff, K., Renemann, H. e.a. Classification of Hodgkin's disease. Fortschr. Röntgenstr. 109, 776 (1968).

Ngu, V. A. The lymphatic drainage of the leg and its implications. Clin. Radiol. 15, 197 (1964).

Nguyen, L. J., Lewin, J. R. Angiographic demonstration of fistula between abdominal aorta and thoracic duct. K. A. M. A. 211, 499 (1970).

Nixon, G. W. Lymphangiomatosis of bone demonstrated by lymphography. Amer. J. Roentg. 110, 3, 582 (1970).

Noriega, L. J., José, R. S. M. G. and Falco, J. Intra-osseus phlebography and lymphadenography in carcinoma of the cervix and other pelvic neoplasia. Radiology 83, 219 (1964).

Patrick, D. A. Lymphography: complications encountered in 522 examinations. Radiology 86, 876 (1966).

Patterson, R. M., Ray, C. T. Lymphangiography. An improved technique of lymphatic cannulation. Amer. Heart J. 69, 229 (1965).

Peak, C. J. and Constantinides, S. G. Lymphangiography in malignant melanoma. Cancer 17, 1586 (1964).

Perez-Tamayo, R. Thonbury, J. R. and Atkinson, R. J. "Second-look" lymphography. Amer. J. Roentg. 90, 1078 (1963).

Peters, M. V. Prophylactic treatment of adjacent areas in Hodgkin's disease. Cancer Res. 29, 1232 (1966).

Pfahler, G. E., A demonstration of the lymphatic drainage from the maxillary sinuses. Amer. J. Roentg. 27, 352 (1932).

Picard, J. D. et Manlot, G. La lymphographie dans le cancer du testicule (à propos de 30 cas). Ann. radiol. 5, 565 (1962).

Picard, J. D., Manlot, G. e.a. La lymphographie chez l'enfant. J. de radiol. d'électrol de méd. nucléaire. 44, 363 (1963).

Picard, J. D. et Arvay, N. Les communications lympho-veineuses. Presse méd. 74, 421 (1966).

Picard, J. D. and Di Maria, G. Les lymphatiques dans les affections arterielles et veineuses des membres inférieures. Abst 3' Int. Congr. of Lymphology, Brussels 166 (1970).

Pilleron, J., Durand, J. C. Lymphocèles pelviennes. Mém. Acad. Chir. 93, 281 (1967).

Pomerantz, M. and Waldmann, T. A. Systemic lymphatic abnormalities associated with gastrointestinal protein loss secondary to intestinal lymphangiectasia. Gastroenterology 45, 703 (1963).

Pomerantz, M. and Jones, W. R. Chyluria with lymphangiographic abnormalities. J. A. M. A. 196, 452 (1966).

Prat, P. P., Abbes, M. Peroperative lymphography as a guide to lymph node dissection. Cancer 17, 850 (1964).

Prokopec, J. und Kilihova, E. Die lymphadenographie in der klinischen Praxis. Fortschr. Röntgenstr. 89, 417 (1958).

References

188

Pujol, H. et Lamarque, J. L. Ilio-cavographie et lymphographie dans la recherche des adénopathies retropéritonéales. Masson et Cie Paris (1964).

Rajaram, P. C. Lymphatic dynamics in filarial chyluria and prechyluric state. Lymphology 3, 114 (1970).

Ravel, R. Histopathology of lymph after lymphography. Amer. J. clin. Path. 46, 335 (1966).

Redman, H. C. Dermatitis as a complication of lymphography. Radiology 86, 323 (1966).

Röder, K. Zusatzuntersuchungen zum Routine-lymphogramm. Rad. diagn. 5, 665 (1972).

Röder, K., and Schmidt, F. Überprüfung von Metastasen Kriterien durch lymphografische Verlaufkontrollen. Rad. diagn. 5, 618 (1972).

Rogers, C. L. and Amory, H. J. Extralymphatic entravasation of ethiodol during lymphography. Radiology 92, 108 (1969).

Ronnen, J. R. von. Lymphografie. Ned. Tijdschr. Geneesk. 109, 1451 (1965).

Roo, T. de. Techniek van de lymphografie. J. Belge Rad. 46, 462 (1963).

Roo, T. de. Lymphatico-veneuze verbinding in de regio iliaca bij primair lymphoedeem, aangetoond door middel van lymphografie. Ned. Tijdschr. Geneesk. 108, 198 (1964).

Roo, T. de. Lymphografie van de arm, met een kritische beschouwing over het gebruik van oliehoudende contrastmiddelen bij het lymphoedeem van de bovenste extremiteiten. Journal Belge Radiologie 47, 58 (1964).

Roo, T. de. Differentieel diagnostische mogelijkheden van lymphografie. Ned. Tijdschr. Geneesk. 108, 739 (1964).

Roo, T. de. A new technique of lymphography. Boerhaave radiology lectures, vol. 1, 101 (1964).

Roo, T. de. Tomography in lymphography. Boerhaave radiology lectures, vol. 1, 11 (1964).

Roo, T. de. Differential diagnosis in lymphadenography. Boerhaave radiology lectures, vol. 1, 120 (1964).

Roo, T. de. Lymphografie, een studie van de diagnostische en therapeutische mogelijkheden in de praktijk. Uitg. van Gorcum, Assen. Thèsis, Leiden (1964).

Roo, T. de Lymphografie. Ned. Tijdschr. Geneesk. 108, 12, 627 (1964).

Roo, T. de. Lymphografie. Jaarboek Kankeronderzoek en Kankerbestrijding, 297 (1964).

Roo, T. de. Lymphografie in de praktijk. Journal Belge radiologie 47, 722 (1964).

Roo, T. de. Enkele praktische mogelijkheden van lymphografie. Ned. tijdschr. geneesk. 108, 2123 (1964).

Roo, T. de. Een nieuwe puncteernaald voor lymphografie. Journal Belge radiologie 47, 836 (1964).

Roo, T. de. Valeur de la tomographie en lymphadénographie. Annales radiologie 8, 17 (1965).

Roo, T. de. Une nouvelle technique simple pour la lymphographie. Annales radiologie 8, 97 (1965).

Roo, T. de. Lymphografie, techniek en pathologisch lymphogram. Ned. tijdschr. geneesk. 109, 2114 (1965).

Roo, T. de. The technique of lymphography. Medicamundi 10, 3, 97 (1965).

Roo, T. de. Differential diagnosis in lymphadenography. Medicamundi 11, 3, 97 (1965).

Roo, T. de., and Minden, S. H. van. Quelques formes rares de communications lymphatico-veneuse. Annales radiologie 8, 797 (1965).

Roo, T. de., Thomas, P. and Kropholler, R. W. The importance of tomography for the interpretation of the lymphographic picture of lymph node metastases. Amer. J. Roentgen. 4, 9, 24 (1965).

Roo, T. de., and Voorthuizen, A. E. van. Gecombineerd lymphografisch en angiografisch onderzoek bij maligne afwijkingen in het lymphevaatstelsel. Ned. Tijdschr. Geneesk. 109, 1102 (1965).

Roo, T. de. Application de l'angiographie comme méthode complémentaire de la lymphographie pour dépister les processus malins et déterminer leur étendue. Annales radiologie 8, 319 (1965).

Roo, T. de., and Voorthuizen, A. E. van. Aanvullend angiografisch onderzoek bij lymphografie. Ned. Tijdschr. Geneesk. 109, 2119 (1965).

Roo, T. de. Lymphografie bij lymphoedemen van de extremiteiten. Ned. Tijdschr. Geneesk. 110, 523,534 (1966).

Roo, T. de. An improved, simple technique of lymphangiography. Amer. J. Roentgen. 4, 98, 948 (1966).

Roo, T. de., and Voorthuizen, A. E. van. The indications for selective supplementary angiographic examination in lymphography. Amer. J. Roentgen. 4, 97, 957 (1966), and Yearbook of Urology, Chicago (1968).

Roo, T. de. The value of lymphangiography in lymphoedema. Surgery, Gynec & Obstet. 124, 755 (1967).

Roo, T. de. Aanvullende onderzoekmethoden, onmisbaar bij lymphografie. Ned. Tijdschr. geneesk. 111, 35, 1515 (1967).

Roo, T. de, and Thomas, P. Lymphography with supplementary tomographic examination in the pre-operative analysis of melanosarcoma. Clin. Radiology 18, 1, 83 (1967).

Roo, T. de, and Huurdeman, J. E. A. Na-onderzoek bij lymphografisch onderzochte patiënten. Ned. tijdschr. geneesk. 111, 305 (1967).

Roo, T. de. L'angiographie sélective supplémentaire, examen indispensable pour l'interprétation correcte de certaines lymphographies. La Grosse Jambe, 93; édit par R. Tournay, l'expans. Scient. Paris (1968).

Roo, T. de. Eine einfache Techniek der Lymphografie. Der Radiologe 8, 7, 197 (1968).

Roo, T. de. Die besondere Bedeutung ergänzerder Untersuchungsmethoden bei der Lymphografie. Der Radiologe 8, 7, 202 (1968).

Roo, T. de. Lymphografie en melanosarcoma. Ned. tijdschr. geneesk. 113, 960 (1969).

Roo, T. de. Methods of additional examination in lymphography. Progress in Lymphology, Ed. by M. Viamonte, 200 Georg Thieme Verlag, Stuttgart (1969).

Roo, T. de. Supplementary angiographic examination in lymphangiography. Progress Clin. et Ther. de la Phlebologie 141. Stenvert & Zn. Apeldoorn (1970).

Roo, T. de., and Minden, S. H. van. Lymphatico- venous communications. Progress Clin. et Ther. de la Phlebologie 604. Stenvert & Zn. Apeldoorn (1970).

Roo, T. de. Lymphography in malignant melanoma. Long term results. Arch. Chir. Neerl. 3, 189 (1970).

Roo, T. de. Lymphography in lymphoedema. Long term results. Medicamundi 16, 3, 152 (1971).

Roo, T. de. Lipiodol accumulations simulating lung-metastases as complication after lymphography. Amer. J. Roentgen. 3, 3, 483 (1971).

Roo, T. de. Op metastasen gelijkende lipiodol ophopingen in de long als complicatie na lymphografie. Ned. tijdschr. geneesk. 115, 34, 1441 (1971).

Roo, T. de Lymphoedema: lymphangiographic studies in a series of 287 patients with limb involvement. Abstr. II Eur. Congress of Radiology, Amsterdam 51, 23 (1971).

Roo, T. de Lymphoedema as first symptom of a neoplasm. Abstr. IV Int. Congress of Phlebology, Luzern 1, 38 (1971).

Roo, T. de., and Minden, S. H. van. Lymphografische bevindingen bij een serie van 216 patienten met een testis tumor. Ned. tijdschr. geneesk. 116, 31, 1332 (1972).

Roo, T. de. Lymphangiographic studies in a series of 55 patients with malignant melanoma. Lymphology 6, 6 (1973).

Roo, T. de. Lymphography in testicular tumours. Abstr. 4'Int. Congress of Lymphology, Tucson, Arizona, 36 (1973).

Roo, T. de. Histological verification of additional examinations in lymphography. Abstr. 4' Int. Congress of Lymphology. Tucson, Arizona, 37 (1973).

Roo, T. de. Additional examinations in lymphography; a radiological-surgical-pathological correlation. Lymphology 7, 45 (1974).

References

Rosenberg, S. A. Contribution of lymphography to our understanding of lymphoma. Cancer Chem. Rep. 52, 213 (1968).

Rouvière, H. Anatomie des lymphatiques de l'homme. Paris, Masson (1932).

Rüttimann, A., Del Buono, M. S. und Cocchi, U. Neue Fortschritte in der Lymphographie. Schweiz. med. Wschr. 91, 1460 (1961).

Rüttimann, A. und Del Buono, M. S. Die Lymphographie mit öligen Kontrastmittel. Fortschr. Röntgenstr. 97, 551 (1962).

Rüttimann, A. Venographie und Lymphographie. Schweiz. med. Wschr. 92, 849 (1962).

Rüttimann, A. Zur Lymphknotenbeurteilung im Lymphogramm. Radiol. clin. 32, 456 (1963).

Rüttimann, A. Die Lymphographie in Ergebnisse der med. Strahlenforsschung. H. R. Schinz, R. Glauner and A. Rüttimann. Band I.S. 248 Georg Thieme Verlag (1964).

Rüttimann, A. Fehlermöglichkeiten bei der Lymphographie. Rad. Austriaca 16, 77 (1966).

Rüttimann, A. International statistics. Progr. in Lymphology; ed. Rüttimann. Georg Thieme Verlag 140 (1967).

Rüttimann, A. Value of locating occult disease in treatment of Hodgkin' disease. Progr. in Lymphology, Thieme Verlag, 119 (1967).

Saito, M. Etude sur la lymphographie chez l'homme. Ann. anat. path. 10, 833 (1933).

Salleras, V. and Pascual, J. Abdominal tumours of lymphatic origin. Abst 3' Int. Congr. of Lymphology. Brussels 144 (1970).

Sayegh, E., Brooks, T., Sacher, E. and Bush, F. Lymphangiography of the retroperitoneal lymph nodes through the inguinal route. J. Urol. 95, 102 (1966).

Schaffer, B., Gould, R. J., Walace, S. e.a. The urologic applications of lymphangiography. J. Urol. 87, 91 (1962).

Schaffer, B., Koehler, P. R., Daniel, C. R. e.a. A critical evaluation of lymphangiography. Radiology 80, 917 (1963).

Schield, P. N., Cose, L. and Mahony, D. T. Anatomic demonstration of mechanism of chyluria by lymphography, with succesful surgical treatment. New England J. Med. 274, 1495 (1966).

Seitzman, D. M. and Halaby, F. A. Lymphangiography: an evaluation of its applications. J. Urol. 91, 301 (1964).

Servelle, M. A propos de la lymphographie expérimentale et clinique. J. Radiol. électrol. 26, 165 (1944/45).

Servelle, M. La lymphangiectomie superficielle totale. Traitement chirurgical de l'éléphantiasis. Rev. chir. 85, 294 (1947).

Servelle, M. Lymphographie. Acta Chir. Belge 63, 678 (1964).

Shaver, W. A., Altman, D. and Viamonte, M. Lymphangiography in children. Amer. Surgeon. 29, 479 (1963).

Shdanow, D. A. Röntgenologische Untersuchungsmethoden des Lymphgefäszsystems des Menschen und der Tiere. Fortschr. Röntgenstr. 46, 680 (1932).

Sheehan, R., Hreshchyshyn, M., Lin, R. K. e.a. The use of lymphography as a diagnostic method. Radiology 76, 47 (1961).

Sieber, F. Indikation und Wert lymphografischer Untersuchungen. Rad. diagn. 5, 651 (1972).

Simon, H., Moquim, R. and Dameshek, W. The inferior vena-cavogram and lymphoproliferative disorders. J. A. M. A. 184, 978 (1963).

Smith, C. J., Carven, J., Meyer, J. Lympho-venography in pelvic cancer. Amer. J. Obstet. Gyn. 89, 732 (1964).

Stricstrock, K. H., Weissleder, H. and Schneidel, E. Computer analysis of lymphographic and histological examination results in cases of Hodgkin's disease. Abst. 3' Int. Congr. of Lymphology. Brussels, 110 (1970).

Takahashi, M. Lymphography in the diagnoses of malignant lymphoma. Nipp. Acta Radiol. 27, 1361 (1968).

Taylor, G. W. and Kinmonth, J. B. The lymphatics. In: G. W. Taylor. Recent advances in surgery. London, Churchill (1959).

Taylor, G. W. Chronic Lymphedema. Brit. J. Surg. 54, 898 (1967).

Teneff, S. and Stoppani, F. A propos de la lymphographie. J. Radiol. électrol. 20, 74 (1936).

Thomson, L. K. and Anlyal, W. C. An angiographic evaluation of swollen limbs. Surg. Gynec. and Obstet. 119, 743 (1964).

Tjernberg, B. F. Lymphography. Stockholm, Acta Radiol. suppl. 214 (1962).

Tjernberg, B. F. Trials of new contrast media for lymphography. Abst. 3' Int. Congr. of Lymphology. Brussels 123 (1970).

Tong, E. C. K. Improved technique of lymphatic cannulation for lymphography. Amer. J. Roentgen. 107, 877 (1969).

References

Tosatti, E. Linfatici, linfedema e linfangiografia dell'acto inferiore. Gazz. sanit. 28, 254 (1957).

Trapp, P. and Feindt, H. R. Zur Differentialdiagnose der malignen Lymphome aus dem Lymphogram. Fortschr. Röntgenstr. 107, 336 (1967).

Uslenghi, C. M, Musumeci, R., Luciani, L. and Chiappa, S. Lymphangiography in gynecology. Abst. 3' Int Congr. of Lymphology. Brussels 170 (1970).

Viamonte, M, Meyers, M. B., Soto, M. e.a. Lymphography. J. Urol. 87, 85 (1962).

Viamonte, M., Altman, D., Parks, R. e.a. Radiographic-pathologic correlation in the interpretation of lymphangioadenograms. Radiology 80, 903 (1963).

Viamonte, M. Jr. Lymphangio-adenography in female genital pathology. Prog. Gynec. 4, 515 (1963).

Viamonte, M. Jr. Advances in lymphangio-adenography. Acta radiol. 2, 394 (1964).

Viamonte, M., Stevens, R. C. A new trocar for lymphatic cannulation. Radiology 86, 934 (1966).

Viamonte, M. Jr. and Viamonte, M. Direct and indirect techniques for the diagnoses of lymph node pathology. Abst. 3' Int. Congr. of Lymphology. Brussels 171 (1970).

Virtama, T. and Helela, T. Lymphography and cavography in retroperitoneal fibrosis. Brit. J. of Radiol. 10, 231 (1967).

Vurksanivuc, M., Viamonte, M. Jr. and Martin, J. E. The place of lymph-angio-adenography in the diagnosis and during the treatment of malignant disease. Amer. J. Roentgen. 96, 205 (1966).

Wahlqvist, L., Hulten, L. and Rosencrantz, M. Normal lymphatic drainage of the testis studied by funicular lymphography. Acta chir. Scand. 132, 454 (1966).

Wallace, S., Jackson, L., Schaffer, B. e.a. Lymphangiograms: their diagnostic and therapeutic potential. Radiology 76, 179 (1961).

Wallace, S., Jackson, L. and Greening R. R. Clinical applications of lymphangiography. Amer. J. Roentgen. 88, 97 (1962).

Wallace, S., Jackson, L., Dodd, G. D. and Greening, R. R. Lymphatic dynamics in certain abnormal states. Amer. J. Roentgen. 6, 1187 (1964).

Wallace, S., Jackson, L., Dodd, G. and Greening, R. R. Lymphangiographic interpretation. Radiol. Clin. North Amer. 3, 467 (1965).

Wallace, S. and Jackson, L. Diagnostic criteria for lymphangiographic interpretation of malignant neoplasia. Cancer Chem. Rep. 52, 125 (1968).

Weissleder, H. Technik und Ergebnisse der Lymphangioadenographie. Röntgenblätter 16, 289 (1963).

Weissleder, H. Retroperitoneale Lymphknotenveränderungen beim Morbus Hodgkin. Fortschr. Röntgenstr. 101, 450 (1964).

Weissleder, H. Röntgenkinematografische Untersuchungen des menschlichen Ductus thoracicus. Fortschr. Röntgenstr. 100, 435 (1964).

Weissleder, H., Obrecht, P. Diagnostische Probleme bei der Lymphangio-denographie. Fortschr. Rontgenstr. 100, 82 (1964).

Weissleder, H. Das pathologische Lymphangiogramm der Ductus thoracicus. Fortschr. Röntgenstr. 101, 573 (1964).

Weissleder, H. und Stops, B. Morbus Hodgkin: Eine Gegenüberstellung klinischer und lymphografischer Untersuchungsbefunde. Fortschr. Röntgenstr. 106, 169 (1967).

Weissleder, H. Metastasenähnliche Symptome im Lymphogramm und ihre diagnostische Einordnung. Rad. diagn. 5, 594 (1972).

Westbroek, D. L., Roo, T. de, Oeberius Kapteyn, J. L. T. Ervaringen met het lymphografisch onderzoek bij de chirurgische behandeling van regionaal gemetastaseerde melanomen. Ned. tijdschr. geneesk. 106, 408 (1965).

Wiljasalo, M., Mustala, O. O. Demonstration of late post-traumatic chyluria by lymphography. Ann. Med. intern. Fenn. 54, 45 (1965).

Wiljasalo, M. Lymphographic differential diagnosis of neoplastic diseases. Acta Radiol. Suppl. 247 (1965).

Wiljasalo, M. and Perttala, Y. Lymphographic changes by radiotherapy. Ann. Med. intern. Fenn. 55, 81 (1966).

Wiljasalo, M. Lymphography in lupus erythematosus disseminales. Abst. 3' Int. Congr. of Lymphology. Brussels 128 (1970).

Wiljasalo, S. A. Lymphographic polymorphism in Hodgkin's disease. Acta Radiol. suppl. 289 (1969).

Wiljasalo, S. A. Follow-up and relymphography in Hodgkin's disease. Abst. 3' Int. Congr. of Lymphology. Brussels 112 (1970).

Wiljasalo, M. and Wiljasalo, S. Ergebnisse mit dem Projektion-Difference-Index. Rad. diagn. 5, 609 (1972).

Wiljasalo, M., Wiljasalo, S. and Rauste, J. Einsatz der Elektronische Datenverarbeitung beim Erarbeiten von Metastasen Kriterien. Rad. diagn. 5, 585 (1972).

Yoffey, J. M., and Courtice, F. C. Lymphatics, lymph and lymphoid tissue. London, Arnold (1965).

Ziedses des Plantes, B. G. Subtraction. Georg Thieme Verlag (1961).

Zieman, St. A. Lymphedema: causes, complications and treatment of the swollen leg. London, Grune and Stratton. (1962).

Zolotukhin, A. Roentgenologic method of examination of the lymphatic system in man and animals. Radiology 23, 455 (1934).